19.50
38779
RSL

Disorders of
Communication:
The Science of Intervention

Second Edition

In Memoriam

It is with a sense of great sadness and loss that I note here the deaths of two colleagues, both of whom contributed to the first edition of the book. Betty Byers Brown died in September 1991 and Jennie Lambert died in February 1995. Jennie had only completed a co-authored version of her original chapter for this second edition a few weeks before her untimely death that has left her family, friends and colleagues numb with grief. That great humoured and optimistic spirit of hers will always remain with us. While their deaths leave us the poorer, the dignity, courage and strength that both Betty and Jennie displayed in their illnesses can only leave us richer. *Requiescant in pace*.

M Leahy

Disorders of Communication: The Science of Intervention

Second Edition

Margaret M. Leahy

School of Clinical Speech & Language Studies
Trinity College, University of Dublin

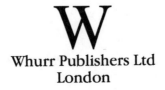

Whurr Publishers Ltd
London

© 1989

Whurr Publishers Ltd
19b Compton Terrace, London N1 2UN, England

First published by Taylor and Francis Ltd 1989.
All rights acquired by Whurr Publishers Ltd 1990.
Reprinted 1992

Second edition 1995

British Library Cataloguing in Publication Data
A catalogue record for this book is available from the
British Library.

ISBN 1-897635-47-8

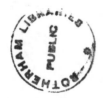

Printed and bound in the UK by Athenaeum Press Ltd, Gateshead,
Tyne & Wear

Contents

Preface

The second edition of *Communication Disorders: The Science of Intervention* presents a series of revised and updated chapters, written by highly respected authors working in the area of communication disorders on both sides of the Atlantic. As with the first edition, the major purpose of the text is to introduce student therapists to the theory and practice of therapy, with a focus on the scientific aspects of the work and on interpersonal skills involved in intervention.

The book is organized in three main sections. Section I provides an overview or framework in which some major professional issues are described and discussed. In Sections II and III, disorders of communication in children and in adults are discussed with a focus on description, assessment and current mainstream treatment approaches to each disorder area. Theoretical underpinnings of therapy and the important topic of therapy effectiveness are integrated throughout the chapters.

Communication disorders associated with hearing and auditory disorders and audiology are considered beyond the scope of this book, because of professional boundaries that exist in some countries. However, this should not be taken as undermining the importance of such subjects in any sense, or to deny their relation to other communication disorders.

Terminology

The terms *client* and *patient* are used variously to describe the person who presents with a communication disorder. The terms *speech and language therapist, speech-language pathologist, therapist* and *clinician* are used to refer to the professional person working with the client. Such terminology is not without disadvantages but is the most appropriate in the view of contributing authors. (Differences in the use of professional names are explained in Chapter 3.) Pronouns *she* and *he* are used to refer to therapist and client respectively, generally reflecting professional preponderances.

vii

Inevitably, there is an amount of repetition in a book of this nature. This allows for each chapter in Sections II and III to be considered as whole, standing alone. Similarities and differences between ways of understanding the nature of communication disorders and therapeutic approaches will be evident when chapters are read in sequence.

It is appropriate to repeat the Irish proverb that was cited in the first edition of the book: *Doras feasa fiafriagh — the door to knowledge is in questioning*. This is an approach which is a basic principle of any science and in acquiring a questioning attitude, the student not only learns from the information read but begins to contribute to the science itself.

It is a great honour to be associated with the authors who present their work in this text. Several new contributors took on the task of writing and submitting chapters with great enthusiasm. The International Association of Logopedics and Phoniatrics (IALP) which is the biggest professional organization of speech and language therapists worldwide, is represented by its President, Dr Marie de Montfort Supple who presents a chapter. The two major professional organizations in the English-speaking world, the American Speech-Language-Hearing Association (ASHA) and the College of Speech and Language Therapists (CSLT) are also well represented and chapters have been written by the current President of ASHA, Dr Jeri Logemann and the current Chair of the CSLT, Dr. Pam Enderby.

Acknowledgements

Gratitude is due to the staff of the School of Clinical Speech and Language Studies at Trinity College Dublin, in particular to Noreen Coyle whose help is invaluable. Technical assistance was provided by Geraldine Loftus and Theresa Logan-Phelan in the Computer Laboratory. Thanks are due also to Harry Purser and Dave Rowley, series editors of the first edition, whose idea it was to produce this book in the first instance. *Mile buiochas*.

Margaret M. Leahy, Feabhra, 1995
Colaiste na Trinoide, Baile Atha Cliath.
(Trinity College Dublin)

List of Contributing Authors

James H. Abbs, University of Wisconsin, Madison, Wisconsin, USA.

Crystal S. Cooper, Tuscaloosa City Schools, Tuscaloosa, AL., USA

Eugene B. Cooper, Department of Communicative Disorders, The University of Alabama, Tuscaloosa, AL., USA

Roxanne DePaul, Center for Communicative Disorders University of Wisconsin, Whitewater, WI., USA

Pamela M. Enderby, Speech and Language Therapy Research Unit, Frenchay Hospital, Bristol, ENGLAND.

Penelope K. Hall, Wendell Johnson Speech and Hearing Center, University of Iowa, Iowa City, IA., USA.

Irmgarde Horsley, Department of Speech, University of Newcastle, Newcastle-upon-Tyne, ENGLAND

Alan G. Kamhi, Memphis Speech & Hearing Center, Memphis State University, Memphis, Tenn., USA

Jennifer Lambert, Faculty of Health & Social Care, Leeds Metropolitan University, Speech & Language Sciences Group, Leeds, ENGLAND.

Margaret M Leahy, Clinical Speech & Language Studies, Trinity College Dublin, IRELAND

Ruth Lesser, Department of Speech, University of Newcastle, Newcastle-upon-Tyne, ENGLAND.

Jerilyn Logemann, Dept. of Communication Sciences & Disorders, Northwestern University, Evanston, IL., USA.

Niklas Miller, Department of Speech, University of Newcastle, Newcastle-upon-Tyne, ENGLAND.

Jane Russell, Speech & Language Therapy Department, The Children's Hospital, Ladywood Middleway, Birmingham, ENGLAND.

Pauline M. Sloane, Clinical Speech & Language Studies, Trinity College Dublin, IRELAND

Joseph C. Stemple, Institute for Voice Analysis and Rehabilitation, Dayton, OH. USA

Marie de Montfort Supple, Clinical Speech & Language Studies, Trinity College Dublin, IRELAND

Anna van der Gaag, University of Strathclyde, Speech & Language Therapy Division, Jordanhill Campus, Glasgow, SCOTLAND

Daphne Waters, Department of Speech & Language Sciences, Queen Margaret College, Edinburgh, SCOTLAND

Part I
Basic Framework of Intervention

Chapter 1
Philosophy in Intervention

MARGARET M. LEAHY

Communication is the means through which people relate to others, maintain contact, learn about the world and interact to exchange information. The ability to communicate through the use of speech and language is regarded as one of the most complex achievements in the development of the child and it is fundamental to personal development throughout life. As we move towards the twenty-first century, communication permeates living. When a person is unable to communicate adequately and effectively, the capacity for relationships is reduced, the achievement of potential inhibited, and the impact on the quality of life may be enormous.

The discipline of speech and language therapy developed in response to society's need and an awareness of the rights of the person to develop potential and strive towards happiness and a good quality of life. The central concern for the welfare of clients with communication disorders is the legacy of speech and language clinicians everywhere and is the single most outstanding unifying aspect of our work. It is this concern that is our *raison d'etre*, that nourishes our motivation and spurs us on to be the best possible clinicians that we can be.

The remit of the speech and language clinician traditionally encompasses the assessment, diagnosis and remediation of the presenting speech and/or language problems. In recent years, the assessment and remediation of swallowing disorders have been added to this brief.

For centuries, atypical patterns of speech and language behaviours have been described, discussed and debated as have methods of remediating speech and language disorders. The early *therapists* were philosophers, biologists, doctors and teachers. Over the centuries, many different disciplines have contributed to the understanding of observed differences in the patterns of speech and language which were considered as deviant or disordered. During the early twentieth century, the disciplines that arguably have contributed more than others are psychology and linguistics. More recently, sciences such as genetics and neurophysiology have been providing the profession with findings that support and, perhaps more importantly, in some cases reject the theories that have been long held by therapists. The fact that the knowledge base which informs speech and language therapy draws from a range of other disciplines has been described as a 'great strength' (Gailey, 1988) and it is this same fact that leads to the diversity of the concerns of the profession, considered by some to be its hallmark (see also Chapter 4) .

Bench (1991: 235) describes speech and language pathology as 'an epistemological hybrid which, *sui generis*, resists conceptual unification and the development of a high paradigmatic consensus'. Furthermore, the indeterminacy of the processes underlying speech and language mean that these processes are open to many different interpretations (Milosky, 1992), as by implication are those processes that underlie disorders. Issues associated with epistemology in the speech and language clinic raise problems that are similar in many ways to the kinds of problems that confront the therapist on a daily basis: the issues are complex, we are aware that there are several different approaches to understanding the problem and therefore to proposing a solution. As a profession however, we are confident in our engagement in a complex problem-solving enterprise, despite an awareness that there are no easy answers. This enterprise, in which the therapist daily engages, is built upon a complex structure of assumptions, which for many may not be specified.

Epistemology

Epistemology – the theory of knowledge – addresses the issues underlying our actions as therapists and 'attempts to specify how particular organisms or aggregates of organisms know, think and decide' (Bateson, 1972). Our thinking and action as therapists are structured to an extent by a range of theories that are not unique to the profession. Such theories are of three main types:

1. *Theories for understanding speech and language*, which derive mainly from linguistics, phonetics, and the biological sciences, particularly neurosciences.
2. *Theories for understanding speech and language disorders*, which derive mainly from medicine (neurology), psychology and linguistics; in recent years, some derive from speech and language therapy.
3. *Theories for intervention and recovery*, which derive mainly from medical and psychological models.

While theories provide us with models, frameworks or principles upon which we can structure therapy, they are replaceable and indeed, part of our role as scientist-practitioners is to question theories and generate new ones, as Perkins (1985) states 'It is by disproving theories that knowledge advances'. The role of theory in therapy is central and will be discussed later, but a cursory glance at some models of practice exploited in the clinic will provide a background for that discussion.

Review of Models of Practice

Current bases for clinical practice of speech and language therapy derive from well respected traditions in health care, which themselves derive from an understanding of disease and disorder, based partly on speculation or intuition and partly on the emergence and interpretation of knowledge. The profession initially tended to follow the medical profession by structuring its body of knowledge in terms of the classification of communication disorders and the stages of therapy. This may be justified if you consider that many of the founder members of the profession in this century were in fact members of the medical profession. The medical model[1] – powerful though it may be – is not necessarily the best model for working with people with communication disorders and it may strengthen the belief that each disorder is treated with a unique technique (Hedge, 1985), a problem that may also be compounded by the organization of college curricula. Student clinicians learn that there are at least 12 subject areas within speech and language pathology, with as many as 30 'diagnostic categories' subsumed therein.

The medical model

The primary objective of the health care professions is the problem-solving activity involving restoration to health and the prevention of the origins, development and recurrence of disease and disorders. In the traditional medical model this problem solving activity demands definition and/or in-depth description of the problem from observing the symptoms or signs that present. Pathology – the branch of medicine that pertains to the origins, nature, and development of changes in the physiology that determine the disease – is linked with the symptoms, on the basis of which the aetiology or causal factors are evaluated. The pathology is the rational basis for treatment and the aetiology the basis of prevention (Kahn and Earle, 1986). Following logical steps, this leads to therapy being structured so that it may proceed in an orderly fashion, leading to improvement or 'cure' and discharge. The profession in the USA and Australia retains pathology in its professional title; in the UK and Ireland the term is retained as the name of the science that we study.

The approach outlined in the medical model is linked to the so-called 'hard sciences', stressing empirical laws. Cause and effect are linked as a unidirectional process based on Newton's model of linear causality, where the changes in movement that occur are (usually) measurable and predictable.

The behaviourist model

The profession's development at the start of the twentieth century coincided with the birth and growth of behaviourism, a model of understanding behaviour that was to have a strong influence in communication disorders. In 1913, Watson proposed the principle of operant conditioning, which considered that behaviour can be shaped and changed according to specified requirements. The concepts of motivation and reward are of central importance and input is directly linked to output.

Like the medical model in many ways, behaviourism stresses empiricism in its methods and the active–passive role is performed by the behaviourist who, having analysed the problem, determines the behaviour(s) of the client to be shaped and changed, and proceeds to do so. Throughout the process there is a strong commitment to objectivity in the analysis and treatment of the problem, with detailed and precise specification of aims and techniques. A major implication of these models is that the more powerful active role is assigned to the expert whereas the client assumes a relatively passive or reactive role.

There are several other models that may have influenced theory and practice of therapy, among others, the models derived from Freudian theory, Gestalt theories, phenomenological humanistic theories etc., but the two presented here have been and continue to be extremely influential for the speech and language therapist, providing an organizational framework for categorizing disorders and a means for approaching treatment (see Hedge, 1985; Van Coppenolle et al., 1993 for detailed application of a behaviourist type approach to speech and language disorders).

Both models outlined may be considered as reductionist models where the dynamics of the whole are understood from the properties of the parts (Kamhi, 1994). In the clinical context, the nature of progress is deterministic and additive, regardless of personal meaning of the client who is reactive.

Circularity or holistic models

There has been increasing realization that the reductionist models cannot adequately account for individual speech and language behaviour patterns or for efficacy in therapy and that there is greater complexity in the nature of interactions and environments affecting the person. This so-called ecological or holistic approach to behaviour focuses on the interrelatedness and interdependence of the elements that comprise our world: physical, biological, psychological, social, and cultural; in Axline's (1989: 10) words: 'The dynamics of life are such that every experience and attitude and thought of every individual is constantly changing in relation to the interplay of psychological and environmental forces upon each and every individual'. This way of thinking demands a shift away from the linear thinking and a move towards circularity, allowing for any item to be defined in terms of its relationship to several other items.

The aetiology of problems is considered more in terms of current interactional patterns that serve to maintain the problem, with symptom and 'cause' operating on one another. In the therapy process, all the parties involved move together and affect one another. This means that the therapist is not 'acting on' the client, as an agent with a relatively passive subject. Rather, the whole system is one where both the therapist and client interact, decisions are made jointly, and therapy becomes part of a process of change, learning and evolution for both the therapist and the client.

Kamhi (1994: 197) compares mechanistic and holistic paradigms and concludes that

> There is nothing wrong with a passionate commitment to a particular theory or paradigm as long as those with such feelings recognize that there may be different ways to achieve the same teaching and learning objectives.

He considers that

> lack of commitment to a particular paradigm may reflect the belief that the use of a plurality of theories from different paradigms is necessary in order to provide the best services for the children we serve.

Knowledge and Science

The question of knowledge in the speech and language clinic is directly associated with the question of practitioner as clinical scientist. In a document from the IALP (1994: 51), logopedics is described as '..a developing profession at the crossroads of pure and applied sciences'. However, in evaluating science in communication disorders, Ringel, Trachtman and Prutting (1984: 34) conclude that since the discipline does not generate unique bodies of knowledge, paradigms or theories that encompass the range of investigations being used and since it lacks a methodological structure, we are bound to use concepts and methods derived from other sciences and therefore cannot qualify as a science. If a science is to be defined only by a particular paradigm that provides a unifying conceptual and methodological structure, then perhaps we are doomed to exist and operate outside of the realm of science. However, Siegel and Ingham (1987) raise the question of whether it is necessary to generate our own conceptual models to be regarded as a science and, more importantly, they question whether we should aspire to be an autonomous science at all. There is no doubt that we share aspects of science with other professionals and neither is there any doubt that we share important non-scientific aspects of relationships with other professions. But questions do arise about the nature of our work that call for scientific reasoning and the application of scientific methods and so perhaps there *is* a need for us to be good scientists in order to be good therapists. For some, it may seem sufficient to recognize that some members of the profession are good scientists, whilst others, e.g. the 'ordinary clinicians' can go about their daily work without considering questions of science (see also, Siegel, 1987). An integral part of the therapist's work is to ensure that the procedures used in therapy are the best possible and to consider the most effective and expedient means to bring about desired change. Kent's (1985: 10) argument, that it is not enough to know that we can change behaviour but that we must be able to document that changes are 'in the right direction and are sufficiently large to warrant the time and energy invested by the clinician and client', calls the ordinary clinician to act as scientist and apply the rigours of scientific thought and methods. In the same sense, Perkins (1985: 14) considers that the therapist not only dispenses therapy, but also actively engages in a scientific endeavour in the clinic:

> Each clinical encounter epitomizes the essence of experimental research. This is the most powerful of the research methods; it is the one used to determine cause-and-effect relationships.

Perkins (1985: 14) expounds further on the similarity between methods used in therapy and science and states:

> ... the clinician is mandated by ethical requirements to use some version of the most rigorous method of science, experimentation on a day-by-day, case-by-case basis in therapy...

Where we, as clinicians, pale in comparison with some other scientists is in our documentation and publication of experiments. This is due in part to the brief of the clinician being limited to working with clients, leaving the questions of documentation to academics, but sometimes this failure may be due to a belief that we cannot adequately document experiments because of a realization of the complex nature of individual patterns and an inability to discern exactly what has caused the changes to occur (in effect, a realization of circularity). Yet, we continue to engage in clinical practice in the belief that what we are doing is effective, in many instances without being in a position to explain why, as indicated by the following authors: 'We are far more certain of the effects of the various treatment procedures used than we are of reasons for these effects' (Perkins, 1985: 15); 'Speech therapists have long been convinced that they can improve children's speech production, and the conviction is largely in accord with the objective evidence' (Howell and McCartney, 1990: 39).

The Role of Theory in Therapy

As long as speech and language disorders have existed, scientists have speculated on the possible reasons for their existence and on the means whereby the problems associated with disorders could be alleviated. In some instances, these early origins of our understanding are reflected in current practice (e.g. the use of relaxation in fluency therapy was recommended in the early Greek therapies), but in many more instances, earlier theories have been disproved if not entirely laid to rest (e.g. linking phonological disorder directly with open auditory discrimination deficits). Some early theories that helped the profession's understanding may not have been coherent theories at all and in many instances were implicit rather than explicit, i.e. a rationale was sought for the effect of what was done and that rationale was called a *theory*. Such a pragmatic approach has guided the profession along an avenue that has led members to use the phrase 'multiple co-existing factors' not only as an explanation for causes of problems, but also as explaining success in therapy. It has also led us to the 'epistemological hybrid' mentioned above, while at the same time providing us with the means of developing creatively and experimentally as clinicians, adapting techniques to suit the individual patterns of behaviour and needs of clients. There are many instances in the literature where therapists report on techniques that are effective, but where there is no theory to support findings adequately, e.g. the use of Auditory Integration Training (Rimland and Edelson, 1994) and techniques used with children having cleft palate. This provokes a *questioning* of rationale that ultimately helps the development of theories and the re-evaluation of therapy methods – an essential aspect of the profession's work. Currently there exists a range of theories in language acquisition, in aphasiology and in motor speech disorders that guide therapy, although in the past therapy techniques have preceded theories. For the most part there is a circular rather than a unidirectional relationship between the two: therapy informs theory, which informs therapy, which informs theory.

A Model of Speech and Language Therapy

When a client seeking change comes to see the speech and language therapist, he generally believes that there is a better way to be, but he recognizes his inability to arrive at that state alone. Fundamental beliefs that the therapist holds include that change is possible and that therapy can help influence change. Such beliefs reflect attitudes that encompass hopefulness and helpfulness and what Darley (1985) calls the 'heart ' of the clinical process.

The theory of change or recovery that the therapist believes in (and there will often be a personal understanding of change) will shape therapy, but where speech and language are concerned some themes are similar and unifying. In order for change to be brought about through therapy, it is desirable that a common understanding is arrived at and made explicit so that therapist and client share common aims in a problem-solving enterprise which demands involvement from both parties. During the early contact with the client, the therapist begins the process of hypothesis testing in order to be able to describe communication behaviours and patterns, defining those that are and are not within normal or appropriate ranges. In doing so, the therapist draws both on the client's expertise, personal knowledge and that of his own communication, and on her own knowledge of theories and experience. So, as well as listening actively to the client's concerns and priorities, the therapist has to listen to her inner self.

During the initial stage of therapy (assessment), defining a cause or aetiology is often not as important as considering the present functioning of the client with the presenting problem and defining those symptoms and factors that interact to maintain present functioning. Just as the processes underlying speech and language are indeterminate, causes of speech and language disorders are often indeterminate and interpretation of causes is linked to a particular theoretical understanding of the processes involved.

Change can only be achieved through changing – by *doing something differently*. Simple as this may sound, we know it is often not simple. It involves hypothesis testing by the therapist and experimenting with behaviours in the clinic setting. While the process of arriving at a change in behaviour may have several possible theoretical explanations, it always involves hypothesis testing by the therapist, who seeks the easiest, most efficient means for the client to attain the desired target behaviour. In turn, the client takes on the experimental procedure. Locke (1994) states that

> Behaviour constantly pushes the young brain around, and it is eminently reasonable to suppose that remediation – undertaken early and pursued rigorously – reorganizes the brain.

This reference to reorganization of the brain in childhood links in with approaches to direct therapy in acquired aphasia, which are described as reactivation, reorganization and substitution. Lesser and Milroy (1993:15) interpret reactivation of function as 'consistent with the claim that neuronal sprouting occurs through stimulation' with recovery of the original behaviour expected. Reorganization implies that language functions are taken over by newly engaged neuronal activity. Substitution implies that alternative means have to be found to achieve the communication target as the original ability cannot be restored in its original form.

In developmental disorders and other non-neurogenic disorders, parallel approaches may be described as activation, where expected functions are achieved through stimulation and/or approximation; organization (or reorganization), where some newly-learned processes produce new pathways; and substitution, where alternative means of communication augment or replace the usual oral/verbal one.

Maintaining change

The change that occurs in the clinic is, however, probably not the solution to the problem, because maintaining change occurs outside of the clinic, when the new behaviour creates some new or different meaning for the client. In this context, those approaches described as *indirect* are important.

Although many attempts have been made to account for the factors that facilitate change, it is difficult to say *with certainty* what has made achieving the difference possible for individual clients. (Indeed it may often be the case that clients themselves cannot specify the factors but echo 'multiple co-existing factors' which may be a euphemism for 'I don't know'.)

Personal warmth and empathy are often listed among therapist's prerequisites, but arguably as important in the problem-solving process is that the therapist's attitude be a questioning one, using the basic experimental method of science. It is the brief of every therapist to question her theories and techniques to help ensure that she is continually acting in the best interests of the client. Kent (1985) suggests that it is necessary for the therapist to learn about new research discoveries, apply selected information to practice, empirically evaluate outcomes and in this way, conduct research in a clinical setting. 'To pose an important question....requires clear thinking' (Perkins, 1985), and for the therapist, it requires *thinking as a therapist*.

Conclusion

The particular expertise of the speech and language therapist that has been described is not meant to be either definitive or all-embracing; rather, it presents a simple model of the structure of a therapist's work, the work of initiating change, helping to make the process of change easy for the client and evaluating outcome.

If the term 'paradigm' is used to designate a world view, representing beliefs (Kamhi, 1994), then perhaps this model may help to make explicit an understanding that is basic to our work as therapists. Recognizing the individuality of the therapist is as fundamental to understanding therapy dynamics as recognizing the individuality of the client. The therapist is informed by a range of theories and we need not expect in the immediate future that one theory will emerge that all therapists will favour, despite recent advances in neurolinguistics and genetics.

Locke (1994: 614) describes the behaviour of clinicians as '...a powerful sociobiological force, conceivably just as powerful as "hard wiring"', (a term he uses to describe the structural neurological basis of language disorder). Drawing on his analogy, I am suggesting that therapists are 'wired' as therapists, their expertise defined by personal attributes which include creativity and flexibility, their way of working following a particular pathway that is aided by the fundamental questioning method of science. Elaboration of the epistemology of the therapist is in the process of being driven forward by describing and understanding the decision-making rules of therapists (see Records and Tomblin, 1994; Roulstone, 1994), understanding our actions as therapists (see, for example, De Bruin and Meijer, 1994) and by analysis of clinical discourse, a theme which Charles Van Riper advocated as early as 1971. As is clearly demonstrated in the chapters that follow, we have the expertise and the means to understand and to specify our understanding and expertise clearly. By so doing and by continuing to question our understanding, we open up the opportunity to develop professionally and thus to serve the community better.

Note

1. It should be noted that these models, like any model, vastly over-simplify the processes that actually occur. Further, it is not implied that any particular professions are faithful to the restricted presentation of the models – in many instances this is clearly not so.

References

Axline V (1989) Play Therapy. Edinburgh: Churchill Livingstone.

Bateson G (1972) Steps to an Ecology of Mind. London: Intertext.

Bench RJ (1991) Paradigms, methods and the epistemology of speech pathology: some comments on Eastwood (1988). British Journal of Disorders of Communication 26(2): 235–43.

Darley FL (1985) The 'Heart' of Clinical Education. Proceedings of 6th Annual conference on Graduate Education. Council of Graduate Programs in Communication Sciences and Disorders, University of Nebraska, Lincoln, NE, USA.

De Bruin D, Meijer M (1994) The therapist's behaviour observed: a way of looking at our own behaviour as therapists. Journal of Fluency Disorders 19: 3. (Abstract of the First World Congress on Fluency).

Gailey L (1988) Competence in Speech Therapy in Ellis R (Ed) Professional Competence and Quality Assurance in the Caring Professions. London: Croom Helm.

Hedge MN (1985) Treatment Procedures in Communicative Disorders. London: Taylor & Francis.

Howell J, McCartney E (1990) Approaches to Remediation. In Grunwell P (Ed) Developmental Speech Disorders. Edinburgh: Churchill Livingstone.

IALP Guidelines for Initial Education in Logopedics (1994) Folia Phoniatrica Logopedica 46: 48–55.

Kahn J, Earle E (1986) The Cry for Help and the Professional Response. Oxford: Pergamon.

Kamhi AG (1994) Paradigm of Teaching and Learning: Is one view the best? Language, Speech and Hearing Services in the Schools 25:194–8.

Kent RD (1985) Science and the clinician: The practice of science and the science of practice. Seminars in Speech and Language 6(1): 1–13

Lesser R, Milroy L (1993) Linguistics and Aphasia. Harlow: Longman Group.

Locke JL (1994) Gradual emergence of developmental language disorders. Journal of Speech and Hearing Research 37(3): 608–17.

Milosky LM (1992) Children listening: the role of world knowledge in language comprehension. In Chapman RS (Ed) Processes in Language Acquisition and Disorders. St Louis: Mosby.

Perkins WH (1985) From clinical dispenser to clinical scientist. Seminars in Speech and Language 6(1): 13–23.

Records NL, Tomblin JB (1994) Clinical decision making: Describing the decision rules of practising speech-language pathologists. Journal of Speech and Hearing Research 37: 144–56.

Rimland B, Edelson SM (1994) The effects of auditory integration training on autism. American Journal of Speech-Language Pathology 3: 16–25.

Ringel RL, Trachtman LE, Prutting C (1984) The science in human communication sciences. ASHA 26(12): 33–7.

Roulstone C (1994) Expertise and Speech and Language Therapy. Paper presented at the CSLT Policy Review Forum, London, UK.

Siegel GM (1987) The limits of science in communication disorders. Journal of Speech and Hearing Disorders 52: 306-19.

Siegel GM, Ingham R (1987) Theory and science in communication disorders. Journal of Speech and Hearing Disorders 52: 99–104.

Van Coppenolle L, Kalf H, Kuipers H, Schade M (1993) Principles of behaviour change applied to communication disorders. In Leahy MM, Kallen JL (Eds) Proceedings of Interdisciplinary Perspectives in Speech and Language Pathology. Dublin: School of Clinical Speech and Language Studies, Trinity College.

Van Riper C (1971) Analyzing the clinician–client interaction. WMU Journal of Speech Therapy 8(3): 7.

Chapter 2
Classification of
Communication Disorders

MARIE DE MONTFORT SUPPLE

The term *communication disorder* emerged gradually in the field of speech and language disorders from about the mid 1960s. In 1966, when in the UK the name of the professional journal changed from *Speech Pathology and Therapy* to *Journal of Disorders of Communication*, the editor, Muriel Morley (1966: 1) stated,

> It has become increasingly apparent that the scope of speech therapy is wider than was initially conceived, and that we are concerned with that aspect of human behaviour which enables one individual to maintain contact with another.

Since that time, and especially since the 1980s, the term has found wider usage, and it is now included in the title of many journals and text books. To date there is no clinical title using the term communication disorders, perhaps because as Byers Brown (1989: 25) suggests such a title 'would signify a field too broad to be mastered by one individual'.

Whilst the terms communication, language and speech are used interchangeably in common usage, there is a professional need to be aware of distinctions that exist between these labels. Communication is the more general term and refers to 'a transfer of knowledge, ideas, opinions, and feelings' (Oyer, Hall and Haas, 1994: 6). These authors state that while the term usually refers to language it can also be used to refer to other forms of interaction such as body language, a powerful communication tool, but of a non-linguistic nature.

Language is a more specific term which is defined as 'a formalized method of communication consisting of (1) the signs and symbols by which ideas can be represented, (2) the rules governing these signs and symbols' (Oyer et al, 1994: 6). A unique feature of language is that it can be used to communicate about the past and future as well as the present. Speech is the narrowest of the terms and refers to 'all vocal or spoken production of language' (Oyer et al, 1994: 6).

The field of communication disorders has seen enormous expansion over the past two decades, this is reflected 'not only in the subdivisions

14

of different specialties but in the incorporation of entirely new procedures' (Byers Brown 1989: 25). A major new role undertaken by speech
and language therapists is the treatment of swallowing disorders. While
such procedures cannot be classified as dealing with communication, it
illustrates the therapist's use of expertise from training and knowledge
of the speech mechanism for a non-communicative function. Another
area which has seen great expansion is the field of augmentative communication, an expansion which is linked to technological developments.

The increase in professional activities of the speech and language
therapist has generated a need for a more comprehensive classification
of communication disorders than could have been envisaged by our
predecessors, in their early attempts to explain and clarify the procedures of the professions involved with speech and language disorders.

The terms *classification* and *terminology* are not synonymous but
there is overlap in meaning and usage. This chapter will deal with classification, the terminologies of specific disorders are dealt with in the
appropriate chapters.

The classification of communication disorders is a complex task
which can be approached from many different perspectives. As Nation
and Aram (1977: 109) state 'there has been a proliferation of nomenclature and classification systems derived from many professional view-
points'. They proceed to list some of the various types of classification
systems attempted including 'aetiologic classifications, behavioural
description classifications, processing classifications and clinical problem – type classifications'.

However Dockrell and McShane (1993: 59), referring specifically to
difficulties with language, state 'There is no agreed-upon system for classifying language difficulties'. This is true for all communication disorders. The problem is a universal one and not confined to English
language countries, as Crystal (1982: 4) points out. Edwards (1985)
refers to the problems experienced by the College of Speech and
Language Therapists (UK) in attempting to develop a terminology and a
classification system. In 1959 a terminology pamphlet was published by
this body which in time became so outdated that a project was funded to
develop a revision. The task proved so difficult that no revised pamphlet
appeared! The more research that was carried out, the more daunting
the task became and the project was eventually abandoned. Sonninen
and Hurme (1989: 7) state that 'The establishment of a scientifically
accurate and internationally recognized terminology is certainly a difficult task in any field'. Referring specifically to the field of communication
disorders and the lack of any agreed classification system they pose the
question: (page 9) 'Could it be that the problem of creating a multi-
lingual terminology simply is too difficult to solve?'.

Possibly nowhere is the difficulty of devising a classification system
seen as clearly as in the efforts of the World Health Organization (WHO)

Collaborating Centre of the Classification of Diseases. The International Association of Logopedics and Phoniatrics (IALP) and the American Speech–Language–Hearing Association (ASHA) have endeavoured to effect changes in the International Classification of Diseases (ICD-10, 1992) from that which appeared in ICD-9 (1980). Specifically they requested the inclusion of the term *language* in addition to *speech*, the inclusion of terms such as dysarthria, hyper- and hypo-nasality and, above all, the removal of developmental speech and language disorders etc. from under the general heading of Mental Disorders. Obviously speech and language therapists had little if any input into ICD-9. It was hoped that ICD-10 would better represent our field, but as we shall see later that was not to be. However, we have to accept that speech and language disorders are but a very minor part of the WHO's Classification System.

The Necessity for a Classification System

Despite the difficulties involved and the perception that it is impossible to arrive at a totally acceptable form of classification of communication disorders, it is essential that some form of classification is attempted and used. The question 'Why label?' can legitimately be asked, as Bishop (1989: 108) does before she justifies the need for labels, in that without them it is not possible to generalize from past experience in developing a treatment schedule or to give a prognosis. She concludes that:

> diagnostic categories provide a structure for gathering information in a clinical setting and are vital if we want to conduct research into the likely causes and appropriate means of treating various disorders.

She notes that a disadvantage in labelling is that once a label is given to a child 'we are likely to have stereotyped expectations and to lose sight of his or her individuality' or indeed of co-existing problems.

Byers Brown (1989: 27) considers that 'professional growth is reflected in the search for a unifying theory of communication disorders' and that, at the same time, there is concern for a 'clear delineation of diagnostic groups for the purpose of treatment and professional accountability'. The more established the profession and the greater its growth, the greater the requirement for a framework for the classification of disorders and procedures.

Byers Brown (1989: 27) gives her reasons for the need of a classification system as follows:

1. Clinical Practice: to establish a code of practice
                              to determine methods of prevention, identification and intervention
                              to determine treatment efficacy

2. Education: to train professional personnel
                            to share information across professions
                            to inform the public
3. Research: to describe subjects in research studies includ-
                            ing epidemiological studies
4. Remuneration: to establish scales of fees for services.

Before attempting to present any form of classification system of communication disorders it is necessary to adequately define what is meant by the term *communication disorders*. Interestingly, there are few definitions of this widely used term. One proposed by ASHA (1993: 40) in their statement on Definitions of Communication Disorders and Variations is the following:

> COMMUNICATION DISORDER is an impairment in the ability to receive, send, process, and comprehend concepts of verbal, non-verbal and graphic symbol systems. A communication disorder may be evident in the processes of hearing, language, and/or speech. A communication disorder may range in severity from mild to profound. It may be developmental or acquired. Individuals may demonstrate one or any combination of communication disorders. A communication disorder may result in a primary disability or it may be secondary to other disabilities.

Byers Brown (1989: 35), commenting on a similar definition in ASHA's (1986) publication, states that such definitions are somewhat cumbersome but that 'it is extremely difficult to be both comprehensive and succinct'. The definition does cover most of the main features of a communication disorder, namely:

1. degree: mild   ↔   profound
2. type: receptive   ↔   expressive
3. time: developmental   ↔   acquired
4. cause: primary   ↔   secondary

These features will be returned to at a later stage in this chapter.

Types of Classification Systems

Aetiological classification

Attempts at classification of communication disorders have generally followed an aetiological model, a behavioural model or an interactive model. In most countries the profession of speech and language therapy has, historically, had close links with the medical profession and therefore it seemed to follow that classification of communication disorders should be based on an aetiological model. Terminology tended to originate specifically with neurologists following the pattern of Graeco-Latin derivation. This accounts for references in the literature to 'cleft palate speech', 'cerebral palsy speech' etc. Thus, as Nation and Aram (1977: 110) state 'The curious practice arose of classifying types of language disorder with little reference to the language behaviour itself'.

While there are obvious merits in an aetiological classification in that in many instances it helps to point out the cause of the communication disorder and aids in communication with our medical colleagues, it can however result in inappropriate placement and management. A child who has a language disorder may be emotionally disturbed, but attaching an 'emotionally disturbed' label does not tell us whether the emotional disturbance was the cause, or the result, of the communication disorder. Stating that a child has cerebral palsy gives no indication as to the type of communication disorders – if any – that the child may have. A further problem with an aetiological classification is that it can obscure the fact that there may be more than one factor causing the communication disorder. A child who has a mental handicap may also have a hearing loss and both factors will be implicated in the resulting communication difficulties. Byers Brown and Edwards (1989: 193) refer to the aetiological term 'developmental dysphasia', which obviously has a neurological connotation but which gives little information regarding the language of the child. They hold that the use of this term has resulted in the definition of this disorder by exclusion – 'not deaf, not mentally handicapped, not behaviourally disturbed, etc.' The term 'developmental dysphasia' has fallen into disuse among speech and language therapists and has been replaced by the term 'specific language impairment' (SLI). It is interesting that the recent subcategories proposed for this disorder originated from a neuropaediatric background. Rapin and Allen (1987) delineated the following subgroups:

1. Verbal Auditory Agnosia
2. Verbal Dyspraxia
3. Phonologic Programming Deficit Syndrome
4. Semantic-Pragmatic Deficit Syndrome
5. Lexical-Syntactic Deficit Syndrome
6. Phonologic-Syntactic Deficit Syndrome.

These categories are descriptive in nature and thus demonstrate a move from the aetiological classification system even within a medical setting.

The aetiological classification system can be useful to the speech and language therapist only when used in conjunction with other classification systems.

Behavioural classification

In 1977 Kleffner (p. 6) remarked that 'The only information which is relevant to the classification of language disorder is information regarding the child's language abilities'. He complained that the majority of reports on children with language disorders provided more information about aetiology and pathology than on language behaviour. Hopefully this situation has changed in the past two decades. Milisen (1957), cited by Nation and Aram (1977), was one of the early writers to move from the aetiological classification to a more behavioural descriptive model. This initial model was crude in that it basically looked at disorders in terms of receptive or expressive deficits. At this same time the influence of linguists began to be felt in the domain of speech and language disorders. Detailed descriptions of language behaviour were published and became an integral part of assessment techniques. Bloodstein (1979: 6) refers to this mode of classification as reporting the symptoms we observe, while he considers that in aetiological classifications we describe the causes of those symptoms. It soon became evident that linguistic descriptions alone were inadequate to classify a communication disorder. The increased emphasis on pragmatics was a major influence in this regard. These considerations led to the next stage in classification systems, which has been termed the process-based or interactive model.

Process-based classification

The Processing Classification System, is an extension of the Behavioural Classification System. Systems based on this form of classification go beyond describing the characteristics of the disorder by providing insight into the basis of the disorder. 'Process-based Classification includes cognitive and linguistic factors as well as a consideration of possible neurological correlates of language pathology' (Byers Brown and Edwards, 1989: 194). This form of classification was used by Rapin and Allen (1987) in their presentation of sub-types of Specific Language Impairment previously referred to.

Byers Brown and Edwards (1989: 194) provide a table (Table 2.1) which admirably compares the three main classification systems. None of the classification systems outlined in the table has proved entirely satisfactory, nor is it possible to classify communication disorders totally under any one of the headings. Each system has to include aspects of the other. The most that can be stated, when classifying disorders under any of the systems, is that one is following a predominately processing system or a predominately behaviourist system etc.

Categories of Communication Disorders

In the first edition of this book, Byers Brown (1989: 28) referred to four basic 'surprisingly robust' categories of disorders.

Table 2.1 Three classifications of language disorder

Aetiological	Behavioural	Process-based
Receptive aphasia	Limited expressive language	Auditory imperception
Central auditory dysfunction	Semantic disability	Failure to access semantic memory
		Limited production
Expressive aphasia (Broca type)	Word-finding difficulty	Phonological-syntactic disorder
	Syntactic limitation	Some comprehension problems
	Phonological-prosodic disability	Impaired connection between higher order schemata of linguistic
units		and peripheral motor planning

Byers Brown and Edwards (1989: 194).

Such categories have been used in the majority of speech and language pathology text books. Official reports, on both sides of the Atlantic, have used the terms which are:

1. Voice and Resonance: abnormalities or phonation and vocal modulation
2. Articulation: abnormalities in the production or use of the sounds of speech
3. Language: abnormalities in the comprehension and/or use of verbal or written symbols
4. Fluency or Rhythm: abnormalities in the rate, timing and flow of speech.

She added two principal modifiers:

ORGANIC	versus	FUNCTIONAL
the cause lying in pathology of organs or systems		where the mechanism appears to be capable of working normally but fails to do so

and the division by

ACQUIRED	versus	DEVELOPMENTAL/ CONGENITAL
where established function is lost or impaired		where the disorder is present at birth or becomes apparent during development.

See for example, *Communicating Quality* (1991) and the 1993 *Definitions of Communication Disorders and Variations* of the American Speech-Language-Hearing Association. Because these terms were already in use in medical practice they were therefore more easily subsumed into general terminology:

> the interrelation of the four basic categories and the two basic modifiers allowed for a useful and flexible form of classification with an increasing number of sub-classifications and then cross classifications (Byers Brown 1989: 28).

Other modifiers could usefully be included

PRIMARY versus SECONDARY
MILD versus PROFOUND

In addition to these modifiers Crystal and Varley (1993) consider the inclusion of the following:

PRODUCTION versus RECEPTIVE DISORDERS
LANGUAGE DEVIANCE versus LANGUAGE DELAY.

The ASHA (1993) definitions, while listing a number of sub-classifications which could be listed under the four broad categories, reflect current theory in the format used. Under the heading Speech Disorder are included Articulation, Fluency and Voice Disorders, whilst Language is subdivided under the headings, Form (including Phonology), Content and Function. It is interesting that 'Hearing Disorder', with the subdivisions of Deaf and Hard of Hearing, is listed following the first two categories of 'Speech Disorder' and 'Language Disorder'. This is a clear example of mixing classification systems, the *speech and language* aspect fitting best into the behaviour system whilst *deafness* would be more appropriate within an aetiological classification system. A further category listed by ASHA (1993) is Central Auditory Processing Disorders (CAP). The inclusion of this category is unique in such a classification. Increasingly, in the past decade, CAP has become recognized as a *cause* of speech and language disorders. Therefore, as with deafness, this category falls within an aetiological classification system.

International Classification Systems

International Statistical Classification of Diseases and Related Health Problems (ICD-10)

Byers Brown (1989: 29) refers to the International Classification of Diseases (ICD) stating that this system was developed by the WHO 'as a statistical tool to enable comparison between countries at the same point in time and between countries over time.' She makes the point that 'it was neither intended to be a clinical classification of medicines nor a nomenclature of diseases'. The tenth revision of the classification (ICD-10), issued in ten languages, came into effect in January 1992. In previous editions disorders of communication were presented under the chapter heading *Mental Disorders and Diseases of the Nervous System*. In the current edition the chapter heading has been altered to *Mental and Behavioural Disorders*. A number of subheadings are used including Disorders of Psychological Development and included under this heading are given ten categories coded from F80 to F89 and including *Specific Developmental Disorders of Speech and Language*, which is coded as F80. Ten categories of Speech and Language Disorders are then listed under this heading.

In the preamble to the section (F80) it is stated that these are disorders 'in which normal patterns of language acquisition are disturbed from the early stages of development' and it is further stated that these disorders are not the result of sensory impairments, mental retardation, etc. Associated problems such as difficulties in reading and spelling, emotional and behavioural disorders are referred to. So far, most speech and language therapists would agree. However, the comment that 'The conditions are not directly attributable to neurological or speech mechanism abnormalities' would not produce the same consensus.

An example of an entry (p.371) is as follows:

F80.0 Specific speech articulation disorder
A specific developmental disorder in which the child's use of speech sounds is below the appropriate level for his mental age, but in which there is a normal level of language skills.
Developmental:
* phonological disorder
* speech articulation disorder
Dyslalia
Functional speech articulation disorder
Lalling
Excludes: speech articulation impairment (due to):
    * aphasia NOS (R47.0)
    * apraxia (R48.2)
    * hearing loss (H90-H91)
    * mental retardation (F70-F79)
    * with language developmental disorder:
        * expressive (F80.1)
        * receptive (F80.2)

(The figures in parenthesis are for cross referencing).

Most practitioners would consider the terms *dyslalia*, *functional speech articulation disorder* and *lalling* as totally out-moded terms, and we would not accept that a phonological disorder excludes the co-existence of a 'language developmental disorder.'

In her reference to earlier editions of this classification system, Byers Brown (1989: 30) states that those professions that deal entirely with disorders of communication, would find such classifications unsatisfactory, but she reminds us that the major purpose of the WHO relates to the underlying conditions affecting mortality and the spread of disease. Communication disorders, as previously stated, form a very small section of the publication.

Efforts were made both by the International Association of Logopedics and Phoniatrics (IALP) and the American Speech-Language-Hearing Association (ASHA) to influence the direction of ICD-10. Some improvements from ICD-9 are noted, but the classification system, as far as communication disorders are concerned, is still not satisfactory.

A main concern of IALP and ASHA was the inclusion of communication disorders in the chapter on mental disorders. ASHA specifically recommended that 'specific developmental disorders of speech and language' be classified in the chapter titled *Diseases of the Nervous System*. IALP made a similar recommendation. These recommendations were not acted upon but, as stated above, the chapter heading was changed to include *Behavioural Disorders*.

International Classification of Impairments, Disabilities and Handicaps

A further publication of the WHO is the above-named classification published in 1980 in an attempt to deal with the consequences of disease, as opposed to the disease process itself; it was reprinted with corrections in 1993. Byers Brown (1989: 31) states that 'it offers a unifying framework within which the consequences of disease can be considered.' This classification is more relevant to a profession concerned with the remediation and rehabilitation of communication disorders than is the ICD, and it is used extensively by some speech and language therapists (see, for example, Chapter 3).

Each of the categories *Impairments*, *Disabilities* and *Handicaps*, is defined and characteristics are given, together with a rationale for classification. Thus impairment is defined as follows:

In the context of health experience an impairment is any disturbance of or interference with the normal structure and functioning of the body and the person.

Characteristics are stated as being 'a permanent or transitory psychological, physiological, or anatomical loss or abnormality.' Encompassed in the description is 'an abnormality of a functional system or mechanism of the body, including the systems of mental function'.

In the rationale it is accepted that overlap can occur between *Impairment* and *Disability* particularly in certain physiological and psychological impairments which may also constitute a disability by virtue of the associated limitation in function. The disability classification is concerned with the functioning of the individual as a whole. The definition given is:

> In the context of health experience a disability is any loss or reduction in the functional performance of the body or the person that is consequent upon impairment.

As with the ICD, a coding system is used with Impairments of Language Function classified between 30 and 34.

A sample of the coding system is as follows.

30.   *Severe impairment of communication*
        Excludes: impairments classifiable to 31
30.0 *Severe functional impairment of communication*
        Includes: mutism
30.1 *Combined central disorders of speech and visual function*
        with severe impairment of communication
        Includes: autism
30.2 *Impairment of higher centres for speech with inability to*
        communicate
        Includes: severe dysphasia
30.3 *Other dysphasia*
30.4 *Other severe impairment of communication due to cerebral*
        damage
30.5 *Other total or severe interference with communication*
30.8 *Other impairment of higher centres for speech*
30.9 *Unspecified*

Other categories which follow include:

31   *Impairment of language comprehension and use*
32   *Impairment of extralinguistic and sublinguistic functions*
33   *Impairment of other linguistic functions*
34   *Other impairment of learning*
35   *Impairments of speech (this section includes voice)*
36   *Other impairment of voice function*
37   *Impairment of speech form (includes fluency)*
38   *Impairment of speech context*
39   *Other impairment of speech*

Communication disorders are also classified under *Disability* with reference made to speaking, listening, seeing and other aspects of communication.

The final section in this publication deals with *Handicap*:

Definition: A handicap is a disadvantage for a given individual, resulting from an impairment or a disability, that limits or prevents the fulfilment of a role that is normal.

This classification system would seem to be of greater relevance to the speech and language therapist than the ICD-10 (see Chapter 3).

Diagnostic and Statistical Manual of Mental Disorders (DSM III)

DSM III represents efforts by the American Psychiatric Association, a major professional body in the USA, to modify the classification system of WHO (ICD-9); the latest revised edition was published in 1987. Reference is made in the introduction to the manual to the growing recognition of the principles of diagnosis in both clinical practice and research. It is stated that 'Clinicians and Research investigators must have a common language with which to communicate about the disorders for which they have professional responsibility' (p.1). While this statement is relevant for those concerned with communication disorders, Byers Brown (1989: 32) states that 'DSM III cannot be expected to meet the needs of professions concerned with communication since it was created by a different professional group'. It does, however, provide a model for the needs of the speech-language therapist, which ICD-10 does not. It places emphasis 'upon clinical usefulness for making treatment and management decisions in varied clinical settings; reliability of diagnostic categories; acceptability to clinicians and researchers of varying theoretical orientations; and usefulness for educating health professionals' (Byers Brown, 1989: 32).

Law (1992: 24) considers the DSM III 'a definitive classification system.' He refers to the section dealing with Developmental Language Disorders (315, 31) which is divided into the following sections:

1. Failure to acquire any language
2. Acquired language disability
3. Developmental language disorder.

According to Law (1992), the first is normally associated with severe mental handicap, the second with trauma or neurological disorder, whilst the third is further subdivided into expressive and receptive language disorder and clearly deals with specific language impairment and not with language disorder secondary to such factors as hearing loss, mental retardation, etc.

Disorders of Communication (315, 39) are given under the general title *Disorders Usually First Evident in Infancy, Childhood or Adolescence*, with a further sub-heading *Specific developmental disorders*. Throughout the volume a similar format is used for each disorder:

a - description
b - associated features
c - age at onset
d - course
e - prevalence
f - familial pattern
g - differential diagnosis
h - diagnostic criteria.

Information is current and relevant but not unnaturally lacks the detail required by the speech-language therapist.

The American Speech-Language-Hearing Association (ASHA) has not found the DSM III communication codes acceptable and has therefore attempted to design their own coding system.

American Speech-Language-Hearing Association Coding System

A Task Force on Classification Systems was established by ASHA in 1982, which resulted in the ASHA Classification System (ASHACS) published in *ASHA* in December, 1987. This system was used by 'the federal government, the Health Care Financing Administration (HCFA), in establishing the Health Care Financing Administration Common Procedure Coding System (HCPCS) for speech-language pathology and audiology procedures' (Spahr, 1994, personal communication).

The purpose of developing the ASHACS was to permit a uniform system for describing procedures used, and diagnosis made, by speech-language pathologists and audiologists. It arose out of 'the inadequate conceptualization and misapplication of speech, language, and hearing disorders and procedures in the DSM-III and other coding systems' (ASHA, 1987).

The system is a numerical one divided into sections and the following is an example of some of these 20 divisions, each containing a number of sub-headings:

01.0 – 11.0	Speech-Language Pathology and Audiology – Procedures
20.0 – 26.0	Audiology Procedures
30.0 – 36.0	Speech-Language Pathology Procedures
110.0 – 117.0	Speech-Language and Related Diagnosis

| 120.0 | Cognitive Communication Disorder |
| 130.0 | Speech Articulation Disorder |

In addition to the general coding the system permits entry of time of onset using 1 = unknown, 2 = prelinguistic or developmental, 3 = postlingual or acquired, 4 = not applicable.

While the main purpose of the system is for financial accounting, the breakdown, under each of the major headings, is adequate for record keeping, epidemiological purposes, etc. and is certainly a big improvement on other classification systems.

The Read Codes

The Read Codes originated in the Primary Health Care Service in the UK and, at the present time, work is in progress to develop this system further in order to provide an agreed thesaurus of terms. It is hoped that through this system a common language will be developed to aid communication between all health care professionals.

The Needs of Professions in Communication Disorders

As stated earlier in this chapter, there are a number of functions served by a classification system. A major function is the collection of data to provide information on prevalence and incidence of disorders. In the USA, third party reimbursement sources require a coding system for billing purposes and now make use of the ASHACS for this purpose. To date this need has not existed as a high priority in the UK, but the move to trusts and purchasing of services within the National Health Service will create such a need. In referring to the current position in the UK, Enderby and Davies (1989: 302) state 'There is little detailed information on the size of the speech and language impaired population and less information with regard to those with speech and language handicap'. Some form of reliable coding system is, therefore, essential to facilitate the collection of data to provide such information. While it is feasible for an organization as large as ASHA (current membership approximately 80 000) to produce its own coding system, for The College of Speech and Language Therapists (CSLT), with a current membership of approximately 5000, it would be difficult to mount such a project alone. The collaboration of the CSLT in the development of the Read Coding System will hopefully fulfil these requirements.

It would seem reasonable to expect that the task of providing a European Coding System could be assumed by the Comité Permanent de Liaison des Orthophonistes-Logopéds (CPLOL) – the permanent liaison committee of EU speech therapists and logopedists, founded in 1988 in an effort to bring together the associations in the European Union (EU) concerned with communication disorders. With freedom of movement within the EU, it will become increasingly necessary to have a quick and easy referencing system available to speech and language therapists and their employing authorities throughout the EU.

References

American Speech-Language-Hearing Association (1986) Classification of Speech-Language Pathology and Audiology Procedures and Communication Disorders. Report of the task force on classification.

American Speech-Language-Hearing Association (1993) Definitions of Communication Disorders and Variations. ASHA 35 (Suppl. 10: 40–1).

American Psychiatric Association (1987) Diagnostic and Statistical Manual of Mental Disorders DSM III. Washington.

Bishop D (1989) Autism, Asperger's Syndrome and Semantic – Pragmatic Disorder: Where are the boundaries? British Journal of Disorders of Communication 24(3): 107–21.

Bloodstein O (1979) Speech Pathology: An Introduction. Boston: Houghton Mifflin.

Byers Brown B (1989) Disorders of Communication. The Science of Intervention, Chapter 3. London: Whurr.

Byers Brown B, Edwards M (1989) Developmental Disorders of Language. London: Whurr.

Communicating Quality (1991) College of Speech and Language Therapists, UK.

Crystal D (1982) Terms, time and teeth. British Journal of Disorders of Communication 17: 3–19.

Crystal D, Varley R (1993) Introduction to Language Pathology (3rd ed.). London: Whurr.

Dockrell J, McShane J (1993) Children's Learning Difficulties. Oxford: Blackwell.

Edwards M (1985) Terminology. Good descriptions are needed for clear diagnosis. Speech Therapy Practice 1: 20–1.

Enderby P, Davies P (1989) Communication disorders: Planning a service to meet the needs. British Journal of Disorders of Communication 24(3): 301–32.

International Classification of Impairments, Disabilities and Handicaps (1980) A manual relating to the consequence of disease. Geneva, World Health Organization.

International Statistical Classification of Diseases and Related Health Problems (1992) Vol. 1. Geneva, World Health Organization.

Kleffner FR (1977) Language Disorders in Children. Indianapolis: Bobbs Merrill. London: Chapman and Hall.

Morley M (1966) Editorial, British Journal of Disorders of Communication 1: 1.

Nation J, Aram D (1977) Diagnosis of Speech and Language Disorders. St Louis: C.V. Mosby.

Oyer HJ, Hall BJ, Haas WH (1994) Speech, Language and Hearing Disorders. A Guide for the Teacher. Boston, MA: Allyn & Bacon.

Rapin I, Allen DA (1987) Developmental dysphasia and autism in preschool children. In Proceedings of First International Symposium: Specific Speech and Language Disorders in Children, University of Reading, UK. London: AFASIC.

Shames GH, Wiig EH (Eds) (1982) Human Communication Disorders. Columbus, OH: Merrill.

Sonninen A, Hurme P (1989) Towards multi-lingual voice terminology. Clinical and Related Research in Communication. Helsinki, Finnish Association of Logopedics and Phoniatrics.

Chapter 3
Epidemiology of Communication Disorders and Service Planning

PAMELA ENDERBY

Services for the speech- and language-impaired are, in most countries, noticeably disparate. They have tended to grow on the basis of local argument and history rather than on objective studies of need. If there is to be efficient planning in the health care process, it is essential for there to be information with regard to the size and needs of the populations to be served and the professional skills and abilities required to serve those needs. This chapter offers one approach to calculating the number of speech and language clinicians required to provide an equitable service. The chapter reviews information regarding the epidemiology of speech and language impairment along with information relating to the role of the speech and language clinician with different client groups.

It is recognized that there are weaknesses in the methodology of collating a mixture of information, some of it sound and relating to objective studies and some of it less sound including speculation, and then adding philosophy. Despite this the author feels that even this approach is more appropriate than the traditional *ad hoc* way of deciding on service levels. Finally, the figures will call into question some of our basic premises regarding the provision of service, suggesting that inability to offer an equitable service in one way should lead to consideration of different forms of provision to meet the needs of the speech- and language-disabled population.

Method

Speech and language disorders form a heterogeneous group as they are often either secondary to a variety of underlying medical or surgical problems, or else part of a general or specific developmental disorder. There is little detailed information on the size of the speech- and language-impaired population in its own right and even less information with regard to those with speech and language disability and handicap. For the purposes of this paper the terms 'impairment', 'disability' and 'handicap' will not be used indiscriminately, but as defined by the World Health Organization, as described in Chapter 2:

> impairments are concerned with the loss or abnormalities of body structure and appearance and with organ or system function resulting from any cause; disability reflects the consequence of impairment on functional performance and activity by the individual; handicaps represent disadvantages resulting from any impairment or disability that limits or prevents the fulfilment of normal roles in life.

The reviews of the literature which exist on the prevalence and incidence of communication impairment, in both adults and children, all indicate the problems related to the lack of clarity in the terminology and the difficulties associated with interpreting data which may have been primarily collected for other purposes (Enderby and Phillipp, 1986; Fein, 1983; Healey et al., 1981; Harasty and McCooey, 1994). However, most of the studies show consistently identifiable trends amongst the general population. In the report by Enderby and Phillipp (1986) the main groups of medical developmental and congenital problems that give rise to speech and language disorders were listed and, where possible, the size of the speech and language population was estimated from the population studies and case series cited in the literature. It was recognized that the list was not exclusive and, where some conditions were the subject of several studies, giving rise to a range of results, the median incidence and prevalence rate was selected to estimate the number of speech- and language-disabled people. This method of study was similar to that used in the report of a committee of enquiry into the UK speech therapy services commonly referred to as the Quirk Report (1972). Incidence and prevalence estimates are difficult to derive for several reasons: definitions are not always uniform, available information is sparse and information is often based on specific populations rather than on community based studies. Thus the findings must be considered an approximation. It is expected that the figures err on the side of caution as any difficulties in interpretation have led to exclusion rather than inclusion. The study was based upon the 1983 mid-year population of the UK (56 377 000 persons) which was produced by the Office of Population Census and Surveys, England and Wales (OPCS) (1984).

Clinical experience has led to an opinion, albeit subjective, of the proportions of 'severe' and 'moderate' speech handicap represented in different population groups. In this report the term 'severe' has been applied to persons who have difficulty in making themselves understood by anyone other than their immediate family. This group also includes the non-vocal. The term 'moderate' includes those persons whose speech defect is noticeable to the lay person, but who may nevertheless remain intelligible.

Information on clinical intervention has been gathered in two ways. First, from studying the text books and relevant journals with regard to current thinking about speech and language therapeutic intervention; second, an analysis of intervention by speech and language clinicians within one district health authority has been conducted. The data have been collected on a time recording sheet which allows analysis not only of the clinicians' input, but also of the amount of intervention each patient from each client group receives. In addition, some arbitrary decisions have been made with regard to what seems 'reasonable'. This chapter will try and be clear about what is fact and what is philosophy.

Numbers of patients with speech and language impairment

The study of the literature supports a widely held view that the true incidence and prevalence of speech and language disorders is much higher than previously estimated. This concurs with the more recently gathered information (Harasty and McCooey, 1994). Whilst there is a general acknowledgement that the data gathered are deficient in many respects, the suggested revised estimate for the size of the speech- and language-impaired population in the UK is 2.3 million persons (severe communication disorders – 800 000). Furthermore, these estimates are probably conservative, as some groups of speech and language disorders have not been included. For example, there are no readily available data from which to estimate the likely number of persons with autism, mutism, psychological speech loss, familial dystonias, psychiatric speech disturbance etc. Nevertheless, these estimates suggest that the speech impaired population of 324 180 persons, quoted in the Quirk Report (1972) is a gross underestimate.

Time analysis: the clinicians' input

The computer-based time analysis system of speech and language clinicians showed that Senior II and Senior I clinicians make an average of 5.3 face-to-face contacts each day. Their working day has a mean of seven hours and the length of treatment sessions is 45 minutes. Thus the contact time with patients per clinician day is 3.9 hours. Non face-to-face contact time shows a mean of 0.85 hours. This includes individual patient directed activities such as telephone calls, liaison with associated professionals, discussions with relatives, analysing test results, writing reports, etc. These clinical duties involve general patient-directed activities such as organizing treatment materials, attending case conferences, teaching groups of staff, and so on. Non-clinical professional duties include collection of statistics, ordering equipment, and attending professional staff meetings, accounting for 0.70 hours. If we assume that the working year is 46 weeks for each speech and language clinician, it is easy to deduce that there is the possibility of 897 face-to-face hours per clinician if we continue to pursue this approach to intervention.

Provision of Services

Children requiring speech and language therapy

In the Quirk Report (1972) on speech therapy the available literature concerning children with speech and language disabilities was discussed. This report cited many studies including the pioneering work of Morley (1972) which reported that 14 per cent of young children were unintelligible to their teachers.

Taking into consideration the social class and age variations between populations that have been studied, Quirk suggested that between 2 and 3 per cent of the normal school population have a specific speech defect. However, Ingram (1972) cautions readers that, although in the UK a number of studies of different population samples have become available, the criteria for defining a speech problem were remarkably crude: 'Before estimates of the prevalence of disorders of speech in childhood are accepted the criteria of what constitutes a speech defect and the methods of selection should be reviewed with care...'. Fortunately, detailed information has since become available from the National Child Development Study (Peckham, 1973; Butler, Peckham and Sheridan, 1973). This study was based on a longitudinal survey of over 15 000 seven-year-old children born in one week in 1958. A survey of these children has shown that, at the age of seven years, between 10 and 13 per cent of the children had some degree of speech impairment. These speech-impaired children were more often males and often from manual social backgrounds. Teachers reported 10.7 per cent of the children to be difficult to understand because of poor speech.

Clearly the prevalence of language delay is dependent on the definitions used and the reports vary considerably: 0.07 per cent (Ingram, 1963), 5.3 per cent (Morley, 1965), 8.4 per cent (Silver, 1980). It is interesting that increasing prevalence has been shown in a chronological fashion; this may reflect the fact that recently more sensitive ways of assessing delayed or abnormal speech and language have been perfected, possibly resulting in improved detection.

> The lack of straightforward or strictly defined prevalence figures in communication impairment in children reflects the nature of the phenomena that prevalence research is trying to define. The communication process is dynamic, complex, and interactive; these characteristics contribute to the difficulty in unequivocally identifying impairment (Blum-Harasty and Rosenthal, 1992).

The Office of Population Census and Surveys (OPCS) indicates that children aged between nought and four-years-old account for 6.37 per cent of the general population and children aged between five- and fourteen-years-old account for 13.09 per cent of the population. A midpoint of the prevalence figures would suggest that there are 1091 children per 100 000 population with specific speech and language disorders. The referral of these children to services will tend to bunch at certain ages, usually at three years and then at five years. We would therefore expect 369 referrals per annum per 100 000 population. Most children require at least two hours face-to-face contact with the speech and language clinician so that general behaviour and interaction in play can be observed and communication disorder can be assessed both formally and informally. Thus, 738 hours of assessment would be required per annum to service the estimated population. The average amount of time spent with a child and family following assessment in order to explain and reassure, and to plan a programme of help, is on average 1.5 hours per child.

A significant proportion of the children will not require further intervention from the clinician, thus accounting for the apparently low mean figure of 0.5 hours for reassessment. Thirty per cent of the population referred to speech therapy would therefore require a mean of 30 hours direct intervention, be it individually or in a group situation.

Clinicians will not be surprised that there is a broad range of treatment lengths running from two hours to over 100 hours. For the population we are discussing, this would account for 3690 hours of intervention. Ten per cent of the children referred have profound problems requiring lengthy and regular involvement, accounting for a further 3394 hours of contact. Thus it is possible to deduce that children's services will require 8169 hours clinical contact which, when divided by the 897 hours available to each speech and language clinicians, indicates that 9.10 clinicians per 100 000 population should be available to provide an equitable service for this group.

It should be pointed out that the level of intervention proposed here is not extravagant and is in line with the professional standards for speech and language therapists as published in *Communicating Quality* (1992). If one considers a child who is not speaking by the age of three, or is speaking in a way that is not intelligible to others, it would seem reasonable that he requires a two-hour assessment. In addition, parents are given 1.5 hours counselling and advice and it does not appear to be extravagant to offer the child on average 30 hours treatment to try and remedy this problem.

Learning Difficulty

Although mental handicap constitutes the largest disabled population with associated communication disorders (Ingram, 1972) it is one of the most problematic to review. There is no sharp dividing line between intellectual normality and sub-normality; persons with mental handicap are not impaired equally in functions and may have concomitant specific impairments. At least 2.5 per cent of children have intellectual handicap (IQ less than 70) and 'over half of these show a severe language deficiency or an articulation defect or both' (Rutter, Tizard and Whitmore, 1970). If we consider again the percentage of children in the population, as was done in the previous section, and calculate that 2.5 per cent of these will be intellectually handicapped and of these 50 per cent will have problems with communication, we arrive at a figure of 243 children up to the age of 14 per 100 000 population who will require the speech and language clinicians' consideration. The referral rates again tend to cluster at three years of age, seven years of age and 14 years of age, leading to an average approximation of 50 referrals per 100 000 population.

Learning-disabled patients are notoriously difficult to assess, requiring in-depth formal and long-term informal observation to establish whether communication development is out of line with mental development. Thus these 50 learning-disabled persons will require, on average, a five-hour assessment, resulting in 250 hours of time spent on this activity. Of these persons, half will require full intervention, which, for the purpose of this paper, has been defined as one hour a day for five days a week for 46 weeks a year.

Commitment to intervening with the intellectually impaired needs to be complete as efforts to change the behaviour of those with learning disabilities is only possible if treatment is delivered with sufficient intensity to ensure that not only is the behaviour learned, but that it is generalized and used. Thus, speech and language intervention could lead to 5750 hours of face-to-face contact with these clients. The other 25 patients referred will usually require reassessment, guidance, advice and support.

Additionally, there is a great deal of training that goes on for those who care for the learning disabled in order to ensure that the environment promotes communication. This general training and advice is difficult to quantify but we have suggested that one hour twice a week for 46 weeks appears to be a reasonable average for each of these 25 clients. In reality, the intervention is frequently provided in a group context with teaching programmes being conducted by speech and language clinicians for groups of caring staff and/or relatives. Thus for the purposes of this calculation, and to reflect reality rather than idealism, I shall allot 1150 hours to these clients rather than the 2300 hours which would be required for individual face-to-face input.

Reappraisal, participation in case conferences, and emphasis on changing the general culture towards communication, are difficult to divide up, and as this is not classified in this study as being 'face-to-face time' I shall omit these separate figures. Thus the speech and language clinician is directly involved for 7150 hours. If we divide this by the 897 hours available for each clinician for face-to-face time then we can deduce that we require 7.97 whole-time equivalents per 100 000 population to deliver this level of service.

This accounts for only one section of the intellectually impaired population and ignores the fact that the non face-to-face component is larger for this group than others, and thus these figures are recognized to be another low estimate.

Acquired communication disorders

The adult services can be divided into four main areas: stroke, the progressively ill, head injury, and dysphonia (including laryngectomy).

Cerebral Vascular Disease. Some 200 persons per 100 000 population have a stroke each year (Whisnant, 1976). The occasions of aphasia immediately after stroke range from 21 per cent (Brust et al., 1976) to 48.7 per cent (Hu, Qiou and Zhon, 1990). The survival rate is suggested to be between 63 and 77 per cent (Carter, 1964; Marquardsen, 1969). Excluding those who die, or those whose speech recovers quickly, stroke has an annual incidence of between 0.03 per cent (Bonita and Anderson, 1983) and 0.02 per cent (Gresham and Phillips, 1979; Wade et al., 1986). Prevalence rates are cited between 0.04 per cent (Gresham and Phillips, 1979) and 0.05 per cent (Hopkins, 1975; Matsumoto et al., 1978) and thus we would expect 30 referrals annually with stroke-related speech and language disorders per 100 000 population. A further 15 patients may be re-referred or referred following a second stroke or deterioration. Thus there will be 45 patients to be assessed by this service.

Assessment of aphasia on average takes 2.5 hours requiring 112.5 hours to be spent on this activity. Many of the patients with persisting speech and language disorder will require one of three kinds of intervention:

1 *Regular therapy*. This is defined as 1.5 hours treatment (including reassessment) per day for four days per week for six months.
2 *Guidance*. This covers the group of patients requiring support, reassurance and reassessment amounting to one hour per week for six months.
3 *Stimulation*. Some patients will require exposure to a socially stimulating environment to promote communicative effectiveness. These patients are often seen in a group situation and it would account for five hours intervention per group per week for 46 weeks.

Stroke studies within the Frenchay district over the last five years have shown that approximately 33 per cent of the 45 patients fall into one of the treatment categories outlined above. Thus regular therapy for 15 patients will require 2340 hours of intervention per year. Fifteen patients will require guidance accounting for 390 hours of intervention, and the final 15 patients, who would benefit from stimulation, account for 230 hours of involvement. Therefore the total face-to-face time for stroke population offering this degree of flexibility would add up to 3072.5 hours, this divided by the 897 hours available to each clinician would suggest that 3.42 whole-time equivalents are required to offer this level of service consistently for stroke patients.

Some studies have suggested that intensive intervention for some stroke dysphasic patients is efficacious (Wertz, Collins and Brookshire, 1978; Basso, Capitani and Vignolo, 1979; Vignolo, 1964). A study by Leigh-Smith et al. (1987) indicated that between five and 14 patients per 100 000 per year would meet criteria suggested as being appropriate for inclusion in this form of therapy (four hours therapy five days a week for three months). If intensive therapy is to be pursued, then it is suggested that a further whole-time clinician is allowed, even when accounting for removing that particular group from the regular therapy sessions.

Progressive Neurological Disease. Many of the progressive neurological diseases may lead to a concomitant speech and language disorder. Parkinson's Disease has an incidence rate of 20 cases per 100 000 population and prevalence rate of 100 to 150 cases per 100 000 (Brewis, Pozkanzer and Roland, 1966). The proportion of patients suffering from speech disorders associated with Parkinson's Disease has been reported as low as 3.8 per cent (Hoehn and Yahr, 1967) to 50 per cent in more detailed studies (Logemann, Fisher and Blonsky, 1978; Merritt, 1979). Gibberd, Oxtoby and Jewell (1985) found that only 36 per cent of patients with Parkinson's Disease considered that they had no speech difficulty.

The incidence of Multiple Sclerosis in Britain has been suggested to be three per 100 000 population (Kurtzke, 1982). However, the incidence rate of this disease, with its uncertain onset, is difficult. Prevalence rate may be more accurate and is considered to be between 0.06 and 0.08 per cent within the UK. Approximately half have some degree of speech and language disorder and of these one third have great difficulty (Darley, Brown and Goldstein, 1972).

Motor Neurone Disease has an incidence of 1.6 per 100 000 population (Kurland, 1977) and the prevalence rate is indicated to be six per 100 000. In 25 per cent of cases dysarthria and dysphagia are the first symptoms of Motor Neurone Disease (Garfinkle and Kimmelman, 1982). However, all patients will finally have some degree of speaking and swallowing difficulty as the disease progresses (Bobowick and Brody, 1973).

Patients with Freidrich's Ataxia, muscular dystrophy, myasthenia gravis and Huntingdon's Chorea may also have quite severe communication problems. The suggested incidence and prevalence rates are seen in Table 3.1.

As a result of the insidious nature of many neurological diseases and the usually slow onset of speech problems, the time of referral to speech therapy varies noticeably from district to district, according to the

Table 3.1 Estimates for the size of the UK speech and language handicapped populations associated with certain medical problems* 1985. (Listed in order of decreasing prevalence of the disorder.) Reproduced by kind permission of the *British Journal of Disorders of Communication:* 21, 151–165, 1986 (Aug.)

Disorder	Incidence of disorder per 100,000 population	Prevalence of disorder per 100,000 population	Percent with disorder causing speech or language problem	Number of speech/lang handicapped per 100,000 population	Number of severely speech/lang handicapped per 100,000 population	Number with moderate speech/lang handicap 100,000 population
Mental handicap (all ages)	NK	2,500.0	55.0	1375.0	800.0	575.0
Stammering	3495.0	1,070.0	100.0	1070.0	70.0	1000.0
Pre-school age speech & lang.**	NK	691.2	100.0	691.2	230.4	460.8
School age speech & lang.**	NK	400.0	100.0	400.0	200.0	200.0
CVA	200.0	500.0	30.0	150.0	70.0	80.0
Deafness	1.6	200.0	60.0	120.0	45.0	75.0
Cerebral Palsy***	2.0	175.0	60.0	105.0	20.0	85.0
Cleft Palate***	2.0	NK (>142.0)	40.0	57.0	19.0	38.0
Parkinson's Disease	20.0	125.0	55.0	69.0	23.0	46.0
Multiple Sclerosis	3.0	60.0	55.0	33.0	10.0	23.0
Dysphonia	28.0	28.0	100.0	28.0	10.0	18.0
Muscular Dystrophy	1.2	20.0	25.0	5.0	2.0	3.0
Motor Neurone Disease	1.6	6.0	57.5	3.5	1.2	2.3
Myasthenia Gravis	3.0	6.0	25.0	1.5	0.5	1.0
Huntington's Chorea	0.4	5.0	60.0	3.0	1.0	2.0
Laryngectomy	0.9	3.0	100.0	3.0	2.0	1.0
Friedreich's Ataxia	0.4	2.0	60.0	1.2	0.6	0.6
Head Injury	286.0	NK (800)	20.0	NK (160)	NK (60)	NK (100)

*   *Many of the figures in this table are estimated from references cited in the text. They should be used as a guide rather than a definitive statement.*

**   *The incidence and prevalence estimates are derived from the number of pre-school children per 100,000 general population.*

***   *Based on the numbers per 100,000 new born population.*

NK   *Not known.*

services available and the knowledge of the consultants with regard to the role of the speech and language clinicians with such disorders.

In one health district, studied for this chapter, 16 patients were referred per 100 000 population per annum with speech language and swallowing problems associated with progressive neurological disease. These 16 patients required assessment for a mean of 2.5 hours and they had an average of one hour's intervention per week for six months. Six of the patients required communication aids and each of these required an average of 15 hours direct intervention time. Reassessment plays a high role in the speech clinician's intervention with the progressively ill in order that she can report back to the medical consultants any change in status and that she has a basis for advice. A further 2.5 hours per patient should be set aside for this. This time is used in different ways so that there may be either many short reassessments or a few longer reassessments according to the type of the disorder. Accordingly, a speech clinician can account for 586 hours of face-to-face contact time resulting in a requirement of 0.65 of a whole-time equivalent speech and language clinician per 100 000 population to offer this basic level of intervention.

Head Injury. It is difficult to establish the morbidity associated with head injury. The number of patients suffering head injury is large; in 1972 there were 142 000 admissions to hospital in England and Wales of patients suffering the effects of head injury (Field Research Division of DHSS, 1975). Fortunately, the majority of patients suffering head injury make a full recovery, but there is a small percentage who remain severely and permanently handicapped. Data from the OPCS suggest an annual incidence rate in England and Wales of 1.1 per cent for persistent dysphasia from intra-cranial injury without skull fracture, and an incidence of 1.5 per cent following a fractured skull. The prevalence rate may be estimated broadly as being 160 people per 100 000 who have some degree of dysphasia as the result of head injury. Of course, the prevalence rate covers a very long span of years and therefore it is difficult to speculate what a reasonable referral rate would be.

However, studies of one particular district suggest that a referral rate of 20 patients per 100 000 population is a fair expectation. All patients referred require an assessment and the mean time for assessing head injury patients has been found to be three hours. The range of speech-therapy intervention available to these patients is again varied; some require little input following assessment and guidance, whilst others require literally hundreds of hours of therapy. Again, the broad range in the standard deviation of intervention time suggests that the means are not particularly useful, but it does give some impression of the services that may be needed. The mean of treatment of the head-injured population is 23 hours per case. This would lead to 460 hours to cover the referral rate per year. Thus, the total care of this population would require 520 hours face-to-face contact time leading to 0.57 of a whole-time equivalent speech and language clinician per 100 000 population to offer this basic level of intervention.

Dysphonia (including laryngectomy). Phonatory problems may be a symptom of neurological, organic or functional disorders. Some of the neurological and organic dysphonias have been included in other sections. This section includes those dysphonias related to polyps, nodules, oedema of the vocal cords and dysphonia associated with functional disorders. Aphonia associated with laryngectomy should also be considered. A review of the literature and a study of patterns of referral are detailed by Enderby and Phillipp (1986). They conclude that there is annual incidence of dysphonia of 28 per 100 000 and this is confirmed by a review of 12 studies by Harasty and McCooey (1994). The latter authors warn that the prevalence range not surprisingly varies quite dramatically according to the base population studied. College students show the lowest prevalence, whereas studies of nursing homes show much higher prevalence.

The incidence of laryngectomy per 100 000 population is estimated to be 0.9 and the prevalence 3.0. There appears to be some regional variations with regard to these figures which are possibly associated with the time of detection and availability of radiotherapy.

The amount of treatment that dysphonic patients and laryngectomy patients require is again very varied. The different approaches available, the different philosophies underlying the treatments, have an effect on the intervention. For the purposes of this article we would suggest that there will be 28 referrals per year per 100 000 of people with dysphonia, and one referral per year per 100 000 population for laryngectomy. The speech clinician will be involved with the laryngectomy patient pre- and post-operatively and this will lead to 60 hours of intervention.

Of the dysphonic patients following a 1.5 hour assessment, ten will require limited therapy and guidance averaging two hours each, and 18 will require ten hours of direct treatment, be this to do with counselling, relaxation or direct voice therapy. Thus, dysphonic patients require 142 hours of intervention. This, along with the hours required for laryngectomy, requires 0.22 whole-time equivalent speech and language clinician.

Care of the elderly

Some 14 per cent of the population are over 65 years of age. Many of those requiring therapy will already have been covered in previous sections. However, increasing age gives rise to a greater likelihood of acquired speech and language disorders associated with neurological illness or disease or psychological deterioration. Study of one Care of the Elderly Unit showed that we would expect 50 new referrals per year per 100 000 population. These require on average 2.5 hours of assessment. Twenty had specific treatment on average twice a week for three months leading to 480 hours. A further 30 required support, stimulation and guidance leading to 0.5 hours per week for a year. To offer this flexibility of service we would require 1295 hours leading to 1.4 whole-time equivalent speech and language clinicians.

Conclusion

Quirk (1972) suggested that the speech therapy service should be based on six clinicians per 100 000 population. When considering his suggestion that 324 180 persons in the UK had a speech and language handicap as compared to the present projected figures of 2.3 million, it is not surprising that the profession does not feel that his indications are now valid. One way of speculating how many speech clinicians we require would be to multiply Quirk's figure of six clinicians by seven indicating the acknowledged increase in speech and language impairment in the community. Thus, one could argue for 42 speech and language clinicians per 100 000 population; however, this figure should be questioned as the sparse information on incidence and prevalence of speech and language disorders available to the Quirk Commission was only matched by the sparse information on the role of the speech clinician. Further, we must be aware that there are many more people with speech and language impairment, disability and handicap who do not require the service of speech clinicians. Thus, the analysis that has been discussed here is another way of speculating how to develop speech therapy provision. If an equitable service is to be implemented, and if current methods of intervention are to be pursued, then it would appear that at least 23.37 speech and language clinicians per 100 000 population are justified. Without this level of staffing, service provision is spread thinly and the allocation is not usually made on a rational basis.

If we consider the needs of the population and the reality of funding difficulties, it may be necessary for us to question whether there are other alternatives to solving the provision of services to the speech and language disabled. We must consider whether continuing in our present mould is justified, practical, and/or likely to be resourced.

We have a choice; either we can offer, in an inequitable way, the model of service presently available, rationing our provision to the clients, or we change our concept of the provision dramatically, redefining the role of the speech clinician and the way that we relate not only to patients and their relatives but also to other professionals.

By looking at the current position in some detail and the implications that it poses for the future, we have more information to fuel discussions of the future of the profession.

References

Basso A, Capitani E, Vignolo LA (1979) Influence of rehabilitation in language skills in aphasic patients : a controlled study. Archives of Neurology 36: 190–6.

Blum-Harasty JA, Rosenthal JB (1992) The prevalence of communication disorders in children: a summary and critical review. Australian Journal of Communication Disorders 20(1): 63–79.

Bobowick AR, Brody JA (1973) Epidemiology of motor neurone disease. New England Journal of Medicine 288: 2047–55.

Bonita R, Anderson A (1983) Speech and language disorders after stroke: an epidemiological study. New Zealand Speech and Language Therapy Journal 38: 2–9.

Brewis M, Pozkanzer DC, Rolland C (1966) Neurological disease in an English city. Acta Neurological Scandinavia Supplement. 42(24): 1–89.

Brust J, Shafer S, Richter R, Bruun B (1976) Aphasia in acute stroke. Stroke 7: 167–74.

Butler NR, Peckham C, Sheridan M. (1973) Speech defects in children aged 7 years: a national study. British Medical Journal 3: 253–7.

Carter AB (1964) Cerebral Infarction. New York: MacMillan.

Communicating Quality (1992) Professional Standards for Speech and Language Therapists. Available from The College of Speech and Language Therapy, Bath Place, Rivington Street, London EC2A 3DR.

Darley FL, Brown JR, Goldstein NP (1972) Dysarthria in multiple sclerosis. Journal of Speech and Hearing Research 15: 229–45.

Enderby P, Phillipp R (1986) Speech and language handicap towards knowing the size of the problem. British Journal of Disorders of Communication 21(2): 151–65.

Fein D (1983) The prevalence of speech and language impairments. American Speech and Hearing Association 25: 37.

Field Research Division of DHSS (1975) Epidemiology of head injuries in England and Wales. London: DHSS.

Garfinkle TJ, Kimmelman CP (1982). Neurologic disorders: amyotrophic lateral sclerosis, myasthenia gravis, multiple sclerosis and poliomyelitis. American Journal of Otolaryngology 14: 204–12.

Gibberd FB, Oxtoby M, Jewell PF (1985) The Treatment of Parkinsons Disease: a consumer view. Health Trends 17: 19–21.

Gresham G, Phillips T (1979) Epidemiology profile of long term stroke disability: the Framingham study. Archives of Physical Medicine and Rehabilitation 60: 487–97.

Harasty J, McCooey R (1994) The prevalence of communication impairment in adults: a summary and critical evaluation of the literature. Australian Journal of Human Communication Disorders 21(1): 81–95.

Healey W, Ackerman B, Chappel C, Perrin C, Stormer J (1981) The prevalence of communicative disorders: a review of the literature. American Speech and Hearing Association. Rockville, MD.

Hoehn MM, Yahr MD (1967) Parkinsonism: onset, progress and mortality. Neurology (Minneapolis) 17: 427–42.

Hopkins A (1975) The need for speech therapy for dysphasia following stroke. Health Trends 7: 58–60.

Hu Y, Qiou Y, Zhon G (1990) Crossed aphasia in Chinese: a clinical survey. Brain and Language 39: 347–56.

Ingram TT (1963) Report of the Scottish Dysphasia Subcommittee of the Scottish Paediatric Society. (Unpublished).

Ingram TT (1972) Classification of speech and language disorders in young children.

In Rutter M, Martin J (Eds) The Child with Delayed Speech. London: Spastics International Medicine.

Kurland LT (1977) Epidemiology of amyotrophic lateral sclerosis with emphasis on antecedents events from case control comparisons. In Rose DF (Ed) Motor Neurone Disease. New York: Grune and Stratton.

Kurtzke JF (1982) The current neurological burden of illness and injury in the US. Journal of Neurology, pp 1207–14.

Leigh-Smith JA, Denis R, Enderby P, Wade D, Langton Hewer R (1987) Selection of aphasic stroke patients for intensive speech therapy. Journal of Neurology, Neurosurgery and Psychiatry 50: 1488–92.

Logemann J, Fisher M, Blonsky E (1978) Frequency of co-occurrence of vocal tract dysfunction in a large sample of Parkinson's patients. Journal of Speech and Hearing Disorders 43: 41–57.

Marquardsen J (1969) The natural history of cerebrovascular disease. Acta Neurological Scandinavia Supplement 45: 90–188.

Matsumoto N, Whisnant J, Kurland L, Okasaki H (1978) Natural history of stroke in Rochester Minnesota, 1955–1969 Stroke. 4: 20–9.

Merritt H (1979) A Text Book of Clinical Neurology (6th ed). Philadelphia: Lea and Febiger.

Morley ME (1965) The Development and Disorders of Speech in Childhood (2nd ed), Edinburgh: Churchill Livingstone.

Morley ME (1972) The Development and Disorders of Speech in Childhood (3rd ed), Edinburgh: Churchill Livingstone.

Office of Population Census and Surveys England and Wales (1984). Population Trends. 38: 37.

Peckham CS (1973) Speech defects in a national sample of children aged 7 years. British Journal of Disorders of Communication 8: 2–8.

Quirk R (1972) Speech Therapy Services. London : HMSO.

Rutter M, Tizard J, Whitmore K (Eds) (1970) Education, Health and Behaviour. London: Longmans.

Silver PA (1980) The prevalence, stability and significance of developmental language delay in pre-school children. Developmental Medicine and Child Neurology 22: 768–77.

Vignolo LA. (1964). Evaluation of aphasia and language rehabilitation: a retrospective exploratory study Cortex. 1: 344–67.

Wade D, Langton Hewer R, David R, Enderby P (1986). Stroke: A Critical Approach to Diagnosis, Treatment and Management. London: Chapman and Hall Medical.

Wertz RT, Collins MJ, Brookshire RH (1978) The Veterans Administration Co-operation study on aphasia: a comparison of individual and group treatment. Journal of Speech and Hearing Research 21(4): 652–67.

Whisnant JP (1976) Ninth Pfizer Symposium: stroke. Edinburgh: Churchill Livingstone.

World Health Organization (1980) International Classification of Impairments, Disabilities and Handicaps (ICIDH). Geneva: WHO 1980

Chapter 4
The Profession at Work

ANNA VAN DER GAAG, CRYSTAL COOPER
AND EUGENE COOPER

One of the most challenging and invigorating aspects of the work of speech and language therapy is its diversity. Speech and language therapy serves a wide range of clients with very varied communication needs. The profession offers such clients and their carers advice, assessment, diagnosis, intervention and support. Each of these activities is sustained by a broad base of knowledge and skills in the disciplines of speech and language pathology, linguistics, psychology, medicine, education, health care policy, service and client management (Greenberg and Smith, 1987; Lingwall, 1988; Davies and van der Gaag, 1992a, b; van der Gaag and Davies, 1992a, b, c). This knowledge and skill base is not static, but constantly changing to meet new demands and offer more advanced services. As a result, any description of the profession at work today will not be an accurate description of the profession at work tomorrow.

In addition to the influence of an ever changing knowledge and skill base, the context in which speech and language therapists work also influences the nature and the impact of their craft. Increasingly, health care professionals are aware that their practice is constrained by social, cultural and political influences. Organizational and cultural differences in health care systems, access to training and resources, levels of public awareness in different countries are amongst the factors that determine to a large extent how services like speech and language therapy are delivered. This chapter provides a brief profile of speech and language therapy at work in three countries; the United States, the United Kingdom and the Republic of Ireland. These are by no means representative of speech and language therapy elsewhere in the world, but probably illustrate some of the more established models of service delivery.

Professional Development in the USA

The beginnings of the profession of speech-language pathology in the USA can be traced to the 1880s when a number of private schools devoted to assisting those with speech problems were established (Clark, 1960; Paden, 1970; McLaughlin, 1986). The first speech-language pathology programmes in the American public schools were established in 1910 in Chicago and Detroit (Paden, 1970). By the middle of the twentieth century's second decade, courses dealing specifically with speech disorders were being offered by several universities throughout the USA (Paden, 1970). In December 1925, 11 individuals meeting in New York City in conjunction with the National Association of Teachers of Speech (NATS), formed the American Academy of Speech Correction (Paden, 1970), which, having undergone several name changes in its 70+ year history, has evolved into the 80 000+ member American Speech-Language-Hearing Association (ASHA).

Today, members of ASHA consider themselves to be students of the discipline of communication sciences and disorders. The three primary areas of study within the discipline are audiology, speech-language pathology, and hearing and speech science. Most ASHA members perceive themselves as being practitioners in one of the discipline's two distinct but related professions: audiology and speech-language pathology. Practitioners are referred to as audiologists or speech-language pathologists. Practitioners of speech-language pathology, since the professions' birthing, have been referred to by a number of names including 'speech correctionist,' 'speech therapist', 'speech teacher', and 'speech clinician'. In recent years, primarily as a result of efforts by the professional association and attempts by federal agencies to adopt uniform terminology in legislation affecting the profession, the term 'speech-language pathologist' is now the accepted and universally applied name given to practitioners of the profession of speech-language pathology in the USA, independent of their place of practice.

Standards

A commitment to standards characterizes the American Speech-Language-Hearing Association's development. In 1925, the professional association's founders set membership qualifications that included the requirement that members hold a master's or a doctoral degree and have a professional reputation untainted by unethical practices. The profession continued its development of standards in 1942 by defining three levels of membership. Fellow and Professional Members were defined as those individuals with a broad education in the field of speech correction qualified to work independently. Clinical Members were those with a minimum academic preparation and experience capable of providing speech correction under supervision. An Associate Member category was offered individuals who were students in training in speech correction.

With the Association's significant growth during the late 1940s and early 1950s, with the development of audiology as an area of study, and with the increasing demand for the profession's services in the nation's schools and health care system, the need for more specific standards became evident. No longer could a simple membership categorization provide evidence of a member's academic as well as clinical credentials. In 1951, the professional association adopted the first set of standards, independent of membership requirements, for qualifying an individual to provide clinical services. Two levels of certification were approved: a *Basic Certificate* was awarded those with a bachelor's degree plus one year's experience and *Advanced Certificate* awarded those with a master's or doctoral degree in either speech-language pathology or audiology.

During the same 25 year period (1925–1950) state departments of education throughout the US were also developing standards for speech-language pathologists (Cooper, 1992). Faced with demands for speech and hearing services, with no nationally accepted standards by which the competencies of these practitioners could be identified, state boards and departments of education established standards of their own for this new specialist. By the time the American Speech-Language-Hearing Association matured sufficiently to begin defining and promulgating its own standards in 1951, standards were already set for over three quarters of the discipline's practitioners by state departments of education throughout the nation.

During the 1950s, with the bachelor's degree in the discipline still being the minimal requirement for membership in the ASHA as well as for the receipt of an ASHA certificate of clinical competence, there was little conflict between the standards being promulgated by the professional association and the standards set by state departments of education. In 1962, the ASHA adopted the master's degree as the minimum requirement for membership. The standards for communication disorder practitioners set by the national professional organization were by this time markedly different from those set by state education departments.

The Council of Postsecondary Accreditation and the United States Department of Education formally recognized the ASHA as the agency responsible for the accreditation of master's degree programmes in speech-language pathology and audiology. With these developments, federal and state public and private agencies, as well as the nation's health insurance community began to require that practitioners, in order to be reimbursed for their services, possess the appropriate ASHA certificate of clinical competence. As the 1960s drew to a close, the professional community was energized by its successes in promulgating the standards set by its national association. Professionals in the state of Florida brought the decade to a successful conclusion in 1969 by having their state legislature pass the first state licensure law regulating the practice of speech-language pathology and audiology embodying standards defined by the national professional association (Cooper, 1989). By the end of the 1970s, 30 states had passed similar licensure laws embodying practitioner requirements similar to those required for the ASHA certificate of clinical competence. During the same period, one half of the state departments of education upgraded their standards for the employment of speech-language pathologists to require the master's degree.

In the late 1980s and early 1990s, the discipline's voluntary standards for its practitioners came under assault from several quarters. One half of the nation's 50 state departments of education continued to employ speech-language pathologists educated at the bachelor's level. This was the case despite the passage of laws in the late 1980s and early 1990s amending and extending the historic 'Education for All Handicapped Children Act' of 1975 (PL92-142). These laws (the most recent of which is labelled the Individuals with Disabilities Education Act – IDEA) require state departments of education to employ only 'qualified providers' in serving the disabled. With professionals employed in nation's schools continuing to be employed at the bachelor's level and with professionals employed in health care facilities calling for increased practitioner entry level standards above that of the master's degree, the fractionation of the speech-language pathology work-force into two groups, the healthcare practitioner and the school practitioner, became a potential reality.

In the late 1980s, following prolonged and frequently emotion-laden debate, the ASHA Legislative Council voted to recognize audiology and speech-language pathology as two professions in the single discipline of communication disorders. The American Academy of Audiology (AAA), independent of the American Speech-Language-Hearing Association, was formed. Audiologists began pressing for the development of a professional doctorate in audiology (AuD) as the entry level into the profession of audiology. Demands from speech-language pathologists increased for the development of a continuum of practitioner standards from the pre-baccalaureate technician through to the post-doctoral specialist. Belatedly, in the minds of many, the ASHA responded by establishing special interest groups within the ASHA governance, by adopting guidelines for the use and regulation of support personnel, by establishing a programme for recognizing specialists within the professions, and by acknowledging the development of the professional doctorate in audiology.

In the late 1980s, several ASHA-independent and potentially politically powerful related professional organizations emerged. Among the more than 40 related professional organizations (RPOs) currently active, to mention only a few, are the following: Academy of Aphasia, Academy of Dispensing Audiologists, Academy of Neurologic Communication Disorders and Sciences, American Academy of Audiology, American

Academy of Rehabilitative Audiologists, American Cleft Palate Association, Council of Graduate Programs in Communication Sciences and
Disorders, Council of State Speech and Hearing Association Presidents,
National Council of State Boards of Licensure in Speech-Language
Pathology and Audiology, and the Public School Caucus. The ASHA, to
maintain and enhance its role as *the* professional organization representing the discipline of communication sciences and disorders and its
professions in the USA, is altering its corporate structure. Some envision
the ASHA as becoming an 'umbrella' organization enabling related
professional organizations as well as consumer and support groups to
participate in the governance of the ASHA (Cooper, 1993). These developments are taking place during a time of significant change in the
nation's educational and health care systems.

Professional Development in the UK

Professional development in the UK has followed along similar lines to
developments in the USA. In the UK, the major professional organization
concerned with communication disorders is the College of Speech and
Language Therapists (CSLT). This is a more circumscribed organization
than those in the USA, where audiologists and speech pathologists are
members of the same professional organization. The UK College only
admits to full membership those who are eligible to practise as speech
and language therapists. Audiologists and hearing therapists are not
eligible. Associate membership is offered to speech and language therapy assistants (or support personnel).

The first organized speech and language therapy service began in
Manchester in 1906, followed closely by similar developments in Glasgow. These services worked through the school's service to help children who stammered. In London, the first speech and language therapy
services were established by two of the major teaching hospitals, which
set up clinics for children with speech problems. Steady though sporadic
development occurred in both schools and hospitals throughout the UK
between the first and second world wars. Two professional associations
were formed during the 1930s, one from a nucleus of remedial teachers
and the other with a more medical orientation. The amalgamation of
these two associations did not take place until after the end of the
second world war. In 1947, the College of Speech Therapists was
formed. One of its main functions was to oversee the examination procedures leading to a diploma in speech therapy. The diploma was to be the
sole means of entry into the profession for the next 20 years.

The development of the speech therapy profession under the leader-
ship of its College proceeded alongside the development of the National
Health Service (NHS), a universal health care system free at the point of
delivery and funded entirely through taxation. The many arrangements

to accommodate speech and language therapists within the NHS were chronicled in the report of the Committee of Enquiry into Speech Therapy Services (Quirk, 1972). This committee was set up by four departments of state 'to consider the need for and the role of speech therapy in the field of education and medicine, the assessment and treatment of those specially concerned with this work and to make recommendations'. Among the important recommendations were (1) that all future training of speech therapists should be at degree level and (2) that the organization and delivery of speech therapy services should be unified and administered under the health authorities, although therapists continued to provide services to education authorities and social services establishments. The committee's report was accepted and acted upon by the government of the time. By the mid 1980s, speech therapy was well on its way towards being an all-graduate profession, and the majority of therapists were employed by the NHS.

The impact of welfare service reforms in the 1990s

Health and social services. Since then, many changes have taken place within the NHS. Concern with the economy and efficiency of health care delivery has led to a number of radical reforms. (Department of Health, 1989a, b, 1992). Pollitt (1992) suggests that the changes have come about for a number of reasons. First, changes in the global economy have brought western governments under increasing pressure to examine their public spending policies and reduce expenditure on welfare services. Second, substantial increases in health care expenditure and an ever-increasing demand for health care services has forced the need for a rationalization of services. Third, an increase in consumer understanding of health and illness has brought with it a decline in what Pollitt calls 'the unquestioning acceptance of professional expertise'. Consumers in countries like the UK are no longer prepared to accept that a professional judgement is, by definition, correct. They are more likely now than ever before to challenge the professional viewpoint, to ask more questions and to demand the care which they think they require.

The reforms have brought about major changes in the organization of health and social services. Changes in budgetary control mean that hospital and community services and the purchasers of services are quite separate. Local authorities and social services have been given more responsibility for providing long-term care in the community. In addition, hospital and community services have been given the opportunity to assume more localized control though the creation of health care trusts. Similarly, General Practitioners (GPs) have been given the opportunity to assume budgetary control over their practices as GP 'Fundholders'. They buy services like speech and language therapy from the local hospital or community trust. These reforms constitute the creation of an internal market within the NHS infrastructure, creating more opportunity for localized control and consequently more local variation in the way services are delivered. Although health and social care remain free at the point of delivery and funded through taxation, in all other respects the reforms have radically altered the organization of welfare services in the UK.

Changes in budgetary control have been developed in parallel with attempts to introduce more systematic measurement of the quality of health care. These reforms, known as 'the quality revolution', require health care professionals to be able to demonstrate that they are delivering the best possible care at the least possible cost (Donabedian, 1980).

Vocational training. Vocational training facilities in the UK have also undergone radical changes in their organizational structure. In the past, the sole route to qualification in vocational work was via a university or college off-the-job course. Training provision has now been extended to include distance learning courses, modular training, and on-the-job training. National Vocational Qualifications (NVQs – NCVQ, 1988) are currently available for speech and language therapy assistants, who are trained and assessed in their place of work. Present government policies aim, eventually, to allow on-the-job training and qualifications to contribute to, if not provide an alternative route towards, qualification as a speech and language therapist.

The impact of the reforms on speech and language therapy

The impact of all these reforms on the speech and language therapy profession has been substantial. Speech and language therapists are no longer unified under one employer, the National Health Service, but are employed by individual hospital and community units or trusts, who set their own standards and conditions of employment for their staff. From within these units, the speech and language therapy service will have a variety of customers, many of whom will 'buy' their services from the unit or trust. For example, a speech and language therapy service which is part of a hospital trust will have contracts with education and social services. These contracts are negotiated and agreed upon for fixed time periods, during which the speech and language service will provide an agreed amount of therapy for a school or a day centre.

The skill mix of many speech and language therapy departments has also been subject to changes, brought about by the increasing number of assistants employed by welfare services. Speech and language therapy departments employ assistants to share the clinical as well as the administrative work of the therapist (van der Gaag and Davies, 1993). Some departments also employ bilingual co-workers, which allow them to provide a more effective service to clients from different linguistic backgrounds.

Recent changes in the professional organization in the UK

The College of Speech and Language Therapists (CSLT) has undergone equally radical changes in its recent history. Its function as the regulator and accreditor of professional training courses has been developed and refined. Like the ASHA, its role as a unifying force in the profession has become even more important in the face of increasing fragmentation of services in the UK. The College has responded positively to the changes by providing its membership with the vehicle for maintaining and promoting professional contact. This has been achieved through the creation of local networks, special interest groups, and regional advisers and policy review forums. The College has produced, through its working parties, a series of position papers on all aspects of professional practice. It publishes a quarterly peer-reviewed journal and a monthly bulletin of information. As part of its strategy for maintaining and monitoring the quality of services, it has introduced a comprehensive guide to professional standards for its members (CSLT, 1991), and a handbook on quality assurance and audit methods (CSLT, 1993). The College has also introduced compulsory registration for its membership, requiring members to agree, year by year, to maintaining specific standards of good practice before they can be registered with the College. These initiatives are being overseen by the College's Professional Standards Board, which is responsible for the development and updating of standards within the profession. Collectively, these initiatives represent a level of professional support never before available to therapists in the UK. They are an indication of how far the College has progressed beyond its early aspirations into a progressive, proactive professional organization with over 5000 members. On a world-wide level, the CSLT has fostered stronger links with the European Community and other countries through the EC Working Party, the International Affairs Committee and the Overseas Therapist's Licensing Committee, all of which work together to promote international exchange and to maximize occupational mobility for speech and language therapists.

Professional Development in the Republic of Ireland

Education of speech and language therapists in Ireland celebrated 25 years of its existence in 1994. The first professionally qualified therapists began working in the country during the 1950s and, by the time the educational course was established, there were 19 therapists in the country, the vast majority of whom had been educated in the UK. This meant that a special liaison between the UK and Ireland was developed, one which endures to this day, when the island of Ireland as a whole is regarded as a region of the College of Speech and Language Therapists. Graduates of the only course in the country at Trinity College Dublin enjoy reciprocal recognition with graduates from courses in the UK. Although speech and language therapists are highly regarded in the health services, cutbacks in public spending during the 1980s negatively affected recruitment. Surveys and feedback from therapists have attempted to identify other factors that may have hindered development and indicate the limited opportunity for career development, work with large caseloads and long waiting lists and pay and working conditions as possible factors. The independent body in the Republic representing therapists, the Irish Association of Speech and Language Therapists (IASLT), has taken on the role of specifically addressing the issue of professional development and has established links with the College of Speech and Language Therapists for the mutual benefit of both bodies.

Standards for professional entry in the UK and the Republic of Ireland

Entry into the profession of speech and language therapy in the UK and the Republic of Ireland is through a university programme leading to a bachelor's degree. The majority of these are honours degrees and all have been constructed to incorporate clinical training into the degree structure. A licence to practise is then granted by the CSLT upon gradua-tion and graduates undergo a pre-registration year before applying for full registration as members of the College. An increasing, though small, number of graduates in the UK and Ireland chose not to practise as clini-cians, opting for careers in the academic or commercial sector.

There are few professionals holding doctoral degrees in either Ireland or the UK, although the proportions are increasing. This contrasts with the USA, where a doctoral degree is not only essential for teaching or research, but also for directing many of the larger clinical programmes.

Despite these differences, the fact that the USA, UK and Ireland share the same language means that they use many of the same teaching texts, read the same journals and draw their clinical material from the same sources. Increasingly, this exchange is broadening to other European countries as well. For example, the CSLT Journal, the *British Journal of Disorders of Communication*, recently renamed the *European Journal of Disorders of Communication*, is now read more widely in other parts of Europe than ever before. The first European Congress of Speech and Language Therapists took place in Athens, Greece in 1992 and subse-quent conferences have now taken place in other European countries. These developments have implications for increasing the exchange of research and of fostering a stronger identity and compatibility amongst therapists from different countries.

Clinical Functions

The work of the speech and language therapist

The work of the speech and language therapist falls into four main categories; individual and group work with clients, work with carers, teaching and training, and administration (see Figure 4.1).

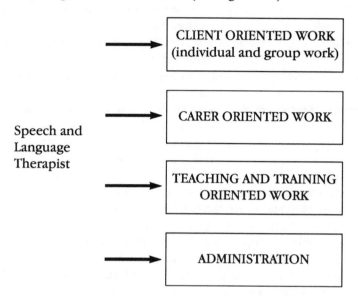

Figure 4.1 The speech and language therapy workload

In the early days of the profession, therapists would spend the majority of their time in face-to-face contact with their clients. Today, the therapist is as likely to use her expertise in working with carers or providing training for other professionals or assistants, as well as seeing clients on an individual basis. Clinical activities continue to include screening, assessment and intervention, but the recognition that therapy is a dynamic, changing process has led to the development of a continuum of service delivery models. For example, in the USA, the traditional 'pull-out' model, used almost exclusively in the past, is now one among a choice of delivery models in schools. In 1993, The ASHA Committee on Service Delivery in the Schools defined four service delivery models:

Collaborative consultation   The speech-language pathologist and teacher or special education teacher and parents work together to facilitate a student's communication and learning.

Classroom-based

This model is also known as integrated services, curriculum-based, transdiscipli-nary or inclusive programming. There is an emphasis on the speech-language pathologist providing direct services to students within the classroom and other environments. Team teaching by the speech-language pathologist and the teacher is frequent with this model.

Pull-out

Services are provided to students individ-ually and in small groups in the speech language therapy room, or within the classroom.

Self-contained programme

The speech-language pathologist is the classroom teacher responsible for provid-ing academic instruction and intensive speech-language remediation.

A variety of service delivery models are also used by therapists working in health care settings. These range from individual sessions delivered in home health-care practices to group work in nursing homes, hospitals and clinics. Further changes may well take place; for example, significant increases are predicted in the use of telecommunications technology in the delivery of services to clients living in isolated areas or incapable of leaving their homes. As in the school services, speech-language patholo-gists are increasingly adopting the consultative approach. They are also working as valued members of interdisciplinary health-care teams.

Depending on location and type of service, the team may be made up of paediatricians, neurologists, otolaryngologists, orthodontists, plastic surgeons, audiologists, psychologists, psychiatrists, physiotherapists, occupational therapists, nurses, classroom teachers, and social workers. More precise examples of the composition of such teams will be discussed in later chapters. The function of these teams is, in general terms, to pro-vide clients with a comprehensive, integrated service in which all their needs are being addressed by a team of professionals working together. Different countries will have different names and terms of reference for their various teams. In the USA, the Child Study team will assess any child thought to be at risk for disability and will advise the parents on the needs of the child. The parent must agree in writing to the programme suggest-ed by the team or it will not be carried out. The parent has the right to ask for re-assessment, or to challenge the programme at any time. Extending the membership of the team of parents and clients themselves is a com-mon pattern in the UK and Ireland as well. Interdisciplinary teams are not only beneficial to the client, they also provide a forum for skills sharing and mutual support between professionals.

Assuming different roles to meet client needs

The descriptions outlined above serve to illustrate how wide ranging the work of the speech and language therapist can be. The settings in which speech and language therapists find themselves are equally wide ranging. They include schools and health centres, hospitals, nurseries, pre-school assessment units, day centres, residential homes and hostels, and visits to clients at home. Increasingly, the therapist will adopt different roles or 'personas' in her work, depending upon the setting in which she finds herself. These roles or 'personas' include those of teacher, carer, resource worker, and team member.

In the school or nursery, for example, the therapist may take on the role of teacher, alongside her educational colleagues. Saunders and Caves (1986) in their study of speech therapists' skills found that therapists were using a broad range of teaching skills in their day-to-day clinical work without necessarily being aware that they were using them. These included skills such as reinforcing, modelling, shaping, cueing, and mirroring particular target behaviours for the client.

Likewise, in the day centre or residential home for the elderly or learning disabled, the primary role of the speech and language therapist may be that of educator of care staff. In this context, the primary focus of intervention will be on teaching carers how best to facilitate communication with their clients. In addition to this role, the speech and language therapist may take on the role of a resource worker, someone who acts as an 'agent' in acquiring a particular service for a client. This is particularly relevant when clients require a communication aid, or a hearing aid, as these are resources which play an important part in securing successful communication.

In the home or hospital setting, the speech and language therapist may assume the role of counsellor. She frequently has a 'supportive' role, both with clients and carers, providing both direct and indirect counselling. In this context, her role is to affirm and encourage. Miller (1990) has highlighted this role in her discussion of the speech and language therapist attending to the emotional and psychological needs of clients. Miller argues that the consequences of a communication difficulty will be linked inextricably with the emotional and psychological balances within the individual. It will also have emotional and psychological consequences for the people who interact with that individual. There can be little doubt that the speech and language therapist has a responsibility to attend to these aspects of the communication difficulty, and that her role as 'carer' in the sense of providing such support is often a vital one.

These roles represent a development from the traditional one to a therapeutic role with clients. They are a response to the increasing complexity and demands of the work. The diversity of clients with communication difficulties requires the application of a more flexible, more diverse range of skills and role than ever before. This is also the case for clinicians involved in teaching and research, who specialize in an ever-increasing range of subjects and interests.

Referral patterns

Another of the consequences of the ever increasing diversity of speech and language therapy work is that the diversity depends on referrals from a range of agents. Medical practitioners are no longer the only source of referral, as they were in the past. Indeed, many communication disorders are first observed by teachers in pre-school or nursery classes, by social workers, health visitors or district nurses in community settings. In the UK, GPs are usually informed that a referral has been made by another professional, but they may have little or no involvement in the referral itself. On both sides of the Atlantic, an open referral system, one which allows referral from any professional, parent, carer or indeed client, is the preferred option from the profession's perspective. Unfortunately, this preferred option may sometimes be hampered by cost factors if a referring agent is a fundholder and is therefore unwilling to use limited resources on the services of a speech and language therapist.

Conclusion

The speech and language therapy profession has undergone substantive changes in both its professional structure and public persona since its emergence as a major service for people with communication difficulties in health, educational and social settings. The future is sure to bring more change and will reflect the dynamic nature of the profession itself. Expanding knowledge and technological advances will undoubtedly have an impact on the nature and practice of speech and language therapy. Economic, social and population changes will also continue to be important influences. It may be that increasing numbers of private clinicians in the USA, and the UK and Ireland will expand their practice to provide evaluation, consultation and intervention in all therapy delivery settings as a result of provider shortages and economic factors. It may be that collaborative work with other professionals becomes the predominant model of service delivery for speech and language therapists. Whatever changes take place in organization structures or models of delivery, the hallmark of the profession will continue to be its commitment to developing ever more rigorous standards of professional practice and its dedication to meeting the individual needs of clients.

References

Clark RM (1964) Our enterprising predecessors and Charles Sydney Bluemel. ASHA 6: 107–14.

College of Speech and Language Therapists (1991) Communicating Quality. London: CSLT.

College of Speech and Language Therapists (1993) Audit: A Manual for Speech and Language Therapists. London: CSLT.

Cooper EB (1989) One lovers quarrel revisited: The state of the profession. ASHA 31: 79–82.

Cooper EB (1992) Standards: who will set: ASHA, state licensure boards, state departments of education? Wellsburg, WV: National Council of State Boards of Examiners in Speech-Language Pathology and Audiology.

Cooper EB (1993) The fractionation of our discipline: A time for action. ASHA 35: 51–7.

Department of Health (1989a) Working for Patients. Cmn 555. London: HMSO.

Department of Health (1989b) Caring of People, Community Care in the Next Decade and Beyond. Cmn 849. London: HMSO.

Department of Health (1992) The Health of the Nation Cmn 1986. London: HMSO.

Davies P, van der Gaag A (1992a) The professional competence of speech therapists: I. Introduction and methodology. Clinical Rehabilitation 6(3): 209–14.

Davies P, van der Gaag A (1992b) The professional competence of speech therapists: III. Skills and skill mix possibilities. Clinical Rehabilitation 6(4): 301–13.

Donabedian A. (1980) Explorations in Quality Assessment and Monitoring, Volume 1 Ann Arbor, MI: Health Administration Press.

Greenberg S, Smith L (1987) Evaluation of the requirements for the certificates of clinical competence of the American Speech Language Hearing Association. ASHA, December 1987.

Lingwall J (1988) Evaluation of the requirements for the certificate of clinical competence in speech language pathology and audiology. ASHA September 1988, p. 76.

McLaughlin, R. M. (1986) Speech-Language Pathology and Audiology. New York: Grune & Stratton.

Miller C (1990) The music behind the words. College of Speech and Language Therapists Bulletin 454: 2–3.

National Council for Vocational Qualifications (NCVQ) (1988) Introducing National Vocational Qualifications: Implications for Education and Training. London: NCVQ.

Paden EP (1970) A History of the American Speech and Hearing Association. Rockville, MD: American Speech-Language-Hearing Association.

Pollitt C (1992) Performance evaluation in the public sector. Paper presented at the National Nursing and Therapy Audit Network. York, UK, November 1992.

Quirk R (1972) Speech Therapy Services. London: HMSO.

Saunders C, Caves R. (1986) An empirical approach to the identification of communication skills with reference to speech therapy. Journal of Further and Higher Education 10(2): 29–44.

Van der Gaag A, Davies P (1992a) The professional competence of speech therapists: II. Knowledge base. Clinical Rehabilitation 6(3): 215–24.

Van der Gaag A, Davies P (1992b) The professional competence of speech therapists: IV. Knowledge base. Clinical Rehabilitation 6(4): 325–24.

Van der Gaag A, Davies P (1992c) The use and value of speech and language therapy assistants; who are they and what do they do? Human Communication 2: 20–3.

Part II
Communication Disorders
In Children

Part II

Communication Disorders in Children

Chapter 5
Childhood Language

ALAN G. KAMHI

Most children acquire their native language without any formal instruction. Because no formal instruction is required, it is sometimes thought that learning a first language is not very difficult. The notion that a first language is easy to learn is, of course, false. In fact, it is arguably the most complex learning task humans accomplish during their lifetimes. The complexities involved in learning language are most readily seen in children who have difficulty learning language. This chapter is about those children. In the first part of the chapter, the dimensions of language and disorders are presented. Causes and correlates of language disorders are then considered. In the second part of the chapter, some general guidelines to assess and remediate child language disorders are presented.

The Nature of Language

The way in which one defines language directly influences who will be classified as language disordered. Current definitions of language are broad-based and highly integrative. An example of such a definition was endorsed by the American Speech-Language-Hearing Association several years ago (ASHA, 1983: 44).

> Language is a complex and dynamic system of conventional symbols that is used in various modes for thought and communication. Contemporary views of human language hold that: (a) language evolves within specific historical, social, and cultural contexts; (b) language, as rule governed behaviour, is described by at least five parameters–phonologic, morphologic, syntactic, semantic, and pragmatic; (c) language learning and use are determined by the interaction of biological, cognitive, psychosocial, and environmental factors; and (d) effective use of language for communication requires a broad understanding of human interaction including such associated factors as nonverbal cues, motivation, and sociocultural roles.

As reflected in the definition, it is generally agreed that there are five dimensions of language. The five aspects of language are described briefly below.

Phonology

Phonology has to do with the way the sounds of a language are organized. It includes a description of what the sounds are and their component features (i.e., phonetics) as well as the distributional rules that
govern how the sounds can be used in various word positions and the
sequence rules that describe which sounds may be combined. For example, the zh sound that occurs in the word 'measure' is never used to
begin an English word. Distributional rules are different in different
languages. In French, for example, the zh sound can occur in the word-
initial position, as in 'je', and 'jouer'. An example of a sequence rule
would be that /ks/ in English can occur in the middle and end of words
(e.g. 'boxer', 'books'), but cannot be used to begin words.

Phonologists have also devised rules to describe how sounds are
produced in certain contexts. There are three general kinds of rules or
processes that govern sound changes (e.g. Ingram, 1976): (1) assimilation processes in which adjacent phonemes or features become more
alike (e.g. gɔg/gɔg); (2) substitution processes in which one segment
is substituted for another (e.g. tek/kek), and (3) syllable structure
processes in which the syllable structure of the word is modified in
some way (e.g. nana/banana). The next chapter will have more to say
about phonology and phonological disorders. It is important to remember, however, that phonological disorders represent a language disorder.

Semantics

Semantics is the aspect of language that governs the meaning of words
and word combinations. Sometimes semantics is divided into lexical and
relational semantics. Lexical semantics involves the meaning conveyed
by individual words. Words have both intensional and extensional meanings. Intensional meanings refer to the defining characteristics or criter-
ial features of a word. A dog is a dog because it has four legs, barks, and
licks people's faces. The extension of a word is the set of objects, entities, or events to which a word might apply to in the world. The set of all
real or imaginary dogs that fit the intensional criteria become the extension of the entity dog.

Relational semantics refers to the relationships that exist between
words. For example, in the sentence 'The Panda bear is eating bamboo',
the word bear not only has lexical meaning, but also is the agent
engaged in the activity of eating. Bamboo is referred to as the 'patient'
(Chafe, 1970) because its state is being changed by the action of the
verb. Words are thus seen as expressing abstract relational meanings in
addition to their lexical meanings.

Morphology

In addition to the content words that refer to objects, entities, and events, there is a group of words and inflections that convey subtle meaning and serve specific grammatical and pragmatic functions. These words have been referred to as grammatical morphemes. Grammatical morphemes modulate meaning. Consider the sentences: 'Elmore is playing tennis', 'Elmore plays tennis', 'Elmore played tennis', and 'Elmore has played tennis'. The major elements of meaning are similar in each of these sentences. What differentiates these sentences are the grammatical morphemes (inflections and auxiliary forms) that change the tense and aspect (temporal contour) of the sentences.

Syntax

Syntax refers to the rule system that governs how words are combined into larger meaningful units of phrases, clauses, and sentences. Syntactic rules specify which word combinations and orders are acceptable and which are not. In English, the sentence 'The boy hit the ball' is a well-formed grammatical sentence, whereas 'Hit the boy ball the' is not.

Pragmatics

Pragmatics concerns the use of language in context. Language does not occur in a vacuum. It is used to serve a variety of communication functions, such as declaring, greeting, requesting information, answering questions, and so forth. Communicative intentions are best achieved by being sensitive to the listener's communicative needs and non-linguistic context. Speakers must take into account what the listener knows and does not know about a topic. Pragmatics thus encompasses rules of conversation or discourse. Speakers must learn how to initiate conversations, take turns, maintain and change topics, and provide the appropriate amount of information in a clear manner. It has become clear recently that different kinds of discourse contexts involve different sets of rules (e.g. Lund and Duchan, 1993). The most frequent kinds of discourse children encounter are conversational, classroom, narrative, and event discourse.

Defining, Classifying and Diagnosing Language Disorders

How one defines language disorders depends in part on the approach one takes to classify and diagnose language disorders. There are three general approaches to the classification and diagnosis of child language disorders: (a) an aetiological (medical) approach, (b) a descriptive-linguistic approach, and (c) a processing approach.

Aetiological approach

The use of aetiological typologies for classification and diagnosis of children with language disorders grew out of the early work of Mykelbust (1954), Morley (1957), and McGinnis (1963). Based on Mykelbust (1954), the aetiologic categories used included (a) deafness and hearing impairment, (b) emotional disturbance and autism, (c) mental retardation, (d) childhood aphasia and apraxia (neurologically-based disorders). Reflecting the socio-political climate of the early 1960s, a fifth category of cultural or social deprivation was added.

There are several advantages to an aetiological approach. Bernstein (1993) points out that aetiology is a convenient way to compare and distinguish among autistic, mentally retarded, and hearing-impaired children. A second advantage of the aetiological approach is that is offers a diagnostic label for a child to receive services in schools and clinics. Special education programmes are often tailored to the primary aetiology of the child, in that many school systems have programmes for the mentally retarded, emotionally disturbed, and hearing-impaired. A third advantage suggested by Bernstein is that aetiologies provide speech-language pathologists with clues about the type of remediation that might be indicated for a particular child. For example, knowing that a child is hearing-impaired will suggest aural rehabilitation procedures and perhaps the use of alternative or augmentative systems to teach language.

The advantages of the aetiological approach are more than outweighed by its disadvantages. Perhaps the most serious problem is that children in each of the aetiological categories are thought to have similar language abilities. A particular diagnostic label, however, provides little information about the child's language abilities. All retarded children, for example, do not have similar language abilities. Indeed, for many years, the assessment procedures used to identify the child's aetiological category did not include specific information about language performance. Another problem with the aetiological approach is that it is rare to find a child who fits neatly into one diagnostic category (Lahey, 1988). For example, many retarded children are hearing-impaired and many autistic children are retarded. A categorical label also implies that there is only one cause for the language disorder. That is, a hearing impairment is the only cause of the language disorder in hearing-impaired children or the cognitive deficit is the only cause of language problems in retarded individuals. Although a single causal factor may be primarily responsible for a language disorder, there are always several contributing factors.

A major unfortunate outcome of the aetiological approach was that it served to divide treatment domains (Aram and Nation, 1982). The mentally retarded and emotionally disturbed were considered to belong to the psychologist or special educator. Hearing-impaired children either were not served or came under the province of educators of the deaf. This left aphasic and culturally deprived children to the speech-language pathologists. Although Bernstein has suggested that different aetiological labels facilitated the provision of services, determining who provides the services often depends more on the aetiological label than on the expertise of the professional. In most instances, the speech-language pathologist is the most qualified professional to treat language disorders, regardless of aetiological type.

Descriptive-linguistic approach

The descriptive-linguistic approach involves describing children according to the language deficit they demonstrate. Although this approach purportedly emphasizes description rather than classification or diagnosis, in practice the distinction between description and classification is difficult to maintain. Unlike the aetiological approach, the descriptive-linguistic approach is a developmental one. Language abilities of disordered children are compared to those of normally developing children. Children's language behaviours are described either in terms of form, content, and use (e.g. Bloom and Lahey, 1978) or in terms of the five language domains (e.g. Lund and Duchan, 1993).

The use of linguistic descriptions to describe children's language disorders can be traced to the early work of Chomsky (1957, 1965). Chomsky provided child-language researchers with a powerful descriptive grammar to capture children's developing proficiency with language. Speech-language pathologists were quick to apply the new developments in linguistics and psychology to the study of language-disordered children. The past 25 years have seen the development of increasingly more precise procedures to describe children's language (see Bernthal and Bankston, 1993; Lund and Duchan, 1993; Nelson, 1993; Retherford, 1993).

Although the descriptive-linguistic approach has clearly placed emphasis on the language behaviours of children with language disorders, the emphasis on language has tended to obscure the aetiological and non-language differences among children. Adherents of this approach sometimes base language therapy solely on the nature of the linguistic handicap without considering age, cognitive, social, and environmental factors. The descriptive-linguistic approach thus often has had a behavioural look, in that only language behaviour is considered in evaluating and treating the language disorder. For example, a syntactic delay would be treated the same way in a retarded child as it would in a child with a specific language disorder.

Processing approaches

Processing approaches provide a means to integrate the best aspects of the descriptive-linguistic approach and the aetiological approach. Generally speaking, processing approaches characterize language disorders in terms of disruptions in language comprehension or formulation processes. A variety of processes have been invoked to account for language disorders, including neurologic, sensory, perceptual, linguistic, and cognitive processes.

One popular processing view is that children with language disorders suffer from an auditory processing deficit (e.g. Eisenson, 1972). Although some children with language problems might have specific auditory processing deficits, this view has more descriptive value than explanatory value. As will be seen in the next section, it is unlikely that language disorders can be explained by a simple processing deficit.

About 10–15 years ago, a number of theorists began to provide processing explanations for child-language disorders that were more comprehensive and integrative. These theorists (e.g. McLean and Snyder-McLean, 1978; Hubbell, 1981; Aram and Nation, 1982; Carrow-Woolfolk, 1988) attempted to build into their models the ways in which constitutional and environmental forces might interact over time to cause language disorders. Although some of these models (e.g. Aram and Nation's Child Language Processing Model) offer considerable explanatory value, the complexity of these models can make them unappealing to most clinicians.

Definition of a Language Disorder

The different approaches to the classification and diagnosis of language disorders exemplify the problems involved in defining a language disorder. Consider, for example, the relatively simple definition proposed by Leonard (1982: 222): 'Children have a language disorder whenever their language abilities are below those expected for their age and their level of functioning.' Leonard notes that a broad-based definition allows one to consider children with differing aetiological histories as language-disordered. Adherents to the aetiological approach, however, would not find this definition very useful. As was noted above, the aetiological approach does not rely heavily on measures of language to make diagnostic classifications. Moreover, the fact that emotionally disturbed and mentally retarded individuals are served primarily by special educators tends to minimize the emphasis that language receives in assessment and treatment. In contrast, the descriptive-linguistic approach classifies children solely on the basis of language performance. Speech-language pathologists frequently use this approach. With such an approach, mentally retarded and autistic children would be considered to have a language disorder.

Broad-based definitions of language disorders are thus the ones preferred by speech-language pathologists. A comprehensive definition of language disorders was provided by ASHA (1980: 317–8).

> A language disorder is the abnormal acquisition, comprehension or expression of spoken or written language. The disorder may involve all, one, or some of the phonologic, morphologic, semantic, syntactic, or pragmatic components of the linguistic system. Individuals with language disorders frequently have problems in sentence processing or in abstracting information meaningfully for storage and retrieval from short- and long-term memory.

It should be apparent that the ASHA definition combines a descriptive-linguistic orientation with a processing orientation. In the next section, the types of language-disordered children are considered. As indicated earlier, it is convenient to use aetiological labels to categorize children with language disorders. As these children are being discussed, it is important to remember that the language abilities of one group of children (e.g. mentally retarded) are not unique to that group.

Children with Language Disorders

Children with specific language impairment

Children with specific language impairment have received considerable attention in the literature (for recent reviews, see Leonard, 1987; Johnston, 1988; Bishop, 1992; Kamhi, 1993; Reed, 1994). Variously labelled as developmentally aphasic, dysphasic, language-impaired, language-disordered or language-delayed, these children acquire language more slowly and often with less success than their age peers. These children are generally defined by the presence of a language impairment in the absence of mental deficiency, sensory and physical deficits, severe emotional disturbances, environmental factors, and brain damage. Language disorders that can be directly attributed to one or more of these predisposing peripheral or central impairments are often considered to be resulting symptoms of more pervasive disorders such as mental retardation, autism, hearing impairment, and frank neurological dysfunction.

Much of the research involving these children with specific language impairments (SLI) has focused on two basic questions: What is the nature of their linguistic deficits and why should children with normal non-verbal intelligence, intact speech and hearing mechanisms, and supportive language-learning environments have difficulty acquiring language? The answer to the first question is considerably more clear cut than the answer to the second question. SLI children's basic deficit is in the grammatical component of language, particularly grammatical morphology. Johnston (1988) provided an extensive review of SLI children's language abilities. Although more recent reviews now exist (e.g. Bishop, 1992; Reed, 1994), Johnston's summary comments still capture the essence of SLI children's language abilities:

> Although further work is needed in each of the areas investigated, there are now sufficient data to make an interim global conclusion. SLI children acquire major grammatical categories and syntactic ordering rules in the same order as normally developing children, albeit more slowly and at a later age. Grammatical morphology also follows the same sequence of development in SLI children, but the acquisition of these forms is markedly protracted. Semantic studies indicate that SLI children follow normal acquisition patterns in most lexical domains and are able to express a variety of relational meanings. Although narrative discourse abilities are clearly delayed, conversational abilities are basically intact. For the most part, SLI children are purposeful and responsive conversationalists, limited only by their relatively poor mastery of grammatical form. (p. 693)

Reviews of causal-based research reveal no clear consensus about why SLI children have difficulty learning language. In the last 25 years, researchers have studied SLI children's performance on a wide range of tasks that tap perceptual, memory, and higher-level cognitive reasoning processes. This research has been reviewed in detail in a number of comprehensive chapters on SLI children (e.g. Leonard, 1987; Johnston, 1988; Bishop, 1992; Kamhi, 1993; Reed, 1994). A brief summary of the major findings from this body of literature is provided below.

SLI children:

1. have difficulty processing rapid, sequenced auditory and visual information (Tallal, 1988);
2. exhibit deficient symbolic, adaptive, and integrative play skills (Terrell, Schwarz and Prelock, 1984; Roth and Clark, 1987);
3. have difficulty generating, maintaining, and interpreting mental images (Johnston and Ellis Weismer, 1983; Savich, 1984);
4. are slower to access items stored in long-term memory (Sininger, Klatzky and Kirchner, 1989);
5. have a reduced capacity to store phonological information (Gathercole and Baddeley, 1990) and perhaps all information (Johnston, 1991);
6. have difficulty solving certain complex reasoning problems (Nelson et al., 1987; Kamhi et al., 1990a; Ellis Weismer, 1991; Masterson, 1993).
7. use age-appropriate reasoning and rule-induction processes to solve problems (Kamhi et al., 1984; Kamhi et al., 1990a; Connell and Stone, 1994);

8. are adept in solving problems that require visual, spatial pattern analyses (e.g. Johnston, 1982; Kamhi, Minor and Mauer, 1990b).

This summary may appear as a hodgepodge of strengths and weaknesses. Although a different reviewer might construct a different list of strengths and weaknesses, all reviewers of this literature would agree that SLI children have strengths and weaknesses. These children do not perform poorly on all measures of perceptual and cognitive processing. This essential characteristic of SLI children, more than any other, provides the best evidence that no single factor or obvious combination of factors can explain the extent and nature of a specific language impairment. The failure to identify the cause of a specific language impairment has led some researchers and clinicians to question the value of continued research and clinical efforts that address causal issues (e.g. Leonard, 1987, 1991). It is my view that 25 years of research has illuminated the problems with simplistic causal accounts of SLI. The fact that causal questions are complex does not mean that they should no longer be addressed. One important benefit from this research is that children with developmental language impairments are being identified much earlier than they used to be. In most cases early intervention will reduce the severity and the impact of the language disorder on other aspects of development. An excellent discussion of the pros and cons of causal issues can be found in a clinical forum entitled 'Specific language impairment as a clinical category', published in the April 1991 issue of *Language, Speech, and Hearing Services in Schools*.

Children with mental retardation

The American Association on Mental Deficiency (AAMD) defines mental retardation as 'significantly subaverage general intellectual functioning existing concurrently with deficits in adaptive behaviour and manifested during the developmental period (Grossman, 1983: 1). There are four categories of mental retardation based on IQ: (a) mild (52–68), (b) moderate (36–51), (c) severe (20–35), and (d) profound (below 20). Around 90 per cent of the population of retarded individuals fall into the mild range.

There are two broad categories of mental retardation: retardation that can be attributed to biological causes and retardation that can be attributed to familial or social-environmental factors. Up until recently, familial factors have been thought to account for the majority of the mentally retarded population. In recent years, many individuals whose retardation was thought to have resulted from familial factors were found to exhibit Fragile X syndrome. Fragile X syndrome refers to a weakness in the female, or X, chromosome. Most males with the Fragile X trait are mentally retarded, compared with only a third of females with the trait (Fryns, 1986, cited in Owens, 1993). If Fragile X syndrome is categorized as a biological-based retardation, the proportion of individuals with biological retardation approaches 50 per cent. However, the Fragile X syndrome has caused some categorization problems because it has both biological and familial characteristics. Though clearly a chromosomal disorder, it also runs in families.

Down's syndrome is the other most common chromosomal disorder. Other than being genetically based, biological causes may be congenital (e.g. metabolic disorders, brain malformation) or related to illness or toxins (e.g. maternal rubella, lead poisoning, foetal alcohol syndrome).

Familial causes are easier to identify than social-environmental ones. Long and Long (1994: 157) in their recent chapter on mental retardation cite research identifying three subtypes of familial retardation:

1. One or both parents of a retarded child are retarded (35 per cent of all individuals with retardation).
2. Parents are not retarded but the retardation is genetically inherited, although not associated with a syndrome (35 per cent of total).
3. Retardation is due to extreme environmental deprivation (5 per cent of total).

The percentages seem to reflect the inclusion of Fragile X as a familial retardation.

All children with mental retardation exhibit some form of language impairment. In other words, language is not commensurate with chronological age. The degree of the language impairment depends in part on the severity of the general mental deficiency. In general, the more severe the mental handicap, the more severe the language deficit. However, the relationship between language and cognition is not always perfect and most theorists now reject the strong cognitive hypothesis associated with the Piagetian view of language and cognition. This hypothesis states that cognitive achievements are prerequisite to the emergence of certain language behaviours (cf. Kamhi and Masterson, 1989; Casby, 1992; Owens, 1993; Long and Long, 1994). It is now thought that language and cognition interact and in some cases language fosters the development of cognition (Vygotsky, 1962).

The interactive nature of language and cognition is reflected in a large scale study by Miller, Chapman and MacKenzie (1981) which examined the relationship between language and cognitive abilities of 130 retarded children between the ages of 7 months and 7 years. Approximately half of the children were functioning at or beyond the language levels associated with cognitive level. Of the remaining children, half exhibited delays in language comprehension and production and half showed delays only in productive syntax. These findings exemplify the heterogeneity of retarded children's language abilities.

In recent years, pragmatic abilities of retarded individuals have been studied extensively. Abbeduto et al. (1991), for example, have found that

children and adolescents with mild to moderate retardation have difficulty varying the linguistic forms of their utterances in response to
contextual cues. Abbeduto et al. also found that the conversational turns
produced by retarded children and adolescents do not add significantly
to the conversation. They have difficulty extending topics by providing
new information or new shading. Retarded children also do a poor job
repairing breakdowns in communication. They rarely seek clarification
when presented with inadequate messages (Abbeduto et al., 1991).
Owens (1993) notes that the conversational role of retarded persons
seems to be one of non-dominance. They are passive conversationalists.
More detailed summaries of retarded individuals' language abilities can
be found in recent chapters by Kamhi and Masterson (1989), Long and
Long (1994), and Owens (1993).

Children with autism

It is generally agreed that autism is one of the most complicated areas of
medical and educational diagnosis. One problem is distinguishing
autism from other emotional and psychotic disorders, such as Asperger's
syndrome, pervasive developmental disorder, and schizophrenia. Long
(1994) provides a thorough table of the definitions of these terms and
behaviours associated with them. Another problem concerns the difference between autism, the noun, which refers to a syndrome and autistic
(or autistic-like), the adjective, which refers to behaviours in children
who often do not meet the criteria for the syndrome of autism. The
DSM-IV (1994) provides a definition of autism that serves as the standard
for many researchers and professionals involved in diagnosing the disorder. Most studies agree that social impairment is the hallmark characteristic, as reflected by a marked lack of awareness of the existence of
feelings of others. Other characteristics that marked most children with
autism were a communicative impairment and a persistent preoccupa-
tion with parts of objects. These social and communicative impairments
lead to difficulties in developing normal relationships with people.
Autistic infants often withdraw from the approach and touch of others
and often become stiff when held or cuddled. They fail to initiate or
maintain eye contact and show no interest in social or co-operative play.
The majority of autistic children function within the mentally retarded
range.

The actual cause of autism is unknown. Long (1994: 236) points out
several methodological problems that make the search for the cause
more difficult. One problem in determining the cause of autism is the
significant variation in the types of severity of problems exhibited by
children with autism. Another problem is that autism is not a discrete
disorder but the most severe form of a pervasive developmental disorder. Thus, the cause of autism must also account for the problems of

children who have related disorders. Despite these problems, some investigators have made suggestions about the nature of the primary deficit in autism. For example, Maurer and Damasio (1982) have implicated the limbic system that is responsible for arousal, attention, and motor responsiveness. Courchesne (1987) has argued that autism is a cerebellar disorder. Fein et al. (1986) speculated that autism reflects dysfunction of cortical and subcortical areas that are responsible for attachment and social behaviour.

The verbal abilities of children with autism range from the total absence of speech to communication that may be accurate in form (syntax and phonology) but reflect semantic and pragmatic abnormalities. It is common for many autistic children to go through a period of mutism sometime early in development. Many autistic children remain mute all of their lives. The incidence of mutism ranges from 28 to 61 per cent (see Tiegerman, 1993). The wide range reflects difficulties with terminology and definitions of mutism. DeMyer et al. (1973) have found that 65 per cent of the children who were mute at age five were still mute several years later. Eisenberg (1956) has posited that if speech has not developed by 6 years of age, there is little likelihood that it will develop at all.

The high incidence of mutism has been challenged in recent years by clinical experiences with facilitated communication (Biklen, 1992). Written messages from individuals with autism suggest that they may have an untapped ability to communicate and much greater social awareness than previously thought. However, the claims made about facilitated communication have been seriously challenged by a number of researchers (e.g. Shane, 1993).

The speech of autistic children who do talk is characterized by severe deficits in the pragmatic and semantic domains, with milder deficits in syntax. Segmental phonology is the least impaired in these children. Children with autism commonly exhibit significant impairment in prosodic aspects of speech. For example, they show unusual fluctuations in vocal intensity, limited pitch range, stereotyped rhythmic patterns ('singsong' speech), frequent whispering, and inappropriate tonal contrasts (cf. Long, 1994).

The high frequency of echolalia is one of the most salient characteristics of autistic children's speech (Prizant and Duchan, 1981; Prizant and Rydell, 1984). Prizant (1982) notes that 75 per cent of verbal autistic children go through a period of echolalia, and 40 per cent of the population are echolalic. Echolalia has been traditionally defined as the meaningless repetition of someone else's sentences. Prizant and Duchan (1981), however, have found that many of the echolalic utterances of autistic children serve communicative functions and carry meaning. In many cases, these children's echoes represent their best attempts to participate in communicative exchanges. Although echolalia may serve various communicative purposes, recent studies have shown that imitating utterances does not help in the acquisition of grammar (Tager-Flusberg and Calkins, 1990). With the possible exception of the early stages of acquisition, autistic children's echolalic utterances are less grammatically complex than their spontaneous utterances.

Children with acquired language disorders

The language-disordered children discussed thus far all have language-learning problems that are noticeable at an early age. There are some children, however, who lose some aspect of their language ability as a result of brain damage. Brain injuries can be either localized or diffuse. Localized or focal lesions are confined to specific areas of the brain. They can be caused by penetrating injuries (e.g. gunshot wounds), vascular lesions (strokes or haemorrhages), or tumours. Diffuse lesions are spread out over several brain regions. These lesions can be caused by traumatic head injuries or poisoning. Closed head injury and traumatic brain injury both refer to diffuse rather than focal brain injury. Traumatic brain injuries can be caused in a number of ways. Infants and toddlers are generally hurt through falls or abuse. Older children suffer injuries through sports and accidents (bike, skating, pedestrian). In adolescents, motor vehicle accidents are the most common cause of injury.

Although strokes and tumours are commonly associated with adults, they do occur infrequently in children. Long (1994) notes that in 1989, the death rate for cerebrovascular disease in the USA was four per 100 000 for children under 15 years of age. More than one third of these strokes occur during the first two years of life. Children who experience damage to the left hemisphere exhibit aphasic symptoms that are comparable to those seen in adults. The most typical causes of stroke in children are cardiac disease, vascular occlusion, sickle cell disease, and haemorrhage. The least frequent cause of acquired aphasia in children is Landau-Kleffner syndrome, which is a convulsive disorder that is associated with a gradual or sudden break-down in language (cf. Long, 1994).

Although adults can suffer the same kinds of brain injuries as children, it is commonly believed that the effect on language is different for young children. In summarizing this literature, Long (1994) notes that children with acquired aphasia are thought to have a lower incidence of aphasia, exhibit different language symptoms, and recover faster and more fully than adults. The lower incidence of aphasia is explained by the fact that fewer children have brain tumours and strokes. With respect to language behaviours, Satz and Bullard-Bates (1981) found that the majority of children with acquired aphasia demonstrate non-fluent aphasia patterns. They tend to be mute immediately following a brain injury. Speech is sparse and effortful when it returns. Like adults, however, children exhibit problems in comprehension, writing, reading, and naming.

Although the language behaviours of children are not remarkably different from those of adults, the prognosis for children is considerably better than it is for adults. Satz and Bullard-Bates (1981) found that about 75 per cent of children showed dramatic spontaneous recovery of language. Long (1994) notes that toddlers and young children appear to recover best because (a) their brains withstand injury better than infants, (b) they have established some degree of language competence prior to injury, and (c) they still have enough plasticity for functional reorganization of the brain to occur.

Given the variability in age, aetiology, severity of injury, and type of aphasia, it is difficult to give a general description of the language characteristics of children with acquired aphasia. Several factors influence the extent of such children's language difficulties, including the severity of the head trauma, the child's age at the time of the trauma, and the child's cognitive abilities before and after the trauma. The language impairment is, of course, most pronounced immediately following the brain injury. After the period of spontaneous recovery during the first year, many children will continue to have residual language difficulties that will affect communication. In most cases, according to many (cf. Long, 1994), the residual language deficits will have their greatest impact on academic performance. For more detailed descriptions of language abilities of children with acquired aphasia and specific assessment and treatment considerations, see the excellent chapter by Long (1994), a recent article by Russell (1993), and Beukelman and Yorkston's (1991) edited volume.

Children with learning disabilities

Any discussion of children with learning disabilities must acknowledge that the field of learning disabilities is characterized by diverse opinions about the nature of the problem, aetiology, definitions, terminology, and methods of assessment and treatment. Every text book on learning disabilities begins with a lengthy discussion of the different definitions that have been advocated (Hallahan, Kauffman and Lloyd, 1985; Bender, 1992; Gerber, 1993; Long and Long, 1994). The definition adopted by the National Joint Committee on Learning Disabilities (1991), which is endorsed by ASHA, is:

> Learning disabilities is a general term that refers to a heterogenous group of disorders manifested by significant difficulties in the acquisition and use of listening, speaking, reading, writing, reasoning, or mathematical abilities. These disorders are intrinsic to the individual, presumed to be due to central nervous system dysfunction, and may occur across the life span. Problems in self-regulatory behaviours, social perception, and social interaction may exist with learning disabilities but do not by themselves constitute a learning disability. Although learning disabilities may occur concomitantly with other handicapping conditions (e.g. sensory impairment, mental retardation, seri-

ous emotional disturbance) or extrinsic influences (e.g. cultural differences, insufficient or inappropriate instruction), they are not the direct result of those conditions or influences.

Like the other disorder types discussed thus far, learning disabilities include a heterogeneous population of children. One defining characteristic of learning-disabled children is the extent of their spoken language impairment. Studies have found that 42 to 46 per cent of children with learning disabilities have significant language deficits (Mattis, French and Rapin, 1975; Lyon and Watson, 1981). Included in this group are children who have previously been identified as having a specific language impairment. Almost all of the remaining 55 per cent of learning-disabled children are identified because they experience difficulty learning to read. Some of these children may have an associated attention deficit disorder (ADD). There is some controversy concerning the relationship between learning disabilities and ADD. Most theorists agree that ADD should not be classified as a learning disability although, practically speaking, many children with ADD have learning problems.

The relationship between dyslexia and learning disabilities has also received considerable attention in recent years (Stanovich, 1988; Kamhi and Catts, 1989; Kamhi, 1992; Long and Long, 1994). It is currently believed that individuals with dyslexia or a specific reading disability have particular problems in automatizing word recognition skills. These problems are caused by deficient phonological processing abilities (Stanovich, 1988). Complicating the picture, however, is the fact that phonological processing abilities tend to be deficient in all children who have difficulty learning to read. Thus, it is often not easy to differentiate the children with a specific reading disability from the garden-variety poor reader (Kamhi, 1992).

Learning disabilities are manifested in different ways as children get older. In young children, the primary deficit is in spoken language abilities and learning to read. In older school-age children, spoken and written language problems continue, but the learning problems now extend to other academic areas. Many children with learning disabilities may also exhibit emotional, social, motivational, attention, and behavioural problems. During adolescence, learning disabilities are seen most often in writing. Reading and some subtle spoken language deficits may still be present (cf. Kamhi and Catts, 1989; Gerber, 1993; Wallach and Butler, 1994). The social consequences of having a learning disability are particularly troublesome for adolescents. Many adolescents with learning disabilities have personal and social adjustment problems. It is important to note, however, that some of the social and emotional problems do not persist into adulthood. Bruck (1986) found that more than half (54 per cent) of the learning-disabled individuals who had social-emotional problems during the school years were well adjusted as young adults.

Causative Factors

Hubbell (1981: 105) begins his chapter on causation in child language disorders as follows:

> If something goes wrong, it's natural to ask why. If the car won't start, you start looking for causes. Out of gas? Battery dead? If a child develops red blotches and a high fever, the physician likewise looks for causes. Similarly, if a child demonstrates impairments in the use of language, we wonder why.

Hubbell goes on to note that the search for causal factors in child language disorders has been frustratingly difficult. A primary reason for this difficulty is that many individuals have assumed that one causal factor could explain the language disorder. Causation, however, is a complex process. This complexity is best seen by contrasting three different views of the process of causation: (a) linear cause-and-effect model, (b) interactional model, and (c) the transactional model. These models are discussed briefly below. For a more detailed discussion, see Hubbell (1981) or Sameroff (1975).

Linear cause-and-effect model

In this model, often referred to as the medical model, there is a direct, one-to-one relationship between cause and effect. The physician, for example, diagnoses the cause of a disease by considering its symptoms or effects. The logic of this model is that for each effect there is a cause and for each cause there is a resulting effect. The term 'linear' refers to the direct connection between cause and effect. There are two contrasting applications of the linear cause-and-effect model, one that emphasizes the child's constitution and the other that emphasizes the child's environment. The term 'constitution' refers to the child's neurophysical make-up and genetic endowment. As Hubbell (1981: 111) notes, both views of the linear cause-and-effect model have a severe shortcoming. A language disorder does not depend solely on constitutional factors or solely on environmental factors. Both constitutional and environmental factors influence language development and thus contribute to language disorders.

Interactional model

The interactional model acknowledges that a child's development results from the interaction between constitutional and environmental factors. The example Hubbell gives (p. 111) is of a child who is born premature and then does not receive adequate medical care. Such a child is at a higher risk than one who suffers from only one of these conditions. The interactional view, however, is still an oversimplification of the process of causation. First, it assumes that constitution and environment do not change over time and, second, it assumes that constitutional and environmental factors do not influence one another. The transactional model addresses both of these concerns.

Transactional model

Unlike the two previous models, the transactional model includes change over time and acknowledges the reciprocal influences of constitutional and environmental factors (Sameroff, 1975; Hubbell, 1981). Consider, for example, two children born with Down's syndrome to two different families. Assume that the intelligence level and other constitutional factors are similar in the two children. In one family, there are two older normal siblings. The family is resentful that they now have a mentally retarded child. They specifically resent the stigma of having such a child and the trouble he will cause them throughout his development. By age five this child is not only mentally retarded, but also has significant behaviour problems. His language abilities are also about one year below his mental age.

In contrast, the family of the other child with Down's syndrome have no other children. Although they are very disappointed that their child was born with Down's syndrome, they try to provide the best possible learning environment for their child. By age five their child is being mainstreamed in a normal kindergarten class. His social behaviour and language abilities are at or above his cognitive level.

This example points out the difficulty in identifying aetiology and causal factors. Neither environmental nor constitutional factors alone can explain the present behaviour of the two five-year-old Down's syndrome children. A number of years ago (Kamhi, 1984), I suggested that the diagnostic process should include clinical hypotheses about the cause-effect relationships that affect children's language learning. The hypotheses should consider the relationship between the structures/mechanisms, processes, and behaviours that impact and characterize language. Although it may be difficult to formulate such hypotheses, it is important for clinicians to ask questions about how perceptual, cognitive, social, and environmental factors impact on specific aspects of language and communication. Leonard (1991) sparked some controversy a few years ago by questioning the clinical benefits of causal-based research. A clinical forum devoted to this topic appeared in the April 1991 issue of *Language, Speech, and Hearing Services in Schools*.

Assessing Children's Language Skills

Much has been written about the assessment of children's language skills (e.g. James, 1993; Lund and Duchan, 1993; Nelson, 1993; Reed, 1994). There is general agreement that the purposes of assessment are to (1) identify children with language disorders, (2) design appropriate language intervention programmes, and (3) monitor changes that result from intervention (James, 1993). There is some disagreement, however, concerning the distinction between the assessment and diagnostic process.

Some theorists, such as Nation and Aram (1977), view assessment procedures as a part of the diagnostic process. The end products of the diagnostic process are clinical hypotheses about pertinent causal factors and recommendations for services based on these hypotheses. Other theorists place little emphasis on diagnosis in their assessment procedures (e.g. Naremore, 1980; James, 1993). Lund and Duchan take a middle ground by including a question about causal factors as one of the five questions that should be answered in assessment. The five questions are:

1. Does the child have a language problem?
2. What is causing the problem?
3. What are the areas of deficit?
4. What are the regularities in the child's language performance?
5. What is recommended for the child?

Nelson (1993: 188-94) provides a more comprehensive series of questions that are appropriate at different stages of the assessment and intervention process. Because assessment is an ongoing process, one must consider the types of assessments that occur during intervention. Some of her questions are listed below:

1. Does the child qualify for services?
2. What kinds of services does the child need?
3. Which speech, language, and communication behaviours and strategies should be changed and what kinds of procedures should be used to effect these changes?
4. Is progress occurring in therapy and are modifications in treatment objectives or procedures necessary?

James (1993: 186) has written that 'the task of assessing children's language would be relatively simple if language were easily quantified like height or weight.' Language, however, is a multidimensional, complex, and dynamic entity involving many interrelated processes and abilities. Although it is possible to group children according to their overall pattern of language performance, to a certain extent every child presents a unique pattern of language abilities. One of the major challenges in assessment is thus to describe the unique pattern of language behaviours that each language-disordered child presents.

Some models of language assessment view language as a self-contained system that is independent from the social world in which people live. In recent years, there has been an increasing awareness that language use is a highly contextualized social activity that is influenced by the participants, situations, language modes (speaking, writing, sign), and socio-cultural factors (cf. Damico, 1992; Kovarsky, 1992; Nelson, 1993). Assessments that are sensitive to this view of language attempt to describe language in as many different contexts as possible (e.g. home, classroom, playground, etc.). Such assessments clearly are more time-consuming than administering a few standardized tests or collecting a language sample in one setting; however, the benefits of such assessments should be obvious if one is interested in obtaining a true picture of someone's language abilities.

To develop competence in the assessment and diagnostic process, I have my students perform an in-depth analysis of a language-disordered child. The purpose of the project is to develop students' competencies in assessing various language and language-related abilities in children and to foster problem-solving skills necessary to think about how structures, processes, and behaviours interact. The guidelines for the project are:

I. LANGUAGE SAMPLE
A. *Sample size* – Try to obtain about 100 spontaneous utterances. The minimum is 50 utterances for children who do not talk too much.
B. *Transcription* – Follow procedures in Retherford (1993).
C. *MLU* – Follow procedures in Retherford (1993).

II. SPEECH SAMPLE
A. *Sample* – 25 utterances from the language sample (100 words) and approximately 35 words from standardized articulation test, such as the Goldman–Fristoe or Fisher–Logemann.
B. *Transcription* – The 25 utterances from your language sample need to be phonetically transcribed. On the left side of the page put the transliterated version of the sentence. On the right side put the phonetically transcribed sentences. Number the sentences according to the way they were numbered in the language sample.
C. *Data reduction* – Alphabetize all of the words from phonetically transcribed sentences and the articulation test. List the words in alphabetical order. In the phonetic column put the phonetic transcriptions of the words. Circle the numbers of the words that are imitated and use dashes to indicate whether a word preceded or followed another word.

III. STORY and EVENT RECALL
A. *Sample* – Have children recall a short story and describe an event (e.g. birthday party, family trip, going shopping, etc.). For the recall

story, describe the picture or series of pictures and then have the child talk about the pictures. If none of this works, we will find you a story to analyse.

B. *Transcription* – Transcribe stories into T-units. All conjoined sentences are treated as separate units. Do not forget to include the full version of the stories you ask the children to recall.

IV. THE DIAGNOSTIC REPORT – PART 1

A. *Developmental history* – Discuss pertinent medical and developmental information, such as motor milestones, feeding behaviour, and significant illnesses. This section may differ some from the comparable section in the clinical report. Do not simply copy the clinical report.

B. *Perceptual and memory processes* – Discuss the child's ability to detect, discriminate, and identify auditory input. Also, discuss child's memory processes (e.g. short-term memory span for verbal and non-verbal information, encoding, storage, and retrieval processes). Is there a difference in the child's ability to process linguistic and non-linguistic information?

C. *Conceptual knowledge* – How much does the child know about the world? Measures of non-verbal intelligence (Leiter, Columbia, TONI), spatial and temporal knowledge, and receptive vocabulary should be reported and discussed in this section. Piagetian measures should also be reported here. In what stage of cognitive development is the child?

D. *Personal-social behaviours and language-learning environment* – Include remarks about the child's emotional maturity, self-image, and motivation to interact and communicate. Does the child have personal-social problems beyond those caused by the language impairment? Discuss the child's language-learning environment.

E. *Problem-solving and attentional behaviours* – Discuss the child's attentiveness, level of activity, and impulsivity/reflectivity. What is the child's general approach to solving problems and learning about the world? Does the child have a particular learning or cognitive style (e.g. analytic vs. Gestalt)?

F. *Receptive language abilities* – Discuss the child's ability to understand language. Can the child carry out commands and follow instructions? Does the child have difficulty understanding certain kinds of discourse?

G. *Summary* – Briefly highlight some of the important findings from the first part of the project.

V. THE DIAGNOSTIC REPORT – PART 2: LINGUISTIC ANALYSES

A. *Phonological analysis* – Includes phonetic and phonological process analyses. Refer to procedures in Ingram (1981), Stoel-Gammon and Dunn (1985), or Grunwell (1985). Optional analyses:

syllable structure, substitution, homonymy, and phonological contrast. Summaries should discuss the impact of phonological system on language abilities and attempt to explain the factors that motivate and sustain the child's phonological problems.

B. *Semantic analysis* – Includes lexical analysis (adverbs and adjectives) (cf. Lund and Duchan, 1993) and semantic relations (Retherford, 1993). Summaries should compare expressive semantic abilities with receptive semantic knowledge and general conceptual knowledge.

C. *Syntactic analysis* – Follow procedures in Retherford (1993) or similar descriptive analysis (e.g. LARSP). Summaries should compare syntactic development across the three domains evaluated: lexical, morphological, and phrase structure.

D. *Pragmatic Analysis* – Includes speech act analysis, one other pragmatic area, and analysis of clarification requests and responses (cf. Brinton and Fujiki, 1991; Retherford, 1993). These analyses should include some proportional data. Summaries should discuss child's pragmatic abilities in relation to social and personal behaviours discussed earlier. Is the child a good communicator and partner in discourse?

E. *Narrative and Event Analyses* – Determine the story and event structures and comment on the guiding scripts and use of various linguistic means to create narratives/events (cf. Nelson, 1993). Summaries should compare narrative and event recalls to conversational abilities.

F. *Summary* – Compare and contrast the child's expressive language abilities in the areas evaluated. This section should be more than just a summary of the previous sections.

VI. WRITTEN LANGUAGE KNOWLEDGE

For pre-school children, evaluate precursors to literacy such as phonological awareness, print knowledge, knowledge of the alphabet, etc. (see Schuele and van Kleeck, 1987; Catts, 1991). For school-age children, note word attack, word identification, and comprehension abilities.

VII. DIAGNOSIS

Generate some hypotheses about cause–effect relationships among physical structures, cognitive processes, and language behaviours. You do not necessarily need to come up with a diagnostic label for the child. However, if there is evidence suggesting such a label (e.g. mental retardation), do not hesitate to use it.

Questions that should be addressed in this section include: (1) Are all language abilities equally delayed? (2) Which deficits seem to be primary and which secondary? (3) What links are there between structural, processing, and linguistic deficiencies?

VIII. RECOMMENDATIONS AND PROGNOSIS

List some short- and long-term objectives for the child as well as other pertinent recommendations. How much progress will the child make in therapy? Will he/she ever be able to function in a normal classroom and eventually become a proficient language user? Will the child be able to attend college at age 18? What might this child be doing in 20 years?

The sections of the diagnostic project provide a framework for assessing children's language and language-related abilities. The project also provides some specific suggestions about how to assess the various areas of language and other related behaviours. It is important to keep in mind that no assessment protocol is a substitute for an informed speech-language pathologist. As Siegel and Broen (1976: 75) have stated,

> The most useful and dependable 'language assessment device' is an informed clinician who feels compelled to keep up with developments in psycholinguistics, speech pathology, and related fields, and who is not slavishly attached to a particular model of language or of assessment.

Principles and Procedures for Language Intervention

Language disorders are associated with a variety of causal factors, involve different aspects of language, and vary in their severity. Faced with such variety, clinicians need to have some basic organizational framework to aid in identifying intervention goals and procedures. At the core of this framework is a theory about what language is, how it is learned, and how it can be taught.

In recent years, there has been much written about the theoretical bases of therapy (e.g. Craig, 1983; Johnston, 1983; McLean, 1985). Johnston and McLean take issue with clinicians who say things like, 'I want something practical – not a lot of theory.' What these clinicians fail to recognize is that all therapy is theoretically based. Acknowledging the theoretical bases of one's language intervention does not mean there is necessarily one proven theory of language and learning. In fact, in a recent article I argued that a plurality of theories guide clinical practice. No one theory can explain the language, cognitive, social, and environmental forces that impact on children's language and communication abilities. It is not sufficient to be knowledgeable about theories of language acquisition. A theory of language acquisition may not help clinicians implement specific therapy procedures and management techniques, comfort concerned parents, collaborate with other professionals, adapt to different clinical settings, and so forth. Clinicians thus need to exploit the plurality of theories that have a direct impact on clinical service.

One's theories about language and learning often lead to a set of principles that guide the intervention process. A number of years ago, Johnston (1985: 132) generated a list of ten principles that can guide intervention for children with language disorders:

1. Teach language that expresses the child's available meanings.
2. Teach language that accomplishes the child's desired purposes.
3. Teach language that the child can interpret given his current knowledge about the language and the world.
4. Teach language recognizing the child's preferred strategies.
5. Teach language while seeming to pursue some other goal.
6. Teach language by providing concentrated, salient examples of a single pattern.
7. Teach language in contexts which clarify meaning.
8. Teach language in natural as well as contrived transactions.
9. Teach language while communicating real messages.
10. Teach language in the child's world.

Perhaps the underlying principle of language intervention is that it is a problem solving process, both for the child learning language and for the clinician who must determine how best to teach language. The use of language involves active problem solving (cf. Hubbell, 1981). One has to figure out what utterances mean, how to initiate turns and topics, how to talk to different people in different contexts, which words and structures to use, how to respond to questions, how to ask questions, and so forth. Language intervention also is a problem solving task. The clinician has to identify language learning problems, determine the factors that are contributing to these problems, and design an intervention programme to treat these problems.

I find it useful to view therapy in terms of three components: context, content (objectives), and procedures. Context refers to the setting, participants, and materials of therapy. Content refers to the goals of the therapy. Procedures are the actual ways or activities used to teach language. These components of therapy are described in more detail below.

Context

The physical setting of therapy is probably the most frequent aspect of context discussed in the literature (cf. Bernstein and Tiegerman, 1993). The influence of physical setting on language therapy, however, seems to be vastly overrated. The principles of language intervention, selection of therapy goals, and procedures should not vary according to the setting in which therapy takes place. In other words, language therapy in a school may not look very different from language therapy in a clinic, hospital, or home. What has more of an influence on language therapy is the type of service delivery model one follows. School-based clinicians who believe in classroom-based intervention and collaborative models approach intervention very differently from clinicians who use a more traditional pull-out model in which children are seen individually or in small groups.

The social context in which treatment is provided is obviously a critical aspect of the language-learning context. As noted above, individual and small group therapy is being gradually replaced by more naturalistic contexts and participants that play an integral role in children's lives (cf. Wilcox, Kouri, and Caswell, 1991; Nelson, 1993). With school-age children, teachers and peers can play an important role in intervention. With infants and very young children, the family and multidisciplinary teams are usually involved in treatment programmes (Ratokalau and Robb, 1993).

The importance of materials is often overlooked in discussions about therapy context. The materials used in therapy constrain what children will talk about and how they will talk about it (Miller, 1981). Using picture books, for example, will encourage the use of descriptive phrases linked by and (e.g. There's a fire engine, and here's a fireman, and this is a policeman). Games tend to elicit phrases such as, 'It's my/your turn' or a narrow set of questions (Miller, 1981). Activities that involve physical manipulation, such as puzzles and drawing, often stifle talking because children become too involved performing the physical activity.

Another concern about materials is that clinicians sometimes begin believing that it is the materials that are doing the teaching rather than the clinician. One way to dispel this belief is to conduct therapy without the usual set of materials. An exercise such as this provides some indication of one's reliance on therapy materials rather than on knowledge of language and the therapy process.

Content

Deciding what it is we want children to be able to do is the question that underlies decisions about language goals (Rees, 1983). Rees adds that oftentimes clinical goals are determined by the availability, attractiveness, or popularity of published tests and materials. For example, for many years it was common to administer the ITPA, teach the skills tapped by the various ITPA subtests, and readminister the test. Although many children presumably became more adept at solving auditory and visual discrimination tasks, there was often not a corresponding increase in communication skills.

It has also been common practice for clinicians to target certain language forms because use of these forms is easily measured by pre-

and post-test instruments. A good example of this practice involves the teaching of auxiliary forms, such as auxiliary *is* in present progressive sentences (e.g. 'He is running'). Language-impaired children have been shown to have considerable difficulty learning auxiliary forms(e.g. Johnston and Schery, 1976; Johnston and Kamhi, 1984). Although these forms add little or no meaning to a sentence (compare 'John is running' with 'John running') and have little communicative value, clinicians spend inordinate amounts of time teaching children to use these forms.

The determination of appropriate language goals is the final step of the assessment process. An important criterion in judging the appropriateness of a goal is the extent to which the attainment of the goal will enhance communicative effectiveness. For young language-disordered children, increasing the frequency with which a child initiates topics or teaching a child how to request clarification clearly enhances communicative effectiveness. In contrast, teaching a young child to use auxiliary forms or to say 'caught' instead of 'catched' has little communicative value and would not be an appropriate language goal if the child has more basic communicative deficits. Teaching auxiliary forms or past tense markers is more likely to be an appropriate language goal for an older language-disordered child (e.g. past 5 years of age) who lacks some of the grammatical niceties of language.

As reflected in Johnston's first three principles, language goals should be determined by the child's available meanings, desired purposes, and conceptual level. In general, therapy with young children should focus on increasing the range of meanings and functions expressed, whereas therapy with older children should place more attention the ways in which language impacts on talking, thinking, reading, and writing. A number of excellent books are now available that address the kinds of goals that should be targeted (Fey, 1986; Bernstein and Tiergerman, 1993; Gerber, 1993; Norris and Hoffman, 1993; Reed, 1994; Wallach and Butler, 1994),

Procedures

I find it useful to think about the actual teaching of speech-language forms in terms of a three-part sequence: (a) the clinician provides a model of communicative behaviour, (b) the child responds in some way to the model, and (c) the clinician provides some kind of feedback to the child about the response. Each of these parts of therapy is discussed below in some detail.

Although there are many different approaches to therapy, ranging from clinician-oriented approaches to child-oriented approaches (see Fey, 1986), and different terminology used to describe the therapy process, the language models children are exposed to during therapy determine what they will learn. In most cases these models are verbal, although non-verbal communicative behaviours (e.g. gestures) and alternative communication systems (e.g. sign language) can also serve as language input. Models can vary in terms of their content and structure as well as in the frequency with which they are produced. The specific language objective determines the structure and content of the language models. The frequency with which a model is produced can be viewed as a continuum that ranges from highly repetitive and systematic modelling of a particular structure (i.e., focused stimulation) at one end to low levels of repetition and unsystematic modelling of structures (general stimulation) at the other end.

Focused stimulation is often used to teach specific syntactic forms. For example, a clinician might have a series of ten picture cards depicting actions that can be described by the same phrase structure rule (NP + Aux + V + ing). The actual models might include sentences such as 'He is running', 'He is jumping', and 'He is swimming'. With general stimulation there is no focus to the language input. Particular language structures are not repeated in any consistent manner. Instead, clinicians attempt to model language forms approximately one level above the child's current level of language functioning. Models at the same level or below the child's current level will not teach the child anything, whereas models more than one level above the child's current level are thought to be too difficult to learn. For example, if a child is currently producing mostly two-word utterances, the clinician should model three-constituent utterances that expand the child's two-word utterances (e.g. child says 'Mummy sock' and clinician responds 'Yes, Mummy has a sock.')

The child's response to the clinician's model can also be viewed on a continuum. In this case the continuum ranges from an elicited exact repetition of the model to no response. Operant approaches often require exact imitations of the models (e.g. Gray and Ryan, 1973; Stremel and Waryas, 1974). An approach to therapy that has come to be called 'modelling' initially requires no response from the child (Leonard, 1975). The child is asked to listen to ten language models before he is given the opportunity to respond. It is important to note that it is the response required from the child that differentiates the operant and modelling approaches rather than the language models provided.

In certain forms of play therapy no response is ever required from the child. The clinician makes no attempt to elicit repetitions of language models. Instead, the clinician may follow the child's lead and comment on what the child is playing with or talking about. Alternatively, the clinician may engage in parallel play and comment on her own activities (see Fey, 1986). The theoretical rationale for this kind of therapy approach is that language is a mental activity that involves rule induction and other reasoning processes. Learning language is thus not necessarily facilitated by repeating language models. The child must induce a language rule from these models and this rule induction is more likely to occur 'off-line' when the child has time to think about language rather than on-line when the child is actually repeating language forms. Connell and Stone (1992, 1994), however, have found that an imitative approach was more effective than a modelling approach in teaching a group of language-impaired children to produce words with an invented morphological suffix. One possible explanation for this finding was that the imitative approach helped to focus attention on the language models to be learned. Connell and Stone (1992) have suggested that children with SLI have difficulty accessing phonological representations of morphemes during on-line naming tasks.

In general, the younger the child, the less stringent the response demands should be. Infants and very young children are often not very responsive to highly directive clinician-oriented approaches that require elicited imitative responses. As children get older and their comprehension and metalinguistic competence increase, they can be more easily directed to produce specific responses.

The final component of therapy sequence is the clinician's response to the child's response. There are two kinds of feedback clinicians can provide to children: evaluative feedback and communicative feedback. Evaluative feedback is when the clinician offers an appraisal of the appropriateness or accuracy of the child's response. Comments that reflect evaluative feedback include, 'Good', 'Good talking/words', 'I like the way you said that', 'No, that wasn't so good.' Clinicians are more likely to give positive evaluative feedback than negative evaluative feedback. For evaluative feedback to be meaningful, however, positive evaluations should follow only appropriate child responses. There are a variety of ways to handle inappropriate responses, including direct negative evaluations (e.g. 'That was not too good', 'You missed that one'); corrective feedback (e.g. 'You said "catched" instead of "caught"'), and neutral feedback (e.g. 'Let's try that one again later').

Importantly, it is neither necessary nor desirable for clinicians to evaluate the appropriateness of every response or utterance a child makes. Responding to children's utterances in communicative rather than evaluative ways also provides feedback to the child. For example, a child might say, 'Hey, there's a spider on the floor' to which the clinician responds, 'Yeah, it's a really big one. Do you like spiders?' Not only is communicative feedback more in line with the kinds of discourse children will encounter outside the therapy context, but expansions and recasts have been shown to facilitate language learning in normal children (Nelson, 1987).

Therapy approaches differ in the extent to which they include evaluative and communicative feedback. Behavioural, clinician-oriented approaches are usually associated with well-defined schedules for providing evaluative feedback. In contrast, client-oriented therapy approaches, such as play therapy, tend to place more emphasis on communicative feedback.

Effectiveness of Therapy

One way to approach questions about therapy effectiveness is through clinical studies in which a specific therapy approach (e.g. modelling vs. imitation) is evaluated in terms of its effectiveness on one or more clients (e.g. Courtright and Courtright, 1976; Connell and Stone, 1992, 1994). Clinical research, however, generally has not examined the effectiveness of a broader treatment regimen. As Schery and Lipsey (1983) point out, a complete treatment regimen consists of many specific therapy treatments and, therefore, its overall effects are probably somewhat different from the effects of any one therapy technique. In a review of clinical treatment studies, Leonard (1981) found that researchers rarely addressed questions about the generality or duration of treatment effects and the range of clients for which a specific approach was appropriate.

Another approach to the question of therapy effectiveness is to consider general programme evaluation, the basic function of which is to provide information for decision making at local, state and federal levels. To do this, Schery and Lipsey (1983) suggest that programme information is needed in four areas: (1) accountability; (2) programme premises; (3) management and administration, and (4) planning. Accountability is usually interpreted as having readily accessible complete records of clients served, along with a justifiable rationale to document need for service. Other accountability issues involve demonstrating that a particular programme serves a need and should continue to be funded. Programme premises include basic assumptions that govern the provision of service, e.g. the assumption that speech-language clinicians with graduate degrees can deliver services more effectively and efficiently that individuals without professional training. As Schery and Lipsey point out, assumptions such as these help determine the programme model under which school and clinic operate.

Management and administration refers to the process rather than the outcome of providing services. The process component of programme evaluation involves keeping track of key operations and activities that constitute the programme (Schery and Lipsey, 1983: 263). A comprehensive programme evaluation would include questions about access, equity and efficiency (Schery and Lipsey, 1983: 264). Programme planning involves foreseeing trends and needs so that the programme can adapt to the changes that might occur in the future.

A different approach to therapy effectiveness that will be considered is reflected in a recent article by Siegel (1987) on the limits of science. Siegel argues that the most important question to ask about therapy is not whether it works, but rather whether it makes sense. Siegel begins with the assumption that it does work. There is no experiment that would convince him otherwise because the definitive treatment experiment cannot be done, there being too many uncontrollable variables relating to the client, clinician setting, therapy method, measures used and so forth. Efficacy studies, therefore, are not needed to demonstrate that therapy works, although they might help influence programme funding decisions. The accountability issue is different and relates to funding decisions and programme evaluation. It is not appropriate to conclude that because a particular programme is not accountable, therapy is ineffective. As Siegel (p. 301) states, 'It seems incontrovertible that all human behaviour is potentially malleable, and that none of us, client or therapist, is working to the absolute limits of his or her ability'. In other words there is no doubt that speech-language clinicians are capable of changing a client's communicative behaviour. Moreover, it is difficult to imagine a speech-language clinician who would knowingly use a therapy procedure that was ineffective in modifying communicative performance. This does not mean, however, that clinicians should not be accountable for what they do.

In recent years, I have become interested in what defines clinical expertise in speech-language pathology (Kamhi, 1994). It has become clear that clinical expertise is defined not only by technical and knowledge-based skills, but also by interpersonal and attitudinal qualities as well (Cornett and Chabon, 1988; DeJoy, 1991; Frattali, 1991). Clinical attitudes include qualities such as confidence, enthusiasm, belief, interest, compassion, and adaptability. Some believe that these qualities may have more of an impact on effective service delivery than technical and knowledge base skills (e.g. Chall, 1983; Gee, 1992). Future studies need to consider the impact these qualities have on clinical decisions and outcomes.

Summary

I began this chapter by noting that learning a first language is the most complex learning task humans accomplish during their lifetimes. These complexities are best seen in children who have difficulty learning language. What this means is that there are no simple answers to the questions most frequently raised about these children, namely: What is a language disorder? What causes it? How are language abilities assessed? How are language abilities taught? Despite the difficulty in answering these questions, I have nevertheless attempted, in this chapter, to provide some answers to each of these questions. Some of my answers may be more satisfactory to you than others. A chapter such as this one is difficult to write because each section must sacrifice detail for brevity. The information provided in this chapter, however, was meant to whet the appetite, not satiate it. Indeed, the complexity of language learning and language disorders ensures that even the most voracious appetite will never be satiated.

References

Abbeduto L, Davies B, Solesby S, Furman L (1991) Identifying the referents of spoken messages: Use of context and clarification requests by children with and without mental retardation. American Journal on Mental Retardation 95: 551–62.

Aram D, Nation J (1982) Child Language Disorders. St Louis, MO: Mosby.

ASHA Committee on Language, Speech and Hearing Services in the Schools (1980) Definitions for communicative disorders and differences. ASHA 22: 317–8.

ASHA Committee on Language (1983) Definition of language. ASHA 25: 44.

Bender, W (1992) Learning Disabilities: Characteristics, Identification, and Teaching Strategies. Boston: Allyn & Bacon.

Bernstein, D (1993) The nature of language and its disorders. In Bernstein L, Tiegerman E (Eds) Language and Communication Disorders in Children (3rd ed). Columbus, OH: Merrill.

Bernstein L, Tiegerman E (Eds) (1993) Language and Communication Disorders in Children (3rd ed). Columbus, OH: Merrill.

Bernthal J, Bankston N (1993) Articulation and Phonological Disorders (3rd ed), Englewood Cliffs, NJ: Prentice-Hall.

Beukelman D, Yorkston K (1991) Communication Disorders Following Traumatic Brain Injury: Management of Cognitive, Language, and Motor Impairments. Austin, TX: Pro-Ed.

Biklen D (1992) Facilitated communication: Biklen responds. American Journal of Speech-Language Pathology 1: 21–2.

Bishop DVM (1992) The underlying nature of specific language impairment. Child Psychology and Psychiatry 33: 3–66.

Bloom L, Lahey M (1978) Language Development and Language Disorders. New York: John Wiley & Sons.

Brinton B, Fujiki M (1991) Conversational Management with Language-impaired Children. Rockville, MD: Aspen.

Bruck M (1986) Social and emotional adjustments of learning disabled children: A review of the issues. In Ceci SJ (Ed) Cognition and the Development of Language. New York: John Wiley & Sons.

Carrow-Woolfolk E (1988) Theory, Assessment and Intervention in Language Disorders: An Integrative Approach. Philadelphia: Grune & Stratton.

Casby M (1992) The cognitive hypothesis and its influence on speech-language services in schools. Language, Speech, and Hearing Services in Schools 23: 198–202.

Catts H (1991) Facilitating phonological awareness: Role of speech-language pathologists. Language, Speech, and Hearing Services in Schools 22: 196–203.

Chafe W (1970) Meaning and Structure of Language. Chicago: University of Chicago Press.

Chall J (1983) Stages of Reading Development. New York: McGraw-Hill.

Chomsky N (1957) Syntactic Structures. The Hague: Mouton.

Chomsky N (1965) Aspects of the Theory of Syntax. Cambridge, MA: MIT Press.

Connell P, Stone CA (1992) Morpheme learning of children with specific language impairment under controlled instructional conditions. Journal of Speech and Learning Research 25: 844–52.

Connell P, Stone CA (1994) The conceptual basis for morpheme learning problems in children with specific language impairment. Journal of Speech and Hearing Research 37: 389–98.

Cornett B, Chabon S (1988) The Clinical Practice of Speech-Language Pathology. Columbus, OH: Merrill.

Courchesne E (1987) A neurophysiological view of autism. In Schopler E, Mesibov GB (Eds) Neurobiological Issues in Autism. New York: Plenum Press.

Courtright J, Courtright I (1976) Imitative modeling as a theoretical base fort instructing language-disordered children. Journal of Speech and Hearing Research 19: 655–63.

Craig H (1983) Applications of pragmatic language models for intervention. In Gallagher T, Prutting C (Eds) Pragmatic Assessment and Intervention Issues. San Diego, CA: College Hill.

Damico J (1992) Systematic observation of communicative interaction: A valid and practical descriptive assessment technique. In Secord W (Ed) Best Practices in School Speech-Language Pathology. New York: Harcourt Brace Jovanovich.

DeJoy D (1991) Overcoming fragmentation through the client-clinician relationship. National Student Speech Language and Hearing Association Journal 18: 17–25.

DeMyer M, Barton S, DeMyer E, Norton J, Allen J, Stelle R (1973) Prognosis in autism: A follow-up study. Journal of Autism and Childhood Schizophrenia 3: 199–216.

Eisenberg L (1956) The autistic child in adolescence. American Journal of Psychiatry 112: 607–12.

Eisenson J (1972) Aphasia in Children. New York: Harper & Row.

Ellis Weismer S (1991) Hypothesis testing abilities of language impaired children. Journal of Speech and Hearing Research 34: 1329–38.

Fein D, Pennington B, Markowitz P, Braverman M, Waterhouse L (1986) Toward a neuropsychological model of infantile autism: Are the social deficits primary? Journal of the American Academy of Child Psychiatry 25: 198–212.

Fey M (1986) Language Intervention with Children. San Diego, CA: College-Hill Press.

Fratalli C (1991) In pursuit of quality: Evaluating clinical outcomes. National Student Speech Language Hearing Association Journal 18: 4–17.

Gathercole S, Baddeley A (1990) Phonological memory deficits in language disordered children: Is there a causal connection? Journal of Memory and Language 29: 336–60.

Gee JP (1992) The Social Mind: Language, Ideology, and Social Practice. New York: Bergin & Garvey.

Gerber A (1993) Language-related Learning Disabilities: Their Nature and Treatment. Baltimore: Paul H. Brookes Publishing Co.

Gray B, Ryan B (1973) A Language Program for the Nonlanguage Child. Champaign, IL: Research Press.

Grossman H (1983) Classification in Mental Retardation. Washington, DC: American Association on Mental Deficiency.

Grunwell P (1985) Phonological Assessment of Child Speech. Austin, TX: Pro-Ed.

Hallahan D, Kauffman J, Lloyd J (1985) Introduction to Learning Disabilities (2nd ed). Englewood Cliffs, NJ: Prentice-Hall.

Hubbell R (1981) Children's Language Disorders: An Integrated Approach. Englewood Cliffs, NJ: Prentice-Hall.

Ingram D (1976) Phonological Disability in Children. New York: Elsevier North-Holland.

Ingram D (1981) Procedures for the Phonological Analysis of Children's Language. Baltimore, MD: University Park Press.

James S (1993) Assessing children with language disorders. In Bernstein D, Tiegerman E (Eds) Language and Communication Disorders in Children (3rd ed). Columbus, OH: Merrill.

Johnston J (1982) The language disordered child. In Lass N, Northern, J, Yoder D, McReynolds L (Eds) Speech, Language and Hearing. Philadelphia: W. B. Saunders Co.

Johnston J (1983) What is language intervention? The role of theory. In Miller J, Yoder D, Schieflebusch R (Eds) Contemporary issues in language intervention. ASHA Reports #12. Rockville, MD: ASHA.

Johnston J (1985) Fit, focus and functionality: An essay on early language intervention. Child Language Teaching and Therapy l: 125–35.

Johnston J (1988) Specific language disorders in the child. In Lass N, McReynolds L, Northern J, Yoder D (Eds) Handbook of Speech-Language Pathology and Audiology. Philadelphia: B.C. Decker.

Johnston J (1991) The continuing relevance of cause: A reply to Leonard's 'specific language impairment as a clinical category'. Language, Speech, and Hearing Services in Schools 22: 75–80.

Johnston J, Ellis Weismer S (1993) Mental rotation abilities in language disordered children. Journal of Speech and Hearing Research 26: 397–403.

Johnston J, Kamhi A (1984) The same can be less: Syntactic and semantic aspects of the utterances of language-impaired children. Merrill-Palmer Quarterly 30: 65–85.

Johnston J, Schery T (1976) The use of grammatical morphemes by children with communication disorders. In Morehead D, Morehead A (Eds) Normal and Deficient Child Language. Baltimore, MD: University Park Press.

Kamhi A (1984) Problem solving in child language disorders: The clinician as clinical scientist. Language, Speech, and Hearing Services in Schools 15: 226–34.

Kamhi A (1992) Response to historical perspective: A developmental language perspective. Journal of Learning Disabilities 24: 48–52.

Kamhi A (1993) Children with specific language impairment: Perceptual and Cognitive Aspects. In Blanten G, Diffman J, Grimm H, Marshall J, Wallesch C (Eds) Linguistics Disorders and Pathologies: An International Handbook NY: Walter de Gruyter. pp 625–40.

Kamhi A (1994) Toward a theory of clinical expertise in speech-language pathology. Language, Speech, and Hearing Services in Schools 25: 115–8.

Kamhi A, Catts H (1989) Reading Disabilities: A Developmental Language Perspective. Boston, MA: College-Hill Press.

Kamhi A, Catts H, Koenig L, Lewis B (1984) Hypothesis testing and nonlinguistic symbolic abilities in language impaired children. Journal of Speech and Hearing Disorders 49: 169–77.

Kamhi A, Gentry B, Mauer D, Gholson B (1990a) Analogical learning and transfer in language-impaired children. Journal of Speech and Hearing Disorders 55: 140–8.

Kamhi A, Masterson J (1989) Language and cognition in mentally handicapped people: Last rites for the difference-delay controversy. In Beveridge M, Conti-Ramsden G, Leudar I (Eds) Language and Communication in the Mentally Handicapped. London: Chapman and Hall.

Kamhi A, Minor J, Mauer D (1990b) Content analysis and intratest performance profiles on the Columbia and the TONI. Journal of Speech and Hearing Research 33: 375–9.

Kovarsky D (1992) Ethnography and language assessment: Toward the contextualized description and interpretation of communicative behavior. In Secord W (Ed) Best Practices in School Speech-Language Pathology. New York: Harcourt Brace Jovanovich.

Lahey M (1988) Language Disorders and Language Development. New York: MacMillan.

Leonard L (1975) Modeling as a clinical procedure in language training. Language, Speech, and Hearing Services in Schools 6: 72–85.

Leonard L (1981) Facilitating linguistic skills in children with specific language impairment. Applied Psycholinguistics 2: 89–118.

Leonard L (1982) Early language development and language disorders. In Shames G, Wiig E (Eds) Human Communication Disorders: An Introduction. Columbus, OH: Merrill.

Leonard L (1987) Is specific language impairment a useful construct? In Rosenberg S (Ed) Advances in Applied Psycholinguistics, Volume I: Disorders of First-language Development. New York: Cambridge University Press.

Leonard L (1991) Specific language impairment as a clinical category, Language, Speech and Hearing Services in Schools 22: 66–8.

Long S (1994) Language and bilingual-bicultural children. In Reed V (Ed) An Introduction to Children with Language Disorders (2nd ed). New York: Macmillan.

Long S, Long S (1994) Language and children with mental retardation. In Reed V (Ed) An Introduction to Children with Language Disorders (2nd ed). New York: Macmillan.

Lund N, Duchan J (1993) Assessing Children's Language in Naturalistic Contexts (3rd ed). Englewood Cliffs, NJ: Prentice-Hall.

Lyon G, Watson B (1981) Empirically derived subgroups of learning disabled readers: Diagnostic characteristics. Journal of Learning Disabilities 14: 256–61.

McGinnis M (1963) Aphasic Children: Identification and Education by the Association Method. Washington, DC: Alexander Graham Bell Association for the Deaf.

McLean J (1985) A language-communication intervention model. In Bernstein D, Tiegerman E (Eds) Language and Communication Disorders in Children (3rd ed). Columbus, OH: Merrill.

McLean J, Snyder-McLean L (1978) A Transactional Approach to Early Language Training. Columbus, OH: Merrill.

Masterson J (1993) The performance of children with language-learning disabilities on two types of cognitive tasks. Journal of Speech and Hearing Research 36: 1026–36.

Mattis S, French J, Rapin I (1975) Dyslexia in children and young adults: Three independent neuropsychological syndromes. Developmental Medicine and Child Neurology 17: 150–63.

Maurer R, Damasio A (1982) Childhood autism from the point of view of behavioral neurology. Journal of Autism and Developmental Disorders 12: 195–205.

Miller J (1981) Assessing Language Production in Children. Baltimore, MD: University Park Press.

Miller J, Chapman R, MacKenzie H (1981) Individual differences in the language acquisition of mentally retarded children. Proceedings of the Second Wisconsin Symposium on Research in Child Language Disorders, University of Wisconsin.

Morley M (1957) The Development and Disorders of Speech in Childhood.

Edinburgh: E. & S. Livingston Ltd.

Myklebust H (1954) Auditory Disorders in Children: A Manual for Differential Diagnosis. New York: Grune & Stratton.

Naremore R (1980) Language disorders in children. In Hixon T, Shriberg L, Saxman J (Eds) Introduction to Communication Disorders. Englewood Cliffs, NJ: Prentice-Hall.

Nation J, Aram D (1977) Diagnosis of Speech and Language Disorders. St Louis: Mosby.

National Joint Committee on Learning Disability (1991) Learning disabilities: Issues on definition. ASHA 35 (suppl. 5): 18–20.

Nelson K (1987) Some observations from the perspective of the rare event cognitive comparison theory of language acquisition. In Nelson K, Van Kleeck A (Eds) Children's Language, Volume 6. Hillsdale, NJ: Erlbaum.

Nelson N (1993) Language intervention in school settings. In Bernstein D, Tiegerman E (Eds), Language and Communication Disorders in Children (3rd ed). Columbus, OH: Merrill.

Nelson L, Kamhi A, Apel K (1987) Cognitive strengths and weaknesses in language-impaired children: One more look. Journal of Speech and Hearing Disorders 52: 36–43.

Norris J, Hoffman P (1993) Whole Language Intervention for School-Age Children. San Diego, CA: Singular Publishing Group.

Owens R (1993) Mental retardation: Difference or delay. In Bernstein D, Tiegerman E (Eds), Language and Communication Disorders in Children (3rd ed). Columbus, OH: Merrill.

Prizant B (1982) Speech-language pathologists and autistic children: What is our role? Part I. ASHA 24: 463–8.

Prizant B, Duchan J (1981) The functions of immediate echolalia in autistic children. Journal of Speech and Hearing Disorders 46: 241–9.

Prizant B, Rydell P (1984) Analysis of functions of delayed echolalia in autistic children. Journal of Speech and Hearing Research 27: 183–92.

Ratokalau N, Robb M (1993) Early communication assessment and intervention: An interactive process. In Bernstein D, Tiegerman E (Eds), Language and Communication Disorders in Children. New York: Merrill.

Reed V (1994) An Introduction to Children with Language Disorders (2nd ed). New York: Macmillan.

Rees N (1983) Language intervention with children. In Miller J, Yoder D, Schiefelbusch R (Eds) Contemporary Issues in Language Intervention. ASHA Reports #12. Rockville, MD: ASHA.

Retherford K (1993) Assessing Children's Language in Natural Contexts (3rd ed). Englewood Cliffs, NJ: Prentice-Hall.

Roth F, Clark D (1987) Symbolic play and social participation abilities of language-impaired and normally developing children. Journal of Speech and Hearing Research 52: 17–29.

Russell N (1993) Educational considerations in traumatic brain injury: The role of the speech language pathologist. LSHSS 24: 67–76.

Sameroff A (1975) Early influences on development: Fact or fancy? Merrill-Palmer Quarterly 21: 267–94.

Satz P, Bullard-Bates C (1981) Acquired aphasia in children. In Sarno MT (Ed) Acquired Aphasia. New York: Academic Press.

Savich P (1984) Anticipatory imagery ability in normal and language-disabled children. Journal of Speech and Hearing Research 27: 494–502.

Schery T, Lipsey M (1983) Program evaluation for speech and hearing services, In Miller J, Yoder D, Schiefelbusch R (Eds) Contemporary Issues in Language Intervention. ASHA Reports #12. Rockville, MD: ASHA.

Schuele CM, van Kleeck A (1987) Precursors to literacy : Assessment and intervention. Topics in Language Disorders 7: 32–44.

Shane H (1993) The dark side of facilitated communication. Topics in Language Disorders 13: ix–xiv.

Siegel G (1987) The limits of science in communication disorders. Journal of Speech and Hearing Disorders 52: 306–13.

Siegel G, Broen P (1976) Language assessment. In Lloyd L (Ed) Communication, Assessment and Intervention Strategies. Baltimore, MD: University Park Press.

Sininger Y, Klatzky R, Kirchner D (1989) Memory scanning speed in language disordered children. Journal of Speech and Hearing Research 32: 289–306.

Stanovich K (1988) Explaining the differences between the dyslexic and the garden-variety poor reader: The phonological-core variable-difference model. Journal of Learning Disabilities 21: 590–612.

Stoel-Gammon C, Dunn C (1985) Normal and Disordered Phonology in Children. Austin, TX: Pro-Ed.

Stremel K, Waryas C (1974) A behavioral-psycholinguistic approach to language training. In McReynolds L (Ed) Developing Systematic Procedures for Training Children's Language. ASHA Monographs, No. 18. Rockville, MD: ASHA.

Tager-Flusberg H, Calkins S (1990) Does imitation facilitate the acquisition of grammar? Evidence from a study of autistic, Down's syndrome and normal children. Journal of Child Language 17: 591–606.

Tallal P (1988) Developmental language disorders. In Kavanagh J, Truss T Jr (Eds) Learning Disabilities: Proceedings of the National Conference. Parkton, MD: York Press.

Terrell B, Schwartz R, Prelock P (1984) Symbolic play in normal and language-impaired children. Journal of Speech and Hearing Research 27: 424–30.

Tiegerman E (1993) Autism. In Bernstein D, Tiegerman E (Eds), Language and Communication Disorders in Children (3rd ed). Columbus, OH: Merrill.

Vygotsky L (1962) Thought and Language. Cambridge, MA: The MIT Press.

Wallach G, Butler K (1994) Language Learning Disabilities in School-Age Children and Adolescents. New York: Merrill.

Wilcox MJ, Kouri T, Caswell S (1991) A comparison of classroom and individual treatment. Language, Speech and Hearing Services in Schools 1: 49–62.

Chapter 6
Childhood Phonological Disorders

JENNIFER LAMBERT AND DAPHNE WATERS

The terms phonological delay and disorder are generally applied to children who, in the absence of known pathology, do not acquire intelligible speech patterns within the usual time scale. The child's main presenting problem is in learning to use speech sounds and sound combinations to signal meaning contrasts between words. Intervention targeting the development of such contrasts is seen as the child's primary therapy need. Such children form a large proportion of the case loads of most community-based speech and language therapists.

In the past 20 to 30 years a great deal of progress has taken place in the provision of assessment and therapy for developmental speech disorders, but there still much to learn. This chapter examines current views on the nature of phonological disability and provides an overview of the principles and techniques of assessment and intervention. There is considerable emphasis on the possible underlying nature and causations of phonological disorder since awareness of these issues is seen as fundamental to the development of well-founded assessment and intervention.

Terminology

The terminology applied to this group of children has undergone several changes in the recent past which have reflected both change in views about the underlying nature of the problem and change in the prevailing model on which the classification of children's speech and language disorders is based. In the UK, before about 1970, children's speech and language disorders were classified according to a medical model and terms reflected supposed underlying aetiology (see Bishop and Rosenbloom, 1987). The terms most commonly used to refer to speech disordered and delayed children were 'dyslalia' (Morley, 1965) and 'articulatory defect'. These terms reflected the view that the disability was centred on the most peripheral level of spoken language encoding – the level of articulator movement. In the USA the term 'functional articulation disorder' was widely used (Powers, 1971; Shelton and McReynolds, 1979). The term 'functional' acknowledged the lack of any known structural or organic cause for the disorder. Nevertheless, in the USA, as well as in the UK, traditional therapy approaches assumed an articulatory basis for the disorder (Grunwell, 1981).

From the late 1960s the influence of linguistic theory and description led to a shift away from an articulation-centred view and towards a view of the disorder as originating at more central levels of processing (see, for example; Beresford and Grady, 1968; Ingram, 1976; Grunwell, 1975, 1981). Terminology derived from a medical model of classification became supplemented by terms derived from a linguistic model and the terms 'phonological delay', 'phonological disorder', and 'phonological disability' came into common usage. The generally accepted understanding of these terms is given by Grunwell:

> A speech disability at the phonological level involves an abnormal, or inadequate or disorganized system of sound patterns evidenced by deviations in the spoken language. ...the disability is a neurolinguistic dysfunction at the phonological level of cortical representation and organization of the language system. (Grunwell, 1987: 272)

The linguistic model is concerned with classification based on 'description of linguistic "output" behaviour at different levels of analysis, i.e. phonetic, phonological, syntactic, semantic, pragmatic' (Stackhouse and Wells, 1993: 332). However the term 'phonological disability' has become absorbed into a classification system based on a medical model and is often used as though it had diagnostic and /or aetiological significance rather than in the sense of describing the linguistic level at which a child's underlying difficulties are manifest to a listener.

More recently, cognitive neuropsychological and psycholinguistic models, which view a child's speech problems in terms of breakdowns in aspects of input processing, output processing and internal representation, have begun to influence terminology and understanding of the nature of developmental speech disorders (Ellis and Young, 1988; Stackhouse and Wells, 1993). This is discussed in more detail below.

Characteristics of Normally Developing Speech

The pronunciation patterns of normally-developing young children are commonly described in terms of 'simplifying phonological processes'. Examples of such processes are 'stopping' in which target fricatives and/or affricates are pronounced as stops ('sea' → [ti] and 'jam' → [dam]); 'consonant cluster reduction' in which initial clusters are realized as single consonants ('spoon' → [pun] and 'glove' → [gʌv]). These simplifications are classified into two broad groups according to whether they reduce the system of sound contrasts or simplify syllable or word structure. For definitions and examples of these simplifying phonological processes see Ingram (1976); Grunwell (1985, 1987) and Hawkins (1984). Grunwell (1985) includes a development chart which gives the estimated order and age of suppression (elimination) of simplifying phonological processes, as well as stages in the expansion of the phonetic inventory in normal development. Description of children's speech characteristics in terms of simplifying processes has proved very useful, not least in the clinical context.

Stampe (1969, 1979) in his *Theory of Natural Phonology* asserted that these simplifying phonological processes reflect natural, universal and innate developmental tendencies and that children gradually learn to suppress these innate processes or 'rules' in order to achieve an ever closer match with the system of speech sound contrasts which operates in their native language. The presumed 'motivation' for the occurrence of these simplifying rules is that they allow children to attempt to reproduce the adult forms they hear within the limitations of their immature articulatory (speech motor) capacities. It is assumed in such a view that young children perceive words in terms of adult surface forms. There has been much debate about the status of simplifying phonological processes: do they reflect mental operations carried out by a child or are they simply a convenient descriptive device for classifying speech output errors in relation to the adult target system?

More recently, non-linear phonological theoretical frameworks have been used as a basis for the description of developing child speech (see, for example, Spencer, 1984; Bernhardt, 1992a). Some clinical implications of this theoretical perspective are highlighted below.

Characteristics of Phonologically-Disordered Child Speech

Typically the pronunciation patterns of children with phonological disorder are characterized by limitations on the number of different speech sounds used (restricted phonetic inventory); limitations on the range of feature combinations which specify these segments; and phonotactic restrictions that limit the range of syllable structure types in the child's output in comparison with normally-developing children of similar age (Grunwell, 1987). As a result of these limitations the child often fails to signal meaning effectively to a listener. When these pronunciation patterns are compared with those of younger, normally-developing children, many similarities are apparent in terms of phonetic inventories, phonotactic constraints and occurrence of simplifying phonological processes (Ingram, 1980; Schwartz et al., 1980; Hodson and Paden, 1981).

As we stated in the previous section, non-linear analytical frameworks are now beginning to be applied to the clinical analysis of disordered phonologies (Bernhardt, 1992b). These frameworks emphasize multi-tiered, hierarchical representation of phonological form which encompasses prosodic (syllabic) information as well as segmental information. Such theories suggest that children come to the language-learning situation with a 'representational framework' or 'set of universal templates' which are used in both decoding and encoding of speech (Menn, 1978; Bernhardt, 1992a). They lead to descriptions of disordered speech development in terms such as restrictions on the number of 'phoneme slots' per syllable and restrictions on the 'content' of onset and rhyme elements within a syllable (Bernhardt and Gilbert, 1992). An alternative syllable theory (*mora theory*) focuses on the notion of 'weight units' within a syllable and on this basis disordered child speech might be characterized in terms of restrictions on the number of weight units (or moras) allowed per syllable, or on the types of phonemes which constitute these weight units (Bernhardt, 1993).

A cross-study survey by Stoel-Gammon and Dunn (1985) uses phonological process analysis to draw together the findings from eight studies which employ a variety of analysis methods. The eight studies, which include both UK and US data, involve a total of 128 phonologically-disordered, English-speaking children between the ages of 3 and 13 years. Nine structural and systemic simplifying phonological processes are identified as having frequent and widespread occurrence across the subjects. These nine processes are: consonant cluster reduction; final consonant deletion; unstressed syllable deletion; stopping of fricatives and affricates; fronting of velar consonants; fronting of palatal consonants; liquid simplification; assimilation; and voicing.

Of these, stopping and liquid simplification have the most consistent occurrence across all subjects. The findings of this cross-study survey are very similar to the findings in two further studies involving Scottish children of pre-school and first year primary school ages (Moss, 1985; Howell, 1989). These nine most commonly occurring processes in the 'disordered' data are all processes which also occur commonly in normal phonological acquisition. However, in addition to these, Stoel-Gammon and Dunn's cross-study data included several other processes which are not commonly found in normally-developing speech and they found a great deal of intersubject variability in the type and frequency of occurrence of particular processes. Such 'non-developmental' features are often referred to as idiosyncratic processes. Examples of processes so labelled are:

* initial consonant deletion in CV syllables;
* replacement of consonants by a glottal stop;
* backing of anterior plosives to velar place of articulation;

- replacement of stops by fricatives;
- atypical reduction of consonant clusters;
- widespread distribution of a 'preferred' or 'favourite' sound.

The labelling of a phonological process as idiosyncratic or as abnormal can only be tentative, since the normal developmental data available are limited, and there is some evidence that these less common processes may in fact occur in normal development but tend to be of very brief duration (Shriberg *et al.*, 1986). However, the notion that two categories of 'normal developmental' and 'abnormal' simplifying phonological processes can be identified is often used as the basis for postulating two categories of phonological disability, 'delayed' and 'disordered/deviant' (Ingram, 1976), and this dichotomy is sometimes suggested as a basis for deciding whether a child requires treatment. Grunwell (1993) lists the characteristics of disordered phonological development as:

1. the persistence of normal processes significantly beyond the usual age of suppression;
2. chronological mismatch in the occurrence of processes, that is, the co-occurrence of processes which are normally eliminated early, for example velar fronting, alongside pronunciation patterns characteristic of much later stages of development, for example the use of consonant clusters;
3. the occurrence of unusual or idiosyncratic processes;
4. systematic sound preference where one type of consonant is used for a large range of target consonants;
5. variable use of processes, where two or more simplifying processes are variably applied to the same target sound.

Research on the speech characteristics of phonological disorder has focused mainly on the consonant system (Stoel-Gammon, 1991). However, both Ingram (1976) and Grunwell (1987) recognize that children with phonological disorders sometimes show vowel system anomalies which are not found in normal development. Reynolds (1990) reports a study of 20 children who were undergoing therapy for phonological disorder. He identifies three groups of vowel system anomalies:

1. Context-free processes
- lowering of the vowels /ɛ, ɛː, ɛɪ/, resulting in neutralizations between pairs of words like 'bad'/'bed';
- fronting of low back vowels (e.g./ɒ/ → [a]);
- diphthong reduction;
- late acquisition of the stressed vowel /ɜ/, in words such as 'girl' and 'purse'.

2. Context-sensitive processes
- lowering or backing of vowels which precede a lateral, as in words such as 'milk', 'hill';

- a tendency for vowels to be more open than usual in the context of a following nasal segment.

3. **Idiosyncratic processes**
   several specific examples are given and Reynolds also includes examples from his data of idiosyncratic vowel neutralizations persisting in children as old as 10 years whose other phonological difficulties have resolved.

Other Linguistic Characteristics of Phonologically-Disordered Children

The results of studies which have investigated other linguistic abilities in phonologically-disordered children such as comprehension vocabulary, sentence comprehension, the use of specific syntactic structures and mean length of utterance, have produced varied results. Overall, there is some indication that some, but not all, phonologically-delayed children do have difficulties with other levels of language. For reviews of such studies see Stoel-Gammon and Dunn (1985); Aram and Kamhi (1982) and Grunwell (1987). Stoel-Gammon and Dunn state that such studies have indicated that 'syntactic deficits co-occurred with phonological problems more frequently than deficits in other linguistic skills' (p. 126). Rapin and Allen (1983) emphasize this link and use the term 'phonologic-syntactic' to designate disordered acquisition of language form as distinct from language meaning and use (semantic-pragmatic disorder). Stoel-Gammon and Dunn suggest the 'some children possibly have difficulty mastering "expressive linguistic form" which might include the form of reading and writing, as well as phonology, morphology and syntax' (p. 126). The issue of relationship between phonological disorder and literacy is discussed briefly below.

A study reported by Bishop and Edmundson (1987) indicates that children whose *only* problems are with phonological acquisition have a much better likelihood of a 'good outcome' than those who have additional grammatical impairments.

Underlying Nature and Causation of Developmental Phonological Disorder and Relationship with Other Disorders

The descriptions of the speech characteristics of phonologically-disordered children given above are derived from perceptually based analyses of speech output. In this section we examine other sources of information and evidence which contribute to our understanding of the underlying nature of phonological disorder. Such sources include evidence from instrumental acoustic measurements of speech output and from psycholinguistic investigations using tasks which tap discrete aspects of speech processing. We have chosen to focus on issues and evidence which, on the basis of clinical experience, we regard as particularly relevant for the development of well founded assessment and intervention procedures.

The acquisition of intelligible speech patterns must involve the successful integration of many aspects of maturation and learning, including development of perceptual abilities, development of neuromotor co-ordination and control for speech, and various aspects of cognitive and linguistic development. When a child fails to develop intelligible speech patterns in the usual way, or at the usual time, any one or any combination of these underlying developmental factors may be implicated. Therefore, children who present with phonological level difficulties are unlikely to constitute a homogeneous group. The classification 'phonologically disordered' must include children with a wide variety of speech processing deficits which underlie their presenting speech output characteristics. We explore some of these issues in this section.

In the latter parts of the section we discuss briefly the relationship between phonological disorder and developmental verbal dyspraxia and refer to the relationship between phonological disorder and literacy acquisition and to phonological problems in the context of various known primary deficits such as cleft palate and hearing impairment.

Speech motor abilities of phonologically-disordered children (instrumental investigations)

Since speech is a motor as well as a linguistic activity, one of the prerequisites for the emergence of adult-like speech patterns must be adequate maturation and functioning of the underlying neuromotor mechanisms upon which speech depends (Hardcastle, 1976). There is much evidence that speech motor control abilities in normal children develop slowly throughout childhood and may not be fully adult-like even as late as 12 years of age (See, for example; Eguchi and Hirsch, 1969; DiSimoni, 1974; Tingley and Allan, 1975; Kent and Forner, 1980. For reviews of these and other related studies see Hewlett, 1990 and Waters, 1992). In common with all other aspects of motor development, there must be individual differences amongst children in the rate at which these speech motor control abilities mature during the speech acquisition period and therefore it is possible that one reason for difficulty in speech acquisition might be delayed or deviant development of speech neuromotor abilities.

Until about 1970 there was a tacit assumption that children's developmental speech disorders had an articulatory/motor co-ordination and control basis and many researchers therefore investigated whether these children might have more widespread motor co-ordination deficits; that is, might have 'less than average precision, speed, strength and control of movement' (Powers, 1971: 733).

Investigators have looked at a wide variety of general motor tasks, especially tasks requiring repeated rapid and/or rhythmical actions, non-speech oral motor tasks, and various diadochokinetic tasks (DDK). For a review of studies up to the 1980s see Bernthal and Bankson (1981). The results of these studies were inconclusive but left open the possibility that differences in performance on co-ordinated, rhythmic motor tasks, particularly oral motor tasks, may exist between normal individuals and those with speech sound difficulties. Interest in the performance of children with speech disorders on rhythmic and DDK tasks has continued (see, for example; McNutt, 1977; Shields, 1981; Henry, 1990). However, the disordered subjects in these studies often have either very severe speech disorders or more widespread language learning problems and it is difficult to relate findings to the group of children labelled as phonologically disordered. A study by Bradford and Dodd (1994) has suggested that a subgroup of phonologically-disordered children, who exhibit inconsistent speech errors, perform poorly on a complex, timed, non-oral, motor-planning task as compared with both other phonologically-disordered children and normal controls.

In the last 20 years or so a number of investigations have used instrumental acoustic measurement techniques to compare speech motor control abilities in normal children and children with speech and language disorders (e.g. Stark and Tallal, 1979; Weismer and Elbert, 1982; Catts and Jensen, 1983; Waters, 1992). These have focused on durational measures, temporal variability and speech rate as indices of level of speech motor control development. Other studies have examined compensatory speech abilities in normal and phonologically disordered children in fixed-jaw (i.e. bite-block) conditions, as a means of comparing maturity of speech motor control (Edwards, 1991). The methodologies and subjects involved in these studies are very varied and it is difficult to draw overall conclusions. However, the weight of evidence seems to point to the likelihood that at least some phonologically-disordered children have poorer speech motor control abilities than their normally-developing peers.

A further group of studies uses instrumental acoustic measurement techniques to examine particular phonological contrasts in the speech of children with phonological disabilities. Instrumental investigations using, for example, electropalatographic (EPG) techniques (Hardcastle, 1984) have shown that, although contrasts may be heard as neutralized, a child may, in fact, be producing a contrast which is not perceptually salient to a listener. Gibbon (1990) used EPG with a phonologically-disordered child who consistently exhibited a 'process' of 'alveolar backing'. The EPG data showed that there was consistently more tongue palate contact for alveolar targets than for velar targets, suggesting that the child was attempting to signal a contrast. Gibbon concluded that the child had specific problems in timing the release of stops. This and other similar investigations demonstrate that, in some instances at least, a speech motor (phonetic level) constraint underlies a child's apparent failure to signal a phonological contrast.

Psycholinguistic profiles of phonologically-disordered children

Cognitive neuropsychological models have been widely applied in the field of adult acquired language disorders, but are only now becoming applied to developmental disorders. The assumptions underlying such models are that language is mediated by an internal information processing system which is modular and consists of discrete subsystems, each responsible for particular processing tasks. The basic framework for such models distinguishes three levels of processing, *input processing*, *internal representations* and *output processing*, each of which include sub-levels of processing. It must be stressed that, to date, most of these models address only single-word processing. A model given by Ellis and Young (1988) is hierarchically organized and conceptualized as 'box and arrow' diagrams and explicitly links phonological processing to the semantic system. A model suggested by Hewlett (1990) focuses on speech production (output) processing. Stackhouse and Wells (1993) suggest a framework which is organized as a series of questions focused on discrete speech processing abilities. The application of such models to the field of developmental speech disorders highlights the diversity of deficits which may underlie children's presenting speech patterns; that is, children with similar speech output characteristics may have very different profiles of deficits and strengths within the speech processing chain.

Metalinguistic abilities of phonologically-disordered children

Metalinguistic abilities are those which involve thinking about and reflecting upon the nature (form) and functions of language, rather than only understanding its meaning (Pratt and Grieve, 1984). Metalinguistic abilities are manifested in a variety of ways. Monitoring the effectiveness of utterances as we speak and making spontaneous speech repairs involves aspects of linguistic and communicative awareness. Young children's spontaneous play with speech sounds and rhyming words and their deliberate practice of sounds and words (Weir, 1962; Cazden, 1983) provide evidence for the very early development of some implicit aspects of metalinguistic ability. Other, more explicit aspects include ability to reflect on the structure of an utterance and make judgements about its semantic or syntactic acceptability or to perform operations on it such as segmentation into word units, syllable units or speech segments. Phonemic synthesis (sound blending) and the abilities to recognize and generate rhymes are skills dependent upon linguistic (phonological) awareness.

Theories of speech acquisition which regard children as 'active discoverers' and 'hypothesis testers' in the learning process (Menn, 1976; Kiparsky and Menn, 1977; Macken and Ferguson, 1983) support the view that linguistic awareness at various levels is implicated in normal acquisition (Howell and Dean, 1994).

The large body of research which has investigated the development of metalinguistic abilities in general, and metaphonological abilities in particular, in normally developing children is reviewed by Howell and Dean (1994), Garton and Pratt (1989), Gombert (1992) and Magnusson (1991). Magnusson reviews studies which compare linguistic awareness in speech-disordered and normally-developing children. These studies have examined word awareness (e.g. Kamhi, Lee and Nelson, 1985), syllable and morpheme awareness (e.g. Fox and Routh, 1975), and various aspects of phonological awareness, including awareness of rhyme (e.g. Magnusson, 1983). Magnusson (1991) concludes that, 'in all comparisons, the phonologically-disordered children managed the metalinguistic tasks less well than the normal children' (p. 106). Bird and Bishop (1992) investigated auditory discrimination for speech and metaphonological abilities (rhyme and alliteration judgement tasks) in 14 phonologically-disordered children aged between 5;0 years and 6;3 years, and 14 normally speaking controls. The phonologically-disordered group had significantly poorer performance on the metaphonological tasks. The extent of the difference could not be explained by differences between the groups on the auditory discrimination tasks and the authors interpret the results as suggesting that the phonologically-disordered children had not progressed to the stage of analysing words at the level of the phoneme. These studies and conclusions, however, relate to group comparisons. Individual results do not always conform to this group trend. It is common to find individual children with apparently normal speech and language abilities who perform very poorly on metalinguistic tasks; conversely some speech-disordered children perform well on such tasks (see, for example, Howell, 1989).

There certainly does not seem to be any straightforward causative relationship between level of metalinguistic ability and phonological disorder. It seems likely that there is a complex inter-relationship amongst speech output characteristics, phonological and communicative awareness and internal representation of phonological form. The great interest in recent years in metalinguistic abilities has led to the development of therapy procedures which utilize and aim to develop these abilities in therapy as a means of stimulating change in phonological knowledge and output.

Relationship between phonological disorder and the acquisition of literacy

The question of whether phonological acquisition difficulties in the pre-school years are predictive of later reading and spelling problems is of great interest to therapists and educationalists. A prospective, longitudinal study by Bishop and Adams (1990) indicated that children who had difficulties *only* with acquisition of the speech sound system, and who were normal with respect to other aspects of language acquisition, and whose phonological problems were substantially resolved by the age of 5;06 years, were no more likely than 'normal' children to encounter literacy problems. Children in the study who had more widespread language learning difficulties were more likely to present with literacy problems (at age 8 years) than either 'normal' children or children with isolated phonological problems. A retrospective study by Lewis and Freebairn (1992) tended to support this finding. However, the possibility remains that more persistent developmental phonological difficulties which extend into the primary school years do have implications for reading and spelling development (Dodd and Cockerill, 1985). There is certainly evidence that some children with severe and persisting intelligibility problems also have severe written language decoding and spelling problems (see, for example, Stackhouse and Wells, 1991).

Many studies have shown that metalinguistic (and particularly metaphonological) abilities are influenced by and have an influence on learning to read and spell (Lundberg, 1978; Tunmer and Nesdale, 1985; Goswami, 1990; Magnusson and Naucler, 1990; Stackhouse, 1990). It may be that an underlying factor in children's written language difficulties relates to poorly developed awareness (knowledge of) phonological form, and that an additional common factor relating to phonological memory may underlie presenting difficulties in speech, phonological awareness and written language.

Relationship between phonological disorder and developmental verbal dyspraxia

The controversy which surrounds the definition of, and terminology relating to, developmental dyspraxia is discussed by Hall (Chapter 7). Hall uses the term 'developmental apraxia of speech' (DAS) and describes the condition as a 'disruption in the motor programming needed for speech production'.

Crary (1993: 51) emphasizes that 'Meaningful speech is a motor phenomenon that is dependent on linguistic input', and proposes a 'motorlinguistic' model of developmental speech disorders based on a continuum of speech motor and language functions. He argues that it is likely that different speech-disordered children have learned 'abnormal' phonological patterns from many different influences: for example, 'some children may demonstrate deviant lexical retrieval and/or phoneme selection processes, others may select the proper phonemes but sequence them inappropriately prior to coding the linguistic message into motor speech specifications...' (Crary, p. 72). Studies by Stackhouse and Snowling (1992) and by Marion, Sussman and Marquardt (1993) indicate that children with developmental dyspraxia may have a variety of speech-processing deficits relating to auditory processing, lexical development and rhyming skills, as well as problems with speech motor programming and co-ordination. Such investigations tend to support a view which designates phonological disorders and developmental dyspraxia of speech in terms of profiles on a continuum of motor execution, motor planning and linguistic aspects of speech processing, rather than as discrete disorders with different aetiologies.

Phonological disability in the context of various primary deficits

Whilst the term phonological disorder is generally applied to children whose speech difficulties are *not* linked to any known pathology, other children experience phonological acquisition difficulties which can be explicitly linked with an identifiable primary deficit. For example, children with hearing impairments (Parker and Rose, 1990); children with cerebral palsy and children with cleft palates (Albery and Russell, 1990; Hewlett, 1990; Sell, Harding and Grunwell, 1994). It is beyond the scope of this chapter to discuss the consequences of these disorders for phonological acquisition, but many of the assessment and intervention strategies discussed in this chapter, with adaptations to meet particular needs, are likely to be relevant to these client groups (see Chapters 7 and 10).

Assessment

The assessment process is informed by the issues discussed above. Assessment procedures enable a clinician to describe a child's pronunciation patterns and to test hypotheses about possible reasons for the child's difficulties. Thorough assessment is, therefore, fundamental to making informed decisions about therapy provision. It is also essential if the child's progress and the effectiveness of therapy are to be objectively evaluated. The assessment process is equally important for the child who is 'kept under review' in order to evaluate developmental progress and for the child who is taken into a therapy programme.

Assessment will include perceptually based, linguistic analysis of speech data (see below) and also investigations of aspects of input, internal and output processing (see below). Information about the child's developmental history will also be sought, with particular attention paid to hearing; oral-motor development, including feeding; pre-speech vocalization (babbling) and to any family history of developmental speech problems/other primary or secondary language difficulties. Often a vocal tract examination will be carried out (Newman, Creaghead and Secord, 1985; Grunwell, 1993). Questioning a parent or carer as to who is able to understand the child can often be revealing. Discussion with a parent about how the child responds to requests for clarification can give insight into the child's awareness of his communicative effectiveness and can give valuable clues as to how to proceed in therapy.

An evaluation of the child's general cognitive abilities and learning 'style' is also of importance and the outcome of such an evaluation is likely to have considerable influence on the way therapy is delivered. It is also necessary to assess whether a child's difficulties are confined to the level of the speech sound system or whether other aspects of language functioning are affected. This will have implications for clinical management of the child and for prognosis. For a school-age child, this evaluation will include information about literacy development; if necessary, liaising with school learning support staff to assess reading and spelling problems in relation to spoken-language difficulties.

Not all these assessments will take place before beginning therapy. Some will be carried out in the context of 'investigative' or 'diagnostic' therapy sessions.

Assessment based on linguistic analysis of speech data

Linguistic analysis procedures form an essential component of assessment. They tell the clinician what a child needs to learn during therapy. That is, they reveal, from a listener's perspective, what changes need to take place in the child's speech patterns in order to increase intelligibility. Such analysis will enable the therapist to decide which particular aspects of a child's speech sound system will become the focus of therapy and will suggest an order of priority in which these various aspects should be targeted.

The choice of a speech sample for linguistic analysis involves several issues: whether it should be a spontaneous or elicited sample, whether it should be a single-word or connected speech sample and the size of the sample. Most published clinical analysis procedures for phonological disorder are based on a mainly single-word sample, usually elicited through the naming of pictures and objects. There is always the danger that the forms a child produces in this 'confrontation naming' situation are not representative of forms in more spontaneous speech; but the difficulties of working with spontaneous speech samples are enormous, especially when dealing with highly unintelligible children. Grunwell (1985) suggests that a single-word sample should include approximately 200–250 items. This large sample is required to ensure a true representation of the child's pronunciation patterns by sampling all target speech sounds and sound combinations in a variety of contexts. It is always desirable to collect multiple tokens of at least some of the words in a sample in order to assess variability. For extensive discussion of these issues, see Grunwell (1985) and Stoel-Gammon and Dunn (1985). In most clinical contexts time constraints dictate that a much smaller data sample is used.

Several published analysis procedures are available which include picture materials for eliciting a speech sample and analysis forms and/or score sheets. Whichever procedure is used, it is essential, at the time of data collection, to make an orthographic 'gloss' and phonetic transcription of all utterances as far as possible. An audio tape recording should always be made against which these 'live' transcriptions can be checked. These published procedures fall broadly into two categories. The first group employs a 'sound by sound' error analysis approach. Some procedures in this group yield a standard score or 'articulation age' score. The group includes the 'Goldman–Fristoe test of articulation' (Goldman and Fristoe, 1972); the Fisher–Logemann test of articulation (Fisher and Logemann, 1971) and the Edinburgh Articulation Test (EAT – Anthony *et al.*, 1971). The EAT is still in widespread use in the UK. It is essentially a test of articulation attainment, based on an error analysis of a single word data set of 41 items, with optional, additional 'qualitative' analysis. It has been standardized on a large group of (Scottish) children and therefore a child's performance on the assessment can be evaluated in comparison with other children of the same age. This is valuable information when deciding whether therapy is required.

Assessment procedures in the second group focus on various forms of phonological analysis (especially phonological process analysis) of a child's speech data. These procedures aim to analyse a child's pronunciation patterns in order to make informed decisions about the precise goals of therapy. Examples of such procedures are the Newcastle Speech Assessment (Beresford, 1986); Phonological Process Analysis (Weiner, 1979); Procedures for the Phonological Analysis of Children's Language (Hodson, 1980); The Metaphon Resource Pack (Dean et al., 1990), and Phonological Assessment of Child Speech (PACS – Grunwell, 1985). PACS is the most comprehensive of these procedures and includes several complementary approaches to analysing a child's data: 'independent analyses' which analyse the child's speech patterns without reference to adult target forms (phonetic inventory, phonetic distribution analysis, analysis of syllable types occurring in the child's output) and 'relational analyses' which compare a child's pronunciations with adult target forms (phonological process analysis, contrastive analysis). It is likely that in the near future additional analysis procedures will become available to clinical practice, based on non-linear analytical frameworks (Shriberg, 1991; Bernhardt 1992b).

The therapist is thus able to make a choice from a wide and increasing variety of procedures by which speech data can be analysed. Different kinds of procedures provide different types of information and therefore fulfil different clinical purposes. Therapy decisions are likely to be influenced by the nature of the analysis which has been carried out and the consequent information which is available about a child's pronunciation patterns. For example an 'error analysis' approach, used in isolation, is likely to lead to a sound-by-sound articulation-training approach to therapy, since that form of analysis reveals very little about 'rules' and constraints that are determining the child's pronunciation patterns. A phonological process analysis will lead to therapy aims expressed in terms of the elimination of particular simplifying phonological processes and this will influence the way therapy is organized (see, for example, Dean et al., 1990). Where non-linear analysis procedures are used, the aims of therapy are likely to be expressed in such terms as 'extending the number and range of segments allowed in the sub-syllabic units of onset and rhyme'.

Most of the procedures mentioned above are concerned almost exclusively with the consonantal system. As pointed out above, phonologically-disordered children may also have deviant vowel systems and it is important that this is borne in mind during assessment. Vowel deviations tend to be very noticeable /salient to the listener and it is unlikely that they will be missed by a vigilant clinician. When particular vowel abnormalities are identified (with reference, of course, to the child's own accent community, not the clinician's), the therapist can then assemble a set of objects or pictures to elicit further items containing the relevant target vowels to allow more systematic evaluation of the problem to be made.

Evaluation of the results of phonetic and phonological analysis, including results of standardized assessment, and considered in relation to results of other aspects of assessment, enables the clinician to make management decisions. *Whether* or not therapy is indicated will be decided on the basis of evaluating the child's speech patterns in relation to developmental expectations. *What* to target in therapy, and in what order, will be decided by evaluating the functional/communicative consequences of various aspects of the child's pronunciation patterns (contrastive analysis; percentage occurrence of each identified simplifying phonological process and degree of variability), and also by considering the current phonetic repertoire of sounds and sound combinations occurring in the child's output.

Psycholinguistic assessment procedures

The aim of such procedures is to reveal specific weaknesses in discrete aspects of speech processing which might be focused on in therapy and, also, areas of strength which might be capitalized upon in therapy. In a sense this form of assessment is not new. In spite of the emphasis on linguistic description as the essential aspect of assessment for phonological disorder, clinicians have continued to carry out other kinds of investigation. In particular, auditory discrimination ability is routinely investigated, as is imitative ability for speech sounds, syllables and words. The application of cognitive neuropsychological/psycholinguistic theory to developmental speech disorders is leading to formalization and extension of these clinical practices. Using a model of single-word processing such as that given by Ellis and Young (1988), assessment tasks can be developed which 'tap' discrete aspects of input and output processing and internal phonological representations, in isolation from other aspects of the speech processing chain. For example, a task involving segmentation, analysis and same/different judgement of non-words could be designed to tap a child's auditory analysis system in isolation from the influence of the semantic system. Investigation of underlying phonological representations might involve asking a child to make 'internal phonological judgements' without reference to their own output and without relying on auditorily presented input. Such a task could be designed around pictures and require the child to say whether two pictured objects start with the same sound (Lewis and Bryan, 1994; Stackhouse and Wells, 1993).

An example of the use of psycholinguistic investigation with a 5-year-old boy, who presented with very deviant phonological production, is reported by Bryan and Howard (1992). The child's output forms were compared under three different conditions: (1) confrontation naming, (2) imitation of real words, (3) imitation of non-words. His performance on (3) was significantly superior to either of the other conditions. Bryan and Howard interpreted this as evidence of a lexical level deficit rather than a lower level output difficulty. They concluded that the child had failed to update his underlying output representations in line with his production capabilities. On the basis of this investigation, therapy goals were targeted explicitly towards increasing the child's awareness and knowledge of the phonological forms of words and towards increasing his ability to analyse and 'manipulate' input and output representations.

Investigation of aspects of output processing might include: specific evaluation of speech motor abilities using DDK rate measures; instrumental investigations of speech rate and temporal variability; and EPG investigation of tongue/palate contact patterns. Such instrumental procedures are not widely available in clinical practice, but are becoming increasingly accessible. Currently, their usefulness is limited by the lack of normative data available for these various measures.

Intervention

Therapy must be based on detailed assessment so that it can be tailored to the needs of the individual child. We have seen that informed interpretation of assessment procedures involving formal, standardized tests and linguistic analysis of speech data tell the clinician whether therapy is indicated; can provide information about what changes in speech output the child needs to achieve; and can suggest priorities for targeting various aspects of a child's speech patterns. Investigation of aspects of speech-processing abilities provides additional information about why a child might present with particular speech patterns and contributes further to the provision of precisely focused intervention. However, although the information obtained from such assessments and investigations is essential to the provision of effective therapy, it is not sufficient. We also need to consider how the child will learn in therapy. That is, what kinds of learning opportunities the clinician will provide for the child and what role the child will be encouraged to play in therapy. The answer to these questions will relate to the particular theoretical view of phonological development which is adopted. For example, behaviourist views of language development will tend to lead to therapy strategies which model target speech patterns and 'shape' the child's responses using reinforcement techniques. This kind of therapy implies a passive role for the child and must specifically target carryover into communicative contexts. In contrast, cognitive and interactionist discovery views of language learning (Menn, 1976; Kiparsky and Menn, 1977; Macken and Ferguson, 1983) will tend to lead to therapy strategies which involve children as active learners who are encouraged to make their own discoveries about language. The therapist also needs to consider individual differences in learning 'style' and creativity and capacity for reflection and independent 'exploration' and discovery. Some children may require and make effective use of opportunities for repeated practice with supportive feedback, while others will learn most effectively through 'talking' and opportunities for discovery.

Howell and McCartney (1990) list five general principles of intervention based on acceptance of a cognitive, interactionist discovery view of language learning. These can be summarized as follows:

1. the therapeutic emphasis should be on learning rather than on teaching, implying equal participation by child and therapist and a shared process of discovery;
2. the child should be encouraged to be an active learner, rather than a passive recipient of information;
3. opportunities should be provided for children to gain knowledge of the phonological system of the adult language and to develop awareness of how their own speech patterns differ from the adult target system;

4. they should be encouraged to develop self-monitoring skills;
5. wherever possible intervention procedures should take place in 'real' communicative contexts so that the child develops awareness of their own communicative effectiveness.

The development of intervention has tended to follow the line of enquiry and discovery about the underlying nature of phonological disability. Approaches to intervention fall broadly into three categories, 'traditional/ behavioural' approaches, 'linguistic' approaches, and 'cognitive/ linguistic' approaches. The most recent, cognitive/linguistic approaches build upon earlier procedures. The 'traditional/behavioural' category includes therapy approaches which centre on articulatory training (see, for example, Mowrer and Case, 1982; Van Riper and Emerick, 1984). Therapy consists of a period of 'ear training' for the target sound followed by 'production training' which is carried out in a step-by-step fashion beginning with production of the target sound in isolation, then in words of increasing length and finally in sentences. These approaches rely largely on error analysis assessment procedures for deciding on therapy targets. The child is largely a passive participant whose responses are gradually changed towards a target imposed by the clinician.

Linguistic approaches, (for example; Weiner, 1981, 1984; Fokes, 1982; Hodson and Paden, 1983) are so named because they are based on analysis of the sound contrasts used by the child in comparison to the system of contrasts in the adult language. They often make use of minimal pairs of words which illustrate the target contrasts. (The term minimal pair refers to words in which meaning difference depends upon only one feature or phoneme. For example, 'sea'/'tea'; 'pin'/'bin'; 'top'/'stop'.) These approaches go some way towards fulfilling the principles of intervention described by Howell and McCartney (1990) since it is assumed that exposure to minimally contrasting words will trigger awareness of the communicative importance of sound differences and prompt the child to make efforts to signal these contrasts more effectively to a listener. However, when the content of therapy is examined, it often seems to be based on a behaviourist view of learning. Hodson and Paden's 'cyclical approach' to intervention has received much attention and is widely used in the USA. This approach, which was developed empirically on the basis of clinical practice, is organized as a series of cycles of therapy targeting sets of speech sounds chosen on the basis of linguistic analysis of speech data. The emphasis is on intensive listening to lists of words containing the target phonemes (auditory bombardment) before a child begins to take part in tasks which require changes in output. Ingram (1986) explores a possible theoretical explanation for the success of this method of therapy, based on cross-linguistic data which emphasizes gradual perceptual learning in normal speech development.

The Metaphon approach to therapy for children's phonological disorders (Dean and Howell, 1986; Howell and Dean, 1994) has been described as a 'cognitive/linguistic' approach since it is based on consideration of learning principles as well as on linguistic analysis of speech output. It centres on the utilization and development of metalinguistic abilities as a means of giving children strategies or 'tools' with which to bring about changes in their speech output. The two-phase therapy procedure first encourages children's awareness of the nature of speech-sound categories and contrasts and second develops their awareness of their own communicative effectiveness, encouraging them to reflect on the reasons for breakdowns in communication when they occur and to use their newly acquired knowledge of the speech-sound system to effect repair. Metaphon was developed on the basis of a view of phonological disorder as a cognitive/linguistic problem in which therapy aims to help a child towards a reorganization of his system of meaningful sound contrasts. It is important also to recognize that some phonologically-disordered children may require opportunities for developing their speech motor (articulatory) skills. A procedure like Metaphon which de-emphasizes articulatory training, can, in fact, provide children with opportunities for exploring, experimenting with and practising new articulatory configurations in a context which meets the principles of intervention listed by Howell and McCartney (see Waters *et al.*, 1995).

It is beyond the scope of this chapter to give detailed accounts of specific therapy procedures. For useful reviews see Newman *et al.* (1985) and Howell and McCartney (1990).

As structured psycholinguistic assessment procedures come into wider use, it is likely that we will see a continuation of the gradual process of adding to, and building upon, previous therapy procedures. Intervention approaches will be published which, in addition to taking account of linguistic evidence and learning theory, also take explicit account of the results of investigations of a child's speech-processing strengths and needs. One interesting issue which is likely to arise as such approaches develop is whether they will focus mainly on developing areas of existing strength in the child's speech-processing skills (with the aim of circumventing and compensating for areas of weakness) or whether they will focus mainly on areas of weakness with the aim of improving processing in those areas.

The context of intervention

Children with phonological disorders are offered therapy in a variety of settings, most usually in schools and nurseries or in community health clinics. The context of therapy will have implications for the involvement of parents and teachers. Ideally the child's parent (or carer) should be involved in therapy as frequently as possible. Teachers should be given as much information as possible about the aims and content of therapy so that their help can be elicited in reinforcing the work in the course of daily classroom routine (including pre-literacy and early literacy activities). A particularly important outcome of parental involvement is likely to be that through observing and taking part in therapy, the parent will modify the way they use clarification requests in their interactions with the child, making them more specific, less 'judgemental' and more sensitively targeted at the child's level of ability to effect repair (McTear, 1985).

Evaluating the effectiveness of intervention

If we are to be able to make informed judgements about choice of therapy approach, it is essential that research is carried out to evaluate the effectiveness of various intervention procedures. Investigations employing large-group experimental designs and investigations using single-case-study approaches both have a role to play in evaluating intervention procedures for phonological disorder (Howell and Dean, 1994). Large-group studies require considerable resources and are therefore undertaken infrequently. Single-case-study investigations make relatively small demands on resources, but cannot yield robust evidence unless it can be shown that results can be replicated with different clients and therapists. It is here that individual clinicians have a vital role to play in efficacy research.

Summary

This chapter has attempted to provide an overview of the nature of childhood phonological disorders and of the principles of assessment and therapy applied to this client group. The focus has been on current practice and the theory which underpins it, while attention has also been drawn to pointers towards future trends. There are many controversial issues in the field of developmental speech disorders and new theoretical perspectives continue to have a challenging impact on clinical practice. The near future is likely to see exciting developments in the provision of effective assessment and therapy for this group of children.

Acknowledgements

The authors wish to thank Fiona Gibbon, Elizabeth Dean and Marysia Nash for helpful information and comments on the text.

References

Albery E, Russell J (1990) Cleft palate and facial abnormalities. In Grunwell P (Ed) Developmental Speech Disorders, Edinburgh: Churchill Livingstone.

Anthony A, Bogle D, Ingram TTS, McIsacc MW (1971) The Edinburgh Articulation Test. Edinburgh: Churchill Livingstone.

Aram D, Kamhi AG (1982) Perspectives on the relationship between phonological and language disorders. Seminars in Speech, Language and Hearing 3: 101–14.

Beresford R (1986) Newcastle Speech Assessment. Department of Speech, University of Newcastle upon Tyne (3rd edition).

Beresford R, Grady PAE (1968) Some aspects of assessment. British Journal of Disorders of Communication 3: 28–35.

Bernhardt B (1992a) Developmental implications of nonlinear phonological theory. Clinical Linguistics and Phonetics, 6: 259–81.

Bernhardt B (1992b) The application of nonlinear phonological theory to intervention with one phonologically disordered child. Clinical Linguistics and Phonetics 6: 283–316.

Bernhardt B (1993) Deriving phonological intervention techniques from theories of syllable structure. Mini-seminar presented at the Annual Convention of the American Speech and Hearing Association, Anaheim, November 1993.

Bernhardt B, Gilbert J (1992) Applying linguistic theory to speech-language pathology: the case for nonlinear phonology. Clinical Linguistics and Phonetics 6: 123–45.

Bernthal JE, Bankson NW (1981) Articulation Disorders. New Jersey: Prentice Hall.

Bird J, Bishop D (1992) Perception and awareness of phonemes in phonologically impaired children. European Journal of Disorders of Communication 27: 289–312.

Bishop DVM, Adams C (1990) A prospective study of the relationship between specific language impairment, phonological disorders and reading retardation. Journal of Child Psychology and Psychiatry 31: 1027–50.

Bishop D, Edmundson A (1987) Language Impaired 4 year olds: distinguishing transient from persistent impairment. Journal of Speech and Hearing Disorders 52: 156–73.

Bishop D, Rosenbloom L (1987) Classification of child language disorders. In Yule W, Rutter M (Eds) Language Development and Disorders. Clinics in Developmental Medicine. London: Mackeith Press.

Bradford, A, Dodd B (1994) The motor planning abilities of phonologically disordered children. European Journal of Disorders of Communication 29: 349–69.

Bryan A, Howard D (1992) Frozen phonology thawed: The analysis and remediation of a developmental disorder of real word phonology. European Journal of Disorders of Communication 27: 343–66.

Catts HW, Jensen PJ (1983) Speech timing on phonologically disordered children: voicing contrast of initial and final stop consonants. Journal of Speech and Hearing Research 26: 501–10.

Cazden CB (1983) Play with language and metalinguistic awareness: one dimension of language experience. In Donaldson M, Grieve R, Pratt C (Eds) Early Childhood Development and Education. Oxford: Blackwell.

Crary MA (1993) Developmental Motor Speech Disorders. London: Whurr Publishers.

Dean EC, Howell J (1986) Developing linguistic awareness: a theoretically based approach to phonological disorders. British Journal of Disorders of Communication 21: 223–38.

Dean E, Howell J, Hill A, Waters D (1990) Metaphon Resource Pack. Windsor: NFER-Nelson.

DiSimoni FG (1974) The effect of vowel environment on the duration of consonants in the speech of 3-, 6- and 9-year-old children. Journal of the Acoustical Society of America 55: 360–61.

Dodd B ,Cockerill H (1985) Phonological coding deficit: A comparison of spelling errors made by deaf, speech disordered and normal children. Beitrage zur Phonetik und Linguistik 48: 405–15.

Edwards J (1991) Compensatory Speech Motor Abilities in normal and phonologically disordered children. Journal of Phonetics 19: 1–19.

Eguchi S, Hirsch I (1969) Development of speech sounds in children. Acta Otolaryngology Supplement, 257: 5–51.

Ellis AW, Young AW (1988) Human Cognitive Psychology. London: Lawrence Erlbaum Associates.

Fisher HB, Logemann JA (1971) The Fisher-Logemann Test of Articulation Competence. Boston: Houghton Mifflin Company.

Fokes J (1982) Problems confronting the theorist and practitioner in child phonology. In Crary M (Ed) Phonological Intervention: Concepts and Procedures. San Diego, CA: College Hill Press.

Fox B, Routh D (1975) Analysing spoken language into words, syllables and phonemes: a developmental study. Journal of Psycholinguistic Research 4: 331–42.

Garton A, Pratt C (1989) Learning to be Literate. The Development of Spoken and Written Language. Oxford: Blackwell.

Gibbon F (1990) Lingual activity in two speech-disordered children's attempts to produce velar and alveolar stop consonants: Evidence from electropalatographic (EPG) data. British Journal of Disorders of Communication 25: 329–40.

Goldman R, Fristoe M (1972) Goldman-Fristoe Test of Articulation. Minnesota: American Guidance Service.

Gombert JE (1992) Metalinguistic Development. New York: Harvester Wheatsheaf.

Goswami U (1990) A special link between rhyming skills and the use of orthographic analogies by beginning readers. Journal of Child Psychology and Psychiatry 31: 301–11.

Grunwell P (1975) The phonological analysis of articulation disorders. British Journal of Disorders of Communication 10: 31–42.

Grunwell P (1981) The Nature of Phonological Disability in Children. London: Academic Press.

Grunwell P (1985) Phonological Assessment of Child Speech (PACS) Windsor: Nfer-Nelson.

Grunwell P (1987) Clinical Phonology (2nd ed). London: Croom Helm.

Grunwell P (1993) Assessment of articulation and phonology. In Beech JR, Harding L, Hilton-Jones D (Eds) Assessment in Speech and Language Therapy. London: Routledge.

Hardcastle WJ (1976) Physiology of Speech Production. London: Academic Press.

Hardcastle W (1984) New methods of profiling lingual palatal contact patterns with Electrpalatography. Speech Research Laboratory Work in Progress, University of Reading, 4: 1–40.

Hawkins P (1984) Introducing Phonology. London: Hutchinson.

Henry C E. (1990) The development of oral diadochokinesia and non-linguistic rhythmic skills in normal and speech-disordered young children. Clinical linguistics and Phonetics 4: 121–37.

Hewlett N (1990) Processes of development and production. In Grunwell P (Ed) Developmental Speech Disorders. Edinburgh, Churchill Livingstone.

Hodson BW (1980) The Assessment of Phonological Processes. Danvill, IL: Interstate.

Hodson BW, Paden EP (1981) Phonological processes which characterise unintelligible and intelligible speech in early childhood. Journal of Speech and Hearing Disorders 46: 369–73.

Hodson BW, Paden EP (1983) Targeting intelligible speech. San Diego, CA: College Hill Press.

Howell J (1989) The metalinguistic awareness of phonologically disordered and normally developing children: a comparative study. Unpublished PhD thesis, University of Newcastle upon Tyne.

Howell J, Dean EC (1994) Treating Phonological Disorders in Children: Metaphon – Theory to Practice (2nd ed). London: Whurr.

Howell J, McCartney E (1990) Approaches to remediation. In Grunwell P (Ed) Developmental Speech Disorders. Edinburgh: Churchill Livingstone.

Ingram D (1976) Phonological Disability in Children. London: Edward Arnold.

Ingram D (1980) A comparative study of phonological development in normal and linguistically delayed children. Proceedings of the First Wisconsin Symposium on Research in Child Language Disorders 1: 23–32.

Ingram D (1986) . Explanation and phonological remediation. Child Language Teaching and Therapy 2: 1–19.

Kahmi AG, Lee R ,Nelson L (1985) Word, syllable and sound awareness in language disordered children. Journal of Speech and Hearing Disorders 50: 207–13.

Kent RD, Forner LL (1980) Speech segment duration in sentence recitations by children and adults. Journal of Phonetics 8: 157–68.

Kiparsky P and Menn L (1977) On the acquisition of phonology. In MacNamara J (Ed) Language Learning and Thought. New York: Academic Press.

Lewis BA, Freebairn L (1992) Residual effects of preschool phonology disorders in grade school, adolescence and adulthood. Journal of Speech and Hearing Research 35: 819–31.

Lewis S, Bryan A (1994) Papers for Developmental cognitive neuropsychological Special Interest Group: Tapping Tasks (Unpublished).

Lundberg I (1978) Aspects of linguistic awareness related to reading. In: Sinclair A, Jarvella RJ, Levelt W (Eds) The Childs Conception of Language. Berlin: Springer Verlag.

Macken M, Ferguson CA (1983) Cognitive aspects of phonological development: model, evidence and issues. In Nelson KE (Ed) Childrens Language, Vol 4. Hillsdale, New Jersey: Lawrence Erlbaum Associates.

McNutt J (1977) Oral sensory and motor behaviours of children with /s/ and /r/ misarticulations. Journal of Speech and Hearing Research 20: 694–703.

McTear M (1985) Childrens Conversations. Oxford: Blackwell.

Magnusson E (1983) The Phonology of Language Disordered Children: Production, Perception and Awareness. Lund: Gleerups.

Magnusson E (1991) Metalinguistic awareness in phonologically disordered children. In Yavas MS (ed) Phonological Disorders in Children. London: Routledge.

Magnusson E, Naucler K (1990) Reading and spelling in language disordered children – linguistic and metalinguistic prerequisites: report on a longitudinal study. Clinical Linguistics and Phonetics 4: 49–61.

Marion MJ, Sussman HM, Marquardt TP (1993) The perception and production of rhyme in normal and developmentally apraxic children. Journal of Communication Disorders 26: 129–60.

Menn L (1976) Evidence for an interactionist-discovery theory of child phonology. Papers and Reports on Child Language Development 12: 169–77. Stanford University.

Menn L (1978) Phonological units in beginning speech. In Bell A, Bybee Hooper J (Eds) Syllables and Segments. Amsterdam: North Holland.

Morley M (1965) The Development and Disorders of Speech in Childhood. Edinburgh, Churchill Livingstone.

Moss FA (1985) A theoretical and experimental investigation of the nature of phonological and phonetic processes in the speech of children with phonological disorders. Unpublished M Phil dissertation: Council for National Academic Awards.

Mowrer DE ,Case JL (1982) Clinical Management of Speech Disorders. Rockville, MD: Aspen.

Newman PW, Creaghead NA, Secord W (Eds) (1985) Assessment and Remediation of Phonological Disorders. Columbus, OH: Charles E Merrill.

Parker A, Rose H (1990) Deaf children's phonological development. In Grunwell P (Ed) Developmental Speech Disorders. Edinburgh: Churchill Livingstone.

Powers MH (1971) Functional disorders of articulation: symptomatology and etiology. In Travis LE (Ed) Handbook of Speech Pathology and Audiology. New York: Appleton-Century-Crofts.

Pratt C , Grieve R (1984) The development of metalinguistic awareness: an introduction. In Tunmer WE, Pratt C, Herriman ML (Eds) Metalinguistic Awareness in Children. Theory, Research and Implications. Berlin: Springer-Verlag.

Rapin I, Allen D (1983) Developmental language disorders: nosologic considerations. In Kirk U (Ed) Neuropsychology of Language, Reading and Spelling. New York: Academic Press.

Reynolds J (1990) Abnormal vowel patterns in phonological disorder: some data and a hypothesis. British Journal of Disorders of Communication 25: 115–48.

Schwartz R, Leonard L, Folger M, Wilcox M (1980) Early phonological behaviour in normally speaking and language disordered children: evidence for a synergistic view of language disorders. Journal of Speech and Hearing Disorders 45: 357–77.

Sell D, Harding A, Grunwell P (1994) A screening assessment of cleft palate speech: Great Ormond Street Speech Assessment. European Journal of Disorders of Communication 29: 1–16.

Shelton RL, McReynolds LV (1979) Functional articulation disorders: preliminaries to treatment. In Lass NJ (Ed) Speech and Language: Advances in Basic Research and Practice, 2. New York: Academic Press.

Shields J (1981) A study of rhythmic abilities and language abilities in young children. First Language 2: 131–40.

Shriberg LD (1991) Directions for research in developmental phonological disorders. In Miller J (Ed) Research on Child Language Disorders. A Decade of Progress. Austin, TX: Pro-ed.

Shriberg LD, Kwiatkowski J, Best S, Hengst J, Terselic-Weber B (1986) Characteristics of children with phonologic disorders of unknown origin. Journal of Speech and Hearing Disorders 51: 140–61.

Spencer A (1984) A nonlinear analysis of phonological disability. Journal of Communication Disorders 17: 325–48.

Stackhouse J (1990) Phonological deficits in developmental reading and spelling disorders. In Grunwell P (Ed) Developmental Speech Disorders, Edinburgh: Churchill Livingstone.

Stackhouse J, Snowling M (1992) Developmental verbal dyspraxia II: A developmental perspective on two case studies. European Journal of Disorders of Communication 27: 35–54.

Stackhouse J ,Wells B (1991) Dyslexia: the obvious and hidden speech and language disorder. Speech Therapy in Practice 7: 12–5.

Stackhouse J, Wells B (1993) Psycholinguistic assessment of developmental speech disorders. European Journal of Disorders of Communication 28: 331–48.

Stampe D (1969) The acquisition of phonetic representation. Paper presented at the Fifth Regional Meeting, Chicago Linguistic Society.

Stampe D (1979) A Dissertation on Natural Phonology. New York: Garland.

Stark R, Tallal P (1979) Analysis of stop consonant production errors in developmentally dyspraxic children. Journal of the Acoustical Society of America 66: 1703–12.

Stoel-Gammon C (1991) Issues in phonological development and disorders. In Miller J (Ed) Research on Child Language Disorders: A Decade of Progress. Austin, TX: Pro-ed.

Stoel-Gammon C, Dunn C (1985) Normal and Disordered Phonology in Children. Baltimore, MD: University Park Press.

Tingley BM, Allen GD (1975) Development of speech timing control in children. Child Development 46: 186–94.

Tunmer WE, Nesdale AR (1985) Phonemic segmentation skills and beginning readers. Journal of Educational Psychology 77: 417–27.

Van Riper C, Emerick L (1984) Speech Correction: an Introduction to Speech Pathology and Audiology (7th ed). New Jersey: Prentice Hall.

Waters D (1992) An Investigation of Motor Control for Speech in Phonologically Delayed Children, Normally Developing Children and Adults. Unpublished PhD thesis, Council for National Academic Awards UK.

Waters D, Reid J, Dean E, Howell J (1995) Metaphon re-examined: A reply to the commentaries. Clinical Linguistics and Phonetics 9: 49-58.

Weiner FF (1979) Phonological Process Analysis (PPA) Baltimore, MD: University Park Press.

Weiner FF (1981) Treatment of phonological disability using the method of meaningful minimal contrast: two case studies. Journal of Speech and Hearing Disorders 46: 97–103.

Weiner FF (1984) A phonological approach to assessment and treatment. In Costello J (Ed), Speech Disorders in Children: Recent Advances. San Diego, CA: College Hill Press.

Weir RH (1962) Language in the Crib. The Hague: Mouton.

Weismer G, Elbert M (1982) Temporal characteristics of functionally misarticulated /s/ in 4–6 year old children. Journal of Speech and Hearing Research 25: 275–87.

Chapter 7
Childhood Articulation Disorders of Neurogenic Origins

PENELOPE K. HALL

Among the most challenging of childhood speech sound disorders are those that are, or appear to be, of neurogenic origin. These disorders fall into two general types: developmental apraxia of speech (DAS) and dysarthria.

Dysarthria

Dysarthria is an articulation disorder marked by neuromotor problems within the musculature of the entire speech-producing system. The child's actual speech attempts may be slow and imprecise owing to weakness of the speech-producing musculature, inco-ordination between the various parts of the speech-producing mechanism, and reduced range of movement within the oral speech-producing mechanism. In addition to the articulatory musculature, other musculature may be involved as well, including that regulating respiration (which provides the breath support needed for speech production), laryngeal function (which provides the phonation or 'voice' involved in speech), and velopharyngeal function (which regulates the air flow into the mouth or nasal cavities). All are important in the task of producing speech.

When speech production is disrupted by dysarthria, the clinician is likely to hear *consistent* errors being made by the child. In other words, the same kind of incorrect productions will be made on repeated speech attempts, from stimulus to stimulus, across uncorrected levels of difficulty (isolation, syllable, words, phrases, sentences, etc.), and from session to session.

Developmental Apraxia of Speech (DAS)

Developmental apraxia of speech is thought to be a disruption in the motor-programming needed for speech production and is characterized by the inability to control the purposeful movements of the articulators during speech attempts. DAS has been a much more controversial entity than is dysarthria. Historically, a central issue has involved whether the disorder even existed. Of those who find the disorder plausible, a point of argument has been in the theoretical nature (e.g. 'motor-programming' vs. 'language') of the disorder (Hall, 1992). Furthermore, the disorder has even been known by a variety of names, such as 'articulatory dyspraxia' (Morley, Court and Miller, 1954); 'developmental articulatory apraxia' (Morley, 1957, 1972); 'congenital articulatory apraxia' (Eisenson, 1972); and 'developmental verbal apraxia' (Aram and Nation, 1982). More recently within the profession there seems to be a cautious agreement that DAS does exist, although there is much that still needs to be known about the disorder.

Currently being explored by clinicians and researchers are attempts to describe what speech characteristics constitute DAS. One of the most important frequently described DAS speech characteristics is that of *inconsistent* errors. Errors may vary in many ways, including across production trials of the same word, across different stimuli for a particular phoneme, and from day to day. Children with DAS produce errors in the sequencing of phonemes, so that phonemes and syllables may be reversed. In addition, more errors occur as the length of the utterance increases, thus multisyllabic words are particularly difficult for children with DAS to produce correctly. Other speech characteristics of DAS include: voicing errors, where voiceless consonants are produced with voicing, and vice versa; vowel and diphthong errors; and 'addition' errors, where phonemes are added to words. Another characteristic is that children with DAS often seem less intelligible (understandable) than one would predict from formal testing, and are less intelligible when an utterance becomes more complex. Additional characteristics of DAS are inconsistent nasal voice quality and nasal emissions, the occurrence of groping and silent posturing of the articulators, and disordered use of stress and inflection within utterances.

Many practising clinicians are comfortable with the concept presented by Jaffe (1984) that DAS consists of a 'cluster' of characteristics that help diagnose the problem. However, within the cluster there is no single characteristic that is essential or mandatory in order to make the diagnosis, nor do all of the characteristics described in the literature need to be present before the diagnosis can be made. Many clinicians find that the characteristics change as they follow children with DAS over time. These changes can be attributed to overall maturation, to continuing development within the speech and language acquisition processes, and to the remediation programmes with which the children have been involved.

Dysarthria and developmental apraxia of speech have many differences, but also share some similarities. For instance, both are considered to be 'motor speech' disorders. The severity range of both disorders is wide, including mild to severe involvement. Some children with these disorders may ultimately approach nearly 'normal' speech skills, whereas others will be so profoundly involved that they will require augmentative communication systems to help them interact with their world. Both disorders should be considered life-long problems, which will often require intensive remediation because the disorders are not simply 'outgrown'. It is also important to remember that *both* dysarthria and DAS can be exhibited within a single child's communication disorder, complicating the clinician's assessment, diagnosis, and treatment tasks. In addition, with these children, clinicians need to be alert to other communication-related problems as well as the obvious speech sound disorder. Children with DAS and/or dysarthria often present co-occurring language disorders and academic learning problems.

Causative Factors

The search for the aetiology of communication problems is important because, if determined, the origins of the problem may be better understood. Aetiology also aids in the identification of the most helpful treatment approaches, as well as what the course and ultimate prognosis for the problem may be.

Dysarthria

Motor speech disorders due to damage in the peripheral or central nervous system are collectively termed as 'dysarthria'. Love (1992) lists five major sites of lesions identified in the presence of childhood dysarthria: muscle, lower motor neuron, upper motor neuron, extrapyramidal, and cerebellar. There are a number of possible causes for the identifiable neurological lesions, such as: prematurity; anoxia, or lack of oxygen to the brain; infections in either the pregnant mother or the child; trauma or accidents of some type to the nervous system, such as a closed head injury; vascular accidents or strokes; ingestion of toxic substances; metabolic disorders; brain tumours; and degenerative diseases. However, the cause may be unknown. The insult can occur before, during, or after birth.

Developmental apraxia of speech

Developmental apraxia of speech is often assumed to have a neurological basis and is usually thought of as a neurogenic disorder. However, this assumption has not yet been supported in medical study. The literature reports on a very small number of children exhibiting DAS who have undergone various types of medical evaluation, including electroencephalography (EEG), computerized tomographic (CT) scans, magnetic resonance imaging (MRI), positron emission tomography (PET), and single photon emission computed tomography (SPECT). So far no focal lesions have been reported. Some children with DAS have exhibited differences in the brain structures; however, these results are dissimilar across children as to the location of the reported anatomical variations.

Another avenue to consider with the possible cause(s) of DAS is that of genetics. There are a growing number of reports indicating that children with DAS often come from families whose members exhibit a wide variety of communication and learning problems (Lewis, 1990). There may be a common genetic denominator, although this is yet undefined.

Thus, at this time, the aetiology of DAS is unknown.

Assessment Considerations

The assessment of children with speech disorders suspected of being neurogenic in origin has two purposes. The first is to obtain baseline descriptions of the child's skills. The second is to facilitate differential diagnosis. Dysarthria and DAS are both speech sound disorders, and they can co-exist. Differential diagnosis is helpful to identify the specific type(s) of disorder the child is presenting so that appropriate intervention plans can logically develop from the assessment information. Then, as intervention is initiated, assessment should continue as an important, on-going, process that allows the clinician to investigate new, or changing, areas of concern.

Throughout the assessment process it is of utmost importance to consider the 'total' child, so that all strengths and weaknesses are identified. While the child's articulation may be of primary interest, other aspects of the child, such as cognitive abilities and potential, hearing status, receptive and expressive language skills, and academic skills, also need to be addressed and considered during the diagnostic baseline assessment process.

Identification of children with neurogenic speech problems, and the differentiation of what type of problem they may be presenting, should be made at the earliest age possible. This allows for the orderly initiation of treatment that addresses the child's needs, potentially reducing the impact of the communication problems upon the educational process and the individual's general abilities to function in the world.

Assessment procedures for children with suspected neurogenic speech disorders cover a number of areas. Some areas should be addressed by the speech-language pathologist, while other areas should be addressed by other 'team' members, e.g. co-operating professionals who also are working with the child in the areas of medicine, audiology, clinical or educational psychology, occupational therapy, physical therapy, and education.

Specific areas to consider when planning a speech assessment with children suspected of exhibiting neurogenic speech disorders follows; additional discussions of assessment techniques can be found in Hardy (1983), Thompson (1988), Love (1992), and Crary (1993).

Feeding and pre-speech skills

With the very young, or very physically involved, client you may need to assess the individual's feeding development. This involves assessing the ability to manage liquids and food in the processes of sucking, drinking, biting, chewing, and swallowing (Alexander, 1987; Mueller, 1972). Not only are these skills needed to sustain the client nutritionally, but many consider these processes to be precursors of speech. During such evaluation the clinician is afforded the opportunity to observe and assess overall muscle tone, head and neck control, respiratory patterns, and phonations/vocalizations. Some clinicians feel comfortable in dealing with these areas, while other clinicians work with occupational and physical therapists to gain the needed assessment information.

Clients with dysarthria, particularly those with cerebral palsy, often have problems in the area of feeding. However, children presenting DAS may also have, or have had, problems with sucking, chewing, and swallowing. Thus, even with the older or less physically involved child exhibiting DAS, a history of feeding and swallowing problems needs to be explored with the primary carers. Current food preferences and dislikes, and present skills in chewing and swallowing various food consistencies and textures need to be discussed as well.

Articulation

A thorough assessment of the child's articulation skills is an essential part of any evaluation in which there is a speech sound disorder. This information is essential to the differential diagnosis as to the *type(s)* of speech sound disorder(s) the child may be exhibiting.

There are a number of commercially published articulation tests worthy of consideration for use; these tests generally assess phonemes at the word level of difficulty. It is suggested that a comprehensive assessment be conducted when DAS or dysarthria is suspected. This includes an evaluation of all consonants and consonant clusters, as well as vowels. After formal testing, the clinician should assess the child's 'stimulability', or ability to produce errored phonemes when provided with a variety of auditory, visual or tactile cues. Also, evaluation of the client's production of specific phonemes and overall articulation should be completed during speech tasks at different levels of complexity. It should be noted if, and how, the complexity of the speech tasks affects the client's ability to correctly produce speech. Testing also will yield information about the *consistency* of errors across task levels that assists in differential diagnosis. Finally, the clinician will need to describe subjectively how intelligible the child is during their speech attempts.

Prosody, or the 'melody' of language, is important to assess because stress and inflection help convey syntactical and emotional information to listeners. It has been noted that individuals with DAS and/or dysarthria may present distorted prosody during speech attempts. Therefore, it is necessary to address prosody in the assessment protocol by determining if the child can ask questions with an upward inflection, and make a statement with a downward inflection. In addition, determine if the child can convey such emotions as gladness, sadness, or anger by the use of word stress within utterances.

Examination of the speech producing mechanisms

The peripheral oral mechanism needs to be examined to determine *structural* and *functional* adequacy for speech. Needing to be examined are the face, lips, teeth, tongue, and velopharyngeal mechanism. There are numerous test forms that can be used as guides for this type of assessment; some are commercially published, but many are clinician-developed. Structural adequacy is assessed by making observations of the structures themselves, as well as the relationships between structures. Functional adequacy is assessed by a variety of techniques involving speech and non-speech tasks, where observations of how consistently, accurately, and rapidly a task is performed may provide helpful information into the nature of the articulation problem. Tasks assessing the strength of the facial, tongue, and lip musculature also can provide helpful diagnostic information in differentiating DAS and dysarthria. The reader is referred to Shipley and McAfee (1992) and Hall (1994) for specific information in conducting evaluation of the speech mechanism.

Children with dysarthria and/or DAS may exhibit 'nasal' resonance due to problems with velopharyngeal function. Thus, clinicians need to attend carefully to determine if actual nasal emissions of air occur during articulation testing and other speech attempts, in addition to visually assessing the structural and functional adequacy of the velopharyngeal port mechanism.

For the child with dysarthria, additional assessment needs to be made of respiration and phonation. Thompson (1988) reports abnormal respiratory patterns including rapid, shallow, or noisy breathing, as well as involuntary movement of the respiratory musculature and 'reverse breathing.' These may result in speech production problems for the child, such as short phrasing, frequent inspiration, and decreased speech rate. A child with dysarthria also may present problems with phonation resulting in an abnormally high or low pitch, reduced pitch range, reduced loudness, and breathy voice quality.

Language

There are a plethora of standardized and non-standardized assessment and analysis procedures that can aid in the assessment of a child's language skills. All aspects of language (morphology, syntax, semantics, discourse, and pragmatics) need to be addressed both receptively and expressively with age-appropriate techniques. Children with neurogenic articulation disorders may present a full range of language skills from normal to severely disordered.

Theoretical Bases of Intervention

Intervention planning for *any* child with *any* form of communication disorder needs to take into account all aspects of the child's needs, and the clinician's focus of remediation should address all aspects of disordered communication as determined through assessment procedures. Speech-language pathologists need to remind themselves that every client is individual and unique. Thus, the development of remedial goals, objectives, and procedures must address the individuality and uniqueness of the child and the child's communication disorder. Additionally, the clinician may need to advocate and facilitate the involvement of professionals from other fields, such as physical therapy, occupational therapy, psychology, and education, as members of a team of professionals working together to best serve the child.

Remediation planning can take different forms depending upon the age of the child and the severity of the communication disorder. The planning needs to reflect short term goals, placed in the context of the probable long-term and intensive services typically needed by children with dysarthria and/or DAS.

Children with neurogenic articulation disorders need to be identified and served at as young an age as possible. Remediation options can have different forms when dealing with infants and pre-school children. For example, speech-language pathologists can be involved with infants, working as a team member with a physical therapist to help develop pre-speech skills. As infants become pre-school children there may be a need to help develop communication systems that are non-verbal so that the child can interact with others in their growing and expanding environments which will soon include formal education. Another advantage of early identification and service is that the parent(s) of the child can receive needed counselling and support for what is often a severe disorder.

Keeping the above treatment philosophies in mind, factors follow that need consideration when developing specific intervention plans for children with neurogenic articulatory disorders.

Dysarthria

As discussed in an earlier section of this chapter, dysarthria is the result of damage in the peripheral or central nervous system. Thus, a number of physiological systems and processes involved in the production of speech may be affected and need to be addressed in a therapy programme. If the child is young or very severely involved, pre-speech and feeding skills may be the focus of remediation. There are often problems with neuromuscular control as evidenced in disordered rate, range, and co-ordination of movements of the articulators for speech purposes. Within the intervention plan the clinician also may need to address difficulties with respiration, phonation, resonance, prosody, and chewing/swallowing as well as the 'obvious' area of articulation.

Developmental apraxia of speech (DAS)

The theoretical bases of intervention with children exhibiting DAS reflect the philosophical differences as to the nature of the disorder (Hall, 1992). Clinicians thinking that DAS is part of a larger 'language' problem use a different approach to remediation than does the author, who is most comfortable with the notion that DAS is a disorder in the motor-programming necessary for the sequences of articulatory movements that result in speech production.

Mainstream Therapy Models

There are numerous therapy models currently purported to facilitate changes in neurogenically based articulation disorders. The author stresses the use of a therapy framework based on motor-programming principles as appropriate for children exhibiting DAS, and a 'systems' approach for children exhibiting dysarthria. However, clinicians are also urged to be eclectic, incorporating into these remedial frameworks additional therapy techniques and approaches, selected to best meet the individual needs of their clients. In addition to those provided below, reviews of specific techniques by Thompson (1988), Love (1992), Crary (1993), and Hall, Jordan and Robin (1993) may be helpful to the reader.

Motor-programming approaches

Therapy based on principles of motor-programming is the author's preferred therapy approach for children exhibiting developmental apraxia of speech. While initially addressed in relation to adults with neurogenic speech disorders, there are now several references that discuss the application of motor-programming principles with the young client presenting DAS (Hall et al., 1993; Haynes, 1985). It should be noted that many of the principles can also be applied to the remediation of some children with dysarthria.

Central to motor-programming-based remediation is the goal that the child acquires *voluntary*, *accurate*, and *consistent* control of the speech articulators. This is important so that the child is able to produce accurately and consistently the phoneme or sequences of phonemes they intend or need to produce. Motor-programming remediation is designed to facilitate the development of the 'memory' for the speech movement patterns, allowing the movements to be accurately performed during future speech attempts.

This author and her colleagues have presented the most salient features of what we consider to be motor-programming therapy (Hall et al., 1993). Included are the following features:

1. *Many* repetitions of the correctly produced speech movements are needed, allowing for habituation of accurate and volitional movement patterns. Often this is best accomplished within sessions that are highly drill oriented with large numbers of responses being achieved each session, particularly with children exhibiting DAS. Conversely, Hardy (1983) cautions clinicians to avoid requiring children with dysarthria to achieve their 'maximum physiological effort' because this may result in 'overflow' movements that are counterproductive to the therapy goal.
2. Motor-programming therapy must progress systematically through carefully detailed hierarchies of task difficulty. The clinician must determine at what level the child can succeed, and then carefully increase the complexity level of the required tasks. Children with DAS are often particularly sensitive to even minute increases in difficulty level of the required speech responses, to which the clinician must be exceedingly sensitive, as well as flexible, in immediately modifying the target to assure client success.
3. Multiple sensory modalities should be used to assist the child in acquiring the skills to produce or sequence phonemes. Visual, tactile, and kinesthetic cues, in addition to the often used auditory cues, can be very helpful to the clinician and child in the teaching–learning process. There are a number of very specific techniques (some of which will be addressed later in this chapter) that can be incorporated, *in toto*, or with modification, into a motor-programming remedial framework.
4. The prosodic features of communication need to be manipulated during the remedial process. The use of rhythm, stress, and intonation should be incorporated as an important component of the remedial programme for children with DAS and/or dysarthria.
5. The overt teaching of compensatory strategies may be a necessary stage of therapy within a motor-programming approach. While a

child with dysarthria or DAS is learning control over their articulators it may be necessary to teach overtly such compensations as slowing the rate, prolonging vowels, including neutral vowels between elements of blends, and increasing the length of pauses between syllables and words. These strategies help the child acquire and stabilize skills, and should be faded and eliminated if, and when, they are no longer needed.

6. Children with neurogenic-based articulation disorders will need intensive services. Progress is slow, thus demanding a great deal of remediation over the short term, and continuation of these intensive services over long periods of time, often for many years. Parents, clinicians, and the child must be prepared for long-term involvement in the remedial process.

Speech-producing 'systems' approach

Hardy (1983) details a management approach for children exhibiting dysarthria, although the information also may be helpful in intervention for some children with DAS. Addressed within the approach are the respiratory, laryngeal, and velopharyngeal systems, as well as rate, articulatory errors, and prosody. The approach advocates simultaneous work on multiple aspects of the child's disordered speech-producing behaviours, while monitoring how the changes in one aspect affect the total system. Management techniques for each system and area are detailed in the original reference; readers may find Love (1992) a helpful reference as well.

Neuro-developmental treatment

The Neuro-Developmental Treatment (NDT) approach to remediation was developed by Karel and Berta Bobath (Bobath and Bobath, 1972). NDT was developed as a comprehensive rehabilitation technique advocating very early intervention in which two factors need to be identified: the pathological patterns that need to be *inhibited*, and the developmental patterns that need to be *facilitated*.

The approach is one that is used with children exhibiting dysarthria, particularly as a component of cerebral palsy. Recently it has also been advocated for use with children exhibiting severe DAS. This treatment philosophy involves interdisciplinary co-operation between physical therapists, occupational therapists, and speech-language pathologists, as well as the child's parent(s).

Neuro-developmental treatment requires training specific to the techniques, that can be received in courses presented by the Neuro-Developmental Treatment Association.

Following NDT Principles, Crickmay (1966) presents stages of NDT specific to speech intervention. The first stage involves the inhibition of the child's pathological and abnormal reflex behaviours that are blocking advancement to the next step of neuromuscular development. Facilitation of more developmentally mature movements is the second stage of treatment. The third stage involves the patient achieving voluntary control over performance movements. Crickmay elaborates specific techniques for each stage.

There are a number of references that deal with intervention based on neurological developmental models, directed at rehabilitation of infants and young children with cerebral palsy. See Mueller (1972) and Alexander (1987) for discussions of pre-speech and feeding intervention, McDonald (1987) for discussions of speech remediation with individuals with cerebral palsy, and the reviews by Thompson (1988).

PROMPT

The Prompts for Restructuring Oral Muscular Phonetic Targets (PROMPT) system was developed by Chumpelik (1984) and described for use with children exhibiting DAS, but the system might also be considered for children with dysarthria. PROMPT is described as a tactile-based method developed to elicit phonemes, but supposedly the prompts can also be administered serially, allowing for assistance with the sequencing of phonemes.

The method is one in which the clinician provides various external prompts to the muscles of the face and under the jaw, as well as to the structures involved with voicing, nasality, and jaw opening. The timing of each prompt is described as crucial. Specific prompts have been developed for all English phonemes and involve the following: place of contact; degree of jaw closure; manner or features, such as duration, continuance, movement, fusion, lateralization, and labialization; muscles used in the production of specific phonemes; amount of tension needed by specific muscles and muscle groups; timing; and stressing patterns.

Gestural cueing systems

Motor-programming approaches to remediation stress the use of multiple modalities to help the child achieve phoneme production or sequences. Some of the preceding remedial methods deal with tactile and kinaesthetic cueing. Gestures can also provide needed helpful production information and 'reminders' about phoneme production features or inclusion, particularly to the child exhibiting DAS. Gestures can be used by both the clinician and the child. In fact, self-cueing may spontaneously occur when a child learns that a particular gesture is helpful in acquiring oral production of the targeted phoneme.

Two gestural systems have been described in the literature. These are Signed Target Phoneme Therapy (STP) (Shelton and Garves, 1985), and the Adapted Cueing Technique (ACT) (Klick, 1985). The former is based on the hand shapes of the American Manual Alphabet, and the latter purports to reflect the shape and movements of the oral cavity during speech.

Sign/total communication

Some children with neurogenically based articulation disorders exhibit severely compromised intelligibility. However, all children need to have a way to communicate. For these children the use of manual communication, such as finger spelling, various sign language systems, and 'total' communication needs to be seriously considered. In fact, the author has dealt with young clients with DAS who have developed their own gestures to help them communicate, and have later welcomed the learning of a formal sign system. A factor to be assessed on an individual basis is to determine if the child, whether they present DAS or dysarthria, has sufficient control of the upper limbs to be able to execute the signs with a reasonable degree of accuracy. There are several formal sign systems presently in use. Therefore, a speech-language clinician must understand the strengths and weaknesses of each in order best to meet the child's needs.

In addition to giving the child with DAS a way to communicate, there is another advantage to the incorporation of a manual communication system – the inherent use of motor sequences needed to perform signs. Thus, signing may help the child acquire the concept and then the opportunity to practise making a series of movements with the upper limbs. This learning may then transfer to making the series of movements by the articulators required for speech production.

Some children may need to use a sign system as their primary communication system, while some may need to use it as an adjunct to their oral communication. Other children ultimately find that use of manual communication is not necessary as the motor control for speech improves and oral communication attempts are increasingly more successful. With these children the use of sign seems to 'fade' in favour of the more efficient oral communication – reassuring to those parents who fear that, if their child is taught a manual communication system, the child will forgo oral speech.

Augmentative and alternative communication (AAC)

Unfortunately, some children with neurogenic-based articulation problems will be so severely involved that the prognosis for oral communication skills is unrealistic. For such children augmentative or alternative communication systems should be considered. The term 'alternative' communication describes systems that can be developed for children who are unable or unlikely to develop oral communication skills, while 'augmentative' communication options are ones that do not replace speech, but can enhance the child's verbal attempts. Augmentative and alternative communication options can be 'aided' or 'unaided.' Aided options are ones that require some type of equipment, some of which are as simple as paper and pencils, to the more complex computerized communication boards. Unaided options do not require anything external to the body and include use of manual communication systems, gestures, etc.

Unaided augmentative and alternative communication systems in the form of sign systems were discussed above in the context of facilitating the progression of a child achieving motor-control of the articulators necessary for speech. Unfortunately, some children may only partially achieve speech skills, so will find manual communication a permanent and necessary adjunct to their oral communication attempts. With these children the use of sign may need to be actively taught as it will become their primary mode of communication.

Aided communication techniques are many, with a rich future, given present and future technology. Aided techniques may be used to enhance a child's communication system or they may be the primary communication system used by the child. There must be a very careful match between the child and the aided system. Many children with DAS are ambulatory and active, thus the device must be highly portable and rugged enough to withstand breakage. Many children will also want to have a system that is as inconspicuous as possible. Most importantly, the child must find the system helpful or it will not be used. The preferences of the child, as well as those of the primary carers and educational teams, must be taken into account.

An aided system that the author has found helpful for active children with DAS is that of a communication book containing plastic-covered pages of categorized pictures or written words. The book is then attached to the child's belt or clothing waistband with a small clip. Although space for vocabulary is restricted, entries to the book can easily be added or deleted, and the system is not expensive.

Technology has allowed a large number of options for children who need more extensive alternative and/or augmentative communication assistance. For instance, children with dysarthria also may exhibit motor problems due to cerebral palsy. These children may require the development of communication boards, either computerized or clinician-made. Because such systems may have a somewhat restricted memory, care must be taken to be sure that the vocabulary programmed into, or included in, the unit is made up of words that are relevant to the child.

The development and use of augmentative and alternative communication systems is becoming a specialized area within the field of speech-language pathology and also draws from many related fields. Changes and advances are rapidly occurring. A clinician without recent experience in this aspect of remediation who is considering such an option for a client with dysarthria or apraxia would be advised to consult a specialist in order to best serve the child's needs.

Effectiveness Measures

All speech-language pathologists want to be 'effective' clinicians with their clients, including those children who exhibit dysarthria or DAS. However, one of the most elusive aspects of the field is to demonstrate that effectiveness; too often effectiveness of treatment is based solely on subjective opinions. Yet, the field is noted for both the art and the science of intervention.

The science of intervention demands that carefully designed methods be used, based on theoretical tenets. The data are objectively gathered and analysed, and conclusions are drawn. The results need to be replicable by others, which establishes the validity of the technique. The art of intervention comes into focus because of a clinician's particular skills and 'style' which may positively (or negatively) influence the outcome of the remediation. However, both the science and the art of intervention must ultimately be measured in the behavioural changes made by the child – and each child will respond in his or her unique way. This requires constant reassessment of both the art and science of remedial planning, and provides challenges, frustrations, and rewards to the clinician.

The literature within the field of children's neurogenic speech disorders reveals that most of the remediation-related articles describe a technique which this author has found helpful. However, some of these lack the detail necessary for another clinician to use the technique. Few contain objective measurements of the behaviours targeted for modification. Many contain clinician's subjective impressions.

Earlier in this chapter several remedial models were presented. The reported efficacy of these approaches is largely non-existent or unknown to the author. However, some attempts have been made to study several of the described remedial approaches objectively. Although more scientific rigour is needed, recognition of the importance of this aspect of careful clinical work should be applauded. Specifically:

- *PROMPT*. Chumpelik (1984), the developer of the system, cited a study she conducted comparing PROMPT with a traditional 'audio-visual' technique. 'Results indicated that for more difficult targets – some vowels, consonants with tension, and timing factors – the PROMPT system was the only way to produce change' (p.150).

However, the actual data from which the results evolved were not reported.

- *Signed Target Phoneme Therapy (STP)*. Shelton and Garves (1985) included a case study of a child with DAS with whom they used STP to achieve correct phoneme production. The two authors alternated conducting 'traditional' therapy with the 5 year old, with one using STP while the other did not. The subject was reported to reach criterion 'more quickly in fewer sessions' when STP was used. However, no data were provided to support this conclusion.

The lack of objective study of remedial techniques includes the author's preferred motor-programming approaches. These approaches have received much attention at the descriptive level, but seem devoid of any published studies on their efficacy with children exhibiting neurogenic speech disorders. Yet clinically, use of motor-programming based remediation has resulted in improved speech skills of the children, as measured and documented by achievement of intervention goals and objectives, and by data from formal and informal assessment tools. The next step is formal study, using scientific methods.

The art of intervention seems to have an important place within the practice of speech-language pathology. However, clinicians need to continue to strive in improving not only this art, but also the science, of intervention. Increasing awareness and practice in the objective assessment of clinical effectiveness needs to be an important goal in professional work with children presenting developmental apraxia of speech or dysarthria.

Summary

Children with neurogenically based articulation disorders are a challenging group with whom to work, as each child presents a unique profile that must be individually addressed through assessment, intervention, and prognosis. Children with DAS and/or dysarthria may be mildly to profoundly affected by the disorder. For some children nearly normal speech skills may ultimately be realistic, while for others the primary use of augmentative and assistive devices must be acknowledged. The children may also present other co-occurring disorders, such as difficulties with language and educational learning, in addition to disordered speech sound production.

Apraxia and dysarthria in children often mean long-term relationships with professionals from many fields, affording the speech-language pathologist the opportunity to work within a team dedicated to providing the best possible overall services to the child. Thus, the challenges of working with this population of children often results in rich rewards as the clinician guides the child's abilities to communicate functionally.

References

Alexander R. (1987) Prespeech and feeding development. In McDonald ET (Ed) Treating Cerebral Palsy: For Clinicians by Clinicians Austin, TX: PRO-ED. pp 133–52.

Aram D M, Nation, JE (1982) Child Language Disorders St Louis, MO: C. V. Mosby. pp 144–249.

Bobath K, Bobath B (1972) The neurodevelopmental approach to treatment. In Pearson PH (Ed) Physical Therapy Services in the Developmental Disabilities. Springfield, IL: Charles C. Thomas, Publisher. pp 114–85.

Chumpelik D (1984) The PROMPT system of therapy: Theoretical framework and applications for developmental apraxia of speech. In Perkins WH, Northern JL (Eds) Seminars in Speech and Language. New York: Thieme-Stratton. pp 139–55.

Crary MA (1993) Developmental Motor Speech Disorders. San Diego, CA: Singular Publishing Group.

Crickmay MC (1966) Speech Therapy and the Bobath Approach to Cerebral Palsy. Springfield, IL: Charles C. Thomas, Publisher.

Eisenson J (1972) Aphasia in Children. New York: Harper and Row. pp 189–202.

Hall PK (1992) At the center of controversy: Developmental apraxia. American Journal of Speech-Language Pathology: A Journal of Clinical Practice 1: 23–5.

Hall, PK (1994) The oral mechanism. In Tomblin JB, Morris HL, Spriestersbach DC (Eds) Diagnosis in Speech-Language Pathology. San Diego, CA: Singular Publishing Group. pp 67–98.

Hall PK, Jordan LS, Robin DA (1993) Developmental Apraxia of Speech: Theory and Clinical Practice. Austin, TX: PRO-ED.

Hardy JC (1983) Cerebral Palsy. Englewood Cliffs, NJ: Prentice-Hall.

Haynes (1985) Developmental apraxia of speech: Symptoms and treatment. In Johns DF (Ed) Clinical Management of Neurogenic Communication Disorders (2nd ed.). Boston: Little, Brown and Company. pp 259–66.

Jaffe MB (1984) Neurological impairment of speech production: Assessment and treatment. In Costello JM (Ed) Speech Disorders in Children. San Diego, CA: College-Hill Press. pp 157–86.

Klick SL (1985) Adapted cueing technique for use in treatment of dyspraxia. Language, Speech, and Hearing Services in Schools 16: 256–9.

Lewis BA (1990) A familial phonological disorder: Four pedigrees. Journal of Speech and Hearing Disorders 55: 160–70.

Love RJ (1992) Childhood Motor Speech Disability. New York: Merrill Macmillan Publishing Company.

McDonald ET (1987) Speech production problems. In McDonald ET (Ed) Treating Cerebral Palsy: For Clinicians by Clinicians. Austin, TX: PRO-ED. pp 171–90.

Morley ME (1957) The Development and Disorders of Speech in Childhood. London: Livingstone.

Morley ME (1972) The Development and Disorders of Speech in Childhood (3rd ed). London: Livingstone.

Morley M, Court D, Miller H (1954). Developmental dysarthria. British Medical Journal 1: 8–10.

Mueller HA (1972) Facilitating feeding and prespeech. In Pearson PH (Ed), Physical Therapy Services in the Developmental Disabilities. Springfield, IL: Charles C. Thomas, Publisher. pp 283–310.

Shelton IK, Garves MM (1985) Use of visual techniques in therapy for developmental apraxia of speech. Language, Speech, and Hearing Services in Schools 16: 129–31.

Shipley KG, McAfee JG (1992) Assessment in Speech-Language Pathology: A Resource Manual. San Diego, CA: Singular Publishing Group.

Thompson CK (1988) Articulation disorders in the child with neurogenic pathology. In Lass NJ, McReynolds LV, Northern JL, Yoder DE (Eds) Handbook of Speech-Language Pathology and Audiology. Philadelphia, PA: B. C. Decker. pp 548–91.

Chapter 8
Voice Disorders in Children

PAULINE M. SLOANE

When a child's voice differs in quality, resonance, loudness, pitch or prosody from that which is considered normal for his age, sex and maturity, the cause of the abnormal voice requires immediate investigation. The recommendation that all children with voice disorders undergo a medical examination is rarely debatable. Although communicative considerations may initially be of secondary importance, one must not lose sight of the fact that voice is a basic component of oral communication. It is regrettable, therefore, that our understanding of, and approach to, childhood voice disorder has been limited by our tendency to consider the disorder as an isolated phenomenon. Traditionally, speech and language therapists have been prepared to view vocal problems as being clearly separate from problems with social, emotional or communicative functioning or, at best, tangentially connected. Textbooks and articles on childhood voice disorders make little reference to vocal incompetence as it might be related to communicative competence. From the birth cry to the onset of adolescent voice change at puberty, and beyond, vocal competence plays a significant role in social interaction. As clinicians we must question the value of separating developmental, social and emotional factors from the assessment and intervention programmes for voice disorders. In one of the earliest definitions of communication disorder, Van Riper (1939) focused on the influence of social and psychological aspects of behaviour in communication breakdown. More recently, Wilson (1987: 2) stated that

> a problem voice may be distracting or unpleasant to the listener, and it may
> be severe enough to interfere with communication.

Current work has extended the concept of vocal competence as an aspect of communicative competence (Champley and Andrews, 1993). The value of considering a voice disorder as an isolated entity can be questioned from a number of perspectives. If clinicians exclude communicative issues from their interest in voice disorders, the result is likely to be an isolation of specific vocal parameters from the environmental context that gives them meaning.

The incidence of clinically significant voice disorders in the school-age population is 5 to 9 per cent (Boone and McFarlane, 1988). Regardless of whether these estimates are accurate, a discrepancy exists between the reported prevalence of voice disorders in this population and the number of children actually receiving voice therapy. A review of relevant literature indicates that children with voice problems constitute 2 to 4 per cent of speech and language therapist's caseloads. There are several reasons for this; poor identification procedures; lack of recognition of voice disorder as a serious or potentially serious communication handicap; lenient sociological responses; uncertainty on the clinician's part about management; and finally a priority system which places these children low in the therapy schedule.

Causative Factors

The nature and causation of commonly diagnosed voice problems in children change across age with vocal-abuse-related problems more common in older children. Voice disorders can be caused by structural anomalies, neurological conditions including paralysis, glottal margin pathologies, trauma, and psychological or physiological dysfunction. Such conditions may lead to abnormal approximation and asymmetrical vibration of the vocal cords, resulting in the vocal quality deviation called hoarseness.

Dobres et al. (1990) reported that structural anomalies of the larynx were amongst the most common voice diagnoses for children aged 0–3 years in a hospital setting. Such laryngeal anomalies are present on a congenital basis and include subglottic stenosis and laryngolmalacia. The latter is a congenital condition caused by failure of the cartilages of the larynx to develop normally. As it ordinarily disappears in early childhood, it may not be called to the attention of the speech and language therapist and voice therapy is rarely the intervention of choice. Congenital laryngeal disorders, such as laryngomalacia, webbing or subglottal stenosis may give rise to a weak and/or hoarse cry are also likely to cause the more serious problem of airway obstruction. Laryngeal webs, which account for 5 per cent of congenital anomalies (Smith and Catlin, 1984) generally involve the anterior portion of the glottis and consist of thin connective tissue. Surgery is the primary form of management. Congenital supraglottic and subglottic stenosis of the laryngeal airway and larynx is generally managed conservatively. Generally the airway requires surgical dilation and ongoing review, until the larynx has matured, is recommended. In more severe cases surgical intervention, in the form of endotracheal intubation, is required for relief of the obstructed airway.

More long-term relief in the form of a tracheostomy – an artificial open-ing created between the cervical trachea and the neck to provide ventila-tory assistance – is required. The clinician must take an active role in the management of children with tracheostomies as these are generally undertaken prior to the development of verbal language skills and consequently communicative maturation can be significantly impaired.

Additionally, the clinician should be aware of other laryngeal malfor-mations and engage in close follow-up of the child as the voice develops. Laryngeal structural anomalies that are earlier regarded as relatively insignificant may become important later as causes for voice disorders.

Neurological conditions including vocal-fold paralysis

Vocal quality may be affected by impaired neurological functioning, either congenital or acquired. The vocal symptoms obviously depend on the nature and severity of the condition and include resonance prob-lems, dysphonia and reduced loudness. Generally speaking, the vocal dysfunction forms part of a larger group of symptoms affecting muscular inco-ordination and voice therapy therefore, of and by itself, is rarely the treatment of choice.

Vocal-fold paralysis that results from recurrent laryngeal nerve damage may be congenital or acquired, unilateral or bilateral and of two types, adductor or abductor. The condition is relatively common in chil-dren and represents about 10 per cent of all congenital anomalies of the larynx and approximately one-third of the paralyses are of undeter-mined aetiology (Wilson, 1987). Other common causes of vocal-cord paralysis include surgical trauma and cardiovascular conditions such as anomalies of the heart and great blood vessels. The symptoms, which can include respiratory and phonatory difficulties, depend on the degree of involvement and the compensations the child has made with regard to closure of the vocal folds. Primary management centres on the assessment and treatment of the cause of the paralysis. Voice therapy in the case of surgical paresis of the vocal cord should be commenced early and emphasis placed on exercises to increase muscular tonus. In cases where the paralysis is unilateral, vocal quality often improves sponta-neously over a period of 6–12 months, with voice therapy enhancing recovery.

Glottal margin pathologies

The incidence and aetiology of benign laryngeal pathologies in the paediatric population are not well known. Perhaps the most common organic change in the laryngeal structures of children is the develop-ment of glottal margin pathologies such as vocal nodules, polyps, oedema and inflammation. Such pathologies are attributed to prolonged abuse and/or misuse of the vocal mechanism and most child-hood dysphonias are thus related. Many authors, including Andrews (1986) and Wilson (1987), have described behaviours related to vocal abuse. Common types of vocal abuse include affective excesses such as prolonged shouting, screaming, yelling and cheering, throat clearing, and talking in the presence of high level noise. Andrews (1986) listed similar behaviours but additionally referred to poor 'interpersonal behaviours' which included talking too much, ignoring feedback, ignor-ing differences between people and situations, ignoring the interests and needs of others and aggressive behaviour. Corroborating this list of interpersonal behaviours, Green (1989) determined through parent report that children with vocal nodules, aged 3-12 years, presented evidence as having a predilection toward aggression, distractibility, disturbed peer relations and immaturity. It must also be noted that adverse physiological and environmental conditions may predispose a child to developing significant changes in vocal cord tissues (Wilson, 1987).

Vocal nodules, which are benign neoplasms resulting from misuse and abuse of the vocal mechanism, are the most frequently occurring laryngeal pathology in school-age children (Miller and Madison, 1984). Nodules are generally sited on the glottal margin, at the junction of the anterior and middle thirds. As nodules result in size–mass changes of the vocal folds, there is a subsequent alteration in the vibratory pattern lead-ing to abnormal vocal quality. The majority of laryngologists consider voice therapy the treatment of choice for children presenting with vocal nodules. Others recommend surgical intervention but the nodule will tend to return if vocal hyperfunctioning practices are not eliminated.

Vocal polyps are rare in children and adolescents. Polyps are fluid-filled sacs of tissue which may result from a single traumatic episode of vocal abuse such as violent screaming or from more prolonged irrita-tion. Polyps may be of two types, pedunculated or sessile, and the vocal characteristics vary according to the size and location of the mass. Surgery is the treatment of choice for polyps, followed by voice therapy to eliminate the source of irritation.

Vocal fold oedema

Oedema, an increase in mass of the membranous tissues of the glottal margin, may produce a mild dysphonia and can be an early warning sign of vocal hyperfunction. Voice therapy, therefore, is the preferred method of management. In untreated cases, continued abuse and misuse of the voice may lead to the development of other glottal margin pathologies. Vocal-fold oedema is also a common acute physical finding in many infections of the upper respiratory tract and, if the voice is not abused or misused during this period of time, hoarseness will seldom persist.

Many miscellaneous glottal conditions also produce dysphonia. Medical and/or surgical intervention is the management of choice in some of these conditions, however the speech and language therapist should be aware of these conditions to be effective in voice management. Among the most common benign laryngeal tumour in children is the squamous cell juvenile papilloma (Ogura and Thawley, 1980). Papillomas are benign neoplasms believed to result from viral infection and the characteristic recurrences and remission are compatible with the behaviour of a viral disease (Sloan, Montague and Buffalo, 1986). Papillomatosis of the larynx has been reported in the neonate. However, it generally becomes symptomatic in children from 3 to 12 years and is reported to undergo remission following puberty. Laryngeal papillomatosis in children is a serious clinical problem, in that the growth can occur in the larynx and obstruct the airway. The voice is often severely impaired and only whispering may be possible. The vocal symptoms cannot readily be distinguished from those produced by less threatening glottal tumours. The long-term complications have yet to be determined and it is by no means certain that voice will be normal following final resolution of the papilloma. Voice therapy in the traditional sense is a questionable form of treatment. The clinician should however, monitor laryngeal and respiratory performance of the child between surgeries and enhance effective communication. Intervention is always medical and/or surgical with repeated surgery being common. When airway obstruction is severe, tracheotomy is necessary.

Trauma

Voice disorders in children may also be associated with laryngeal trauma resulting from prolonged intubation, aspiration of foreign objects, inhalation of toxic substances and direct injuries to the neck. Cartilaginous fractures, inflammation, oedema, ulceration of the vocal folds and enlarging tumours such as granulomas and hemangiomas, leading to dysphonia or aphonia are common sequels of trauma. Surgical intervention is generally the procedure of choice and voice therapy may be indicated following recovery.

Psychological dysfunction

Psychogenic dysphonia may be suspected in the absence of significant laryngeal or other organic findings and when there is evidence for emotional problems that can account more readily for the dysphonia (Aronson, 1985; Morrison et al., 1983). The terms psychogenic or functional should imply that the clinician has isolated an active aetiological agent and that the agent is non-organic. This disorder, which is not common in children, may be viewed as a manifestation of psychological disequilibrium and may be related unconsciously to stress and anxiety in the child's environment. The nature of the relationship between vocal, social and communicative behaviour requires thorough examination in these cases. Assessment of the relationship is not a simple task, particularly as it is likely that the voice problem is transactional in nature, with voice, social and emotional factors influencing each other over time. Some children with functional dysphonia may require help from a clinical psychologist or counsellor.

Physiological dysfunction

Conditions including allergies, infections of the upper respiratory tract, asthma and hearing loss may result in maladaptive vocal compensations that are habituated across time and are significant in predisposing or perpetuating a voice disorder. Medical management is indicated in combination with voice therapy.

Nasal resonance disorders

Vocal resonance is affected primarily by the size, shape, resiliency and posture of the supralaryngeal structures and any deviation from these usually results in a resonance imbalance. Disorders of nasal resonance can be divided into two main categories, characterized by either excessive or insufficient nasality. Hypernasality is characterized by excess nasal resonance perceived during the production of voiced oral sonorants. It is primarily related to excessive coupling between the nasal cavity and oral-pharyngeal tract. All vowel sounds are nasalized and when the condition is severe, the consonants may be affected by the leakage of air pressure out the nose, commonly referred to as nasal escape. Hypernasal voice quality is generally caused by a physiological deficit in the palatopharyngeal mechanism. Hyponasality is characterized by the reduction or absence of expected nasal resonance. It is generally caused by a reduction in the size of the velopharyngeal port.

As many of the supralaryngeal structures responsible for articulation also affect perceived vocal resonance, there is little advantage in considering articulation and resonance independently. The causes and treatment of nasal resonance defects are discussed in Chapter 10.

Voice Disorders of Adolescence

Mutation constitutes the single most important landmark in the vocal history of the male. Mutation falsetto or puberphonia refers to the presence of persistent falsetto voice in the physically normal male. The vocal quality associated with puberphonia is characterized by high pitch and low intensity. A mild dysphonia may be present but often vocal quality is within normal range in terms of laryngeal vibration and resonance. Medical examination reveals normal physical development, sexual maturation and laryngeal growth. Indirect laryngoscopic examination reveals folds of normal adult length and function and any inflammation or oedema present is considered to be the result and not the cause of the deviant vocal quality. In other words, a functional avoidance of vocal mutation has taken place. Authorities do not agree about the reasons for resistance to voice change and have attributed it to several possible aetiologies: a conflicted response to sexual maturity, problems in a relationship with the parent of the same sex (Andrews, 1986), or strong feminine self-identification (Aronson, 1985).

Although incomplete mutation and puberphonia are primarily the result of psychological influences, delayed mutation, according to Aronson (1985) may have an organic basis. Possible causative factors include endocrine imbalance, general debilitating illness during puberty, severe hearing loss, and weakness or inco-ordination of the vocal folds or respiratory system caused by neurological disease during puberty. In such cases the only reasonable treatment is medical.

Voice therapy is the procedure of choice for these disorders and the majority of these cases yield well to direct voice therapy aimed at lowering the pitch to the optimal pitch level. It is imperative, however, that the clinician has an appreciation of the underlying psychological influences in this disorder.

Assessment Considerations

Traditionally, the speech and language therapist has followed the medical model with regard to assessment and diagnosis. This model is based on the assumption that intervention procedures are much more successful if the aetiological correlates have been identified. Thus the vocal disorder is identified as an isolated phenomenon. The use of such a model has led to fragmentation of vocal behaviours and a focus on discrepancies in production as a means of establishing diagnostic criteria. Such fragmentation, by its very nature, forms a conceptual barrier between vocal and communicative competence.

As the clinician's chief concern is to rule out the presence of an underlying serious medical condition, it is standard procedure to refer dysphonic children to the laryngologist for examination before initiating therapy. The laryngological examination and audiological assessment are essential aspects of the voice evaluation process and as such, parental support of the referral process is important. Indirect laryngoscopy allows observations regarding vocal fold colour, thickness, presence or absence of pathology, and symmetry of the vocal folds, both at rest and during phonation.

Clinical evaluation of the voice generally follows and this involves the assembly of pertinent data, such as records of previous investigations by medical or other personnel, case history information directly related to the disorder, and evaluation of specific parameters of vocal and communicative behaviour. Assessment goals should be broad-based enough to address social interactional aspects of vocal use as well as more traditional indices of voice production. During the parental and child interview, the clinician establishes the nature of the presenting problem, onset and possible causes, variations in severity, voice use, related medical problems, and possible family and environmental influences on the problem. Children's phonatory abilities should always be considered in relation to available medical information. The communicative perspective requires the clinician to broaden the scope of the assessment to include an examination of the impact of the child's cognitive, linguistic, emotional and social development on the child's current vocal competence. It becomes a logical extension therefore, to include family and significant caregivers in the assessment of children with voice disorders. The recognition of the coexistence of problems in these areas may depend on the orientation of the clinician. Assessment of the relationship is not a simple task, particularly as it is likely that voice, social and emotional factors influence and interact with each other over time.

The clinical examination of the voice in the school-age child is usually less formal than it is with his older peers and it should be a relatively brief procedure. Assessment relies heavily on parental and sibling reports and observations. A great deal of information can be accessed from listening to the way the child uses his voice spontaneously and in naturalistic settings. Structured assessment tasks however, may be employed which allow the clinician to focus on specific aspects of voice function and control. If such tasks are used, the pre-school and young school-age child needs practice trials, models, visual cues and encouragement in order to respond optimally to most voice assessment tasks. The clinician must pay careful attention to verbal instructions, the level of abstraction required in the tasks, the child's attention span and the appropriateness of the materials employed.

Evaluation of vocal quality is approached subjectively and objectively. Many rating scales are available, such as the Buffalo 111 Voice Profile (Wilson, 1983), which help sharpen the clinician's focus on specific vocal parameters such as, pitch, intensity, range, degree of vocal fold closure, and an overall index of severity. Standardization in terms of elicitation of vocal responses, perceptual judgement scales and acoustic and physiological measures has obvious benefits. Attempts to increase further objectivity in assessment have led to the present emphasis on acoustic analysis of the voice. A variety of auditory analyses of the voice signal have been proposed, including spectrographic and laryngographic

procedures, but presently they are not commonly used in voice assessment of the child and yield little clinically useful information.

A major goal of assessment is to obtain sample behaviours that are
representative of the child's vocal competencies beyond the constraints
of the clinical situation. Vocal abuses should be identified at this time
and the child's vocal behaviour evaluated in the light of the communicative context. Following collection and evaluation of the relevant data, a
hypothesis concerning the aetiology of the disorder may be formed and
this must be checked against medical and laryngological data. Individualized management procedures can then be determined. The astute clinician, however, must be cognizant of the fact that assessment and
intervention form a continuous process.

Mainstream Treatment Practices

Traditionally, the philosophy of intervention for childhood voice disorders was based primarily on a physiological approach, i.e. efforts were
made to alter or influence underlying physiological processes which
were deemed responsible for the existing laryngeal pathological conditions. The approach was based on the rationale that the child's vocal
quality is an audible manifestation of an underlying dysfunction and it is
such dysfunction that should be the clinician's chief consideration and
not the presenting perceptual vocal attributes.

Not all clinicians have a similar procedural approach to voice modification and some authorities believe that the only logical approach to
voice therapy is the behavioural approach (Leith and Johnson, 1986).
The behaviourists' view reflects the idea that it is the child's inability to
perform certain vocal behaviours that results in his voice disorder, with
secondary importance being given to the question of whether this is or is
not due to an underlying medical or structural problem. Behaviourists
base their intervention programme on performance data to identify the
behaviour change goal and on learning theory to teach a new, or modify
an existing, vocal behaviour (Leith and Johnson, 1986; Wilson, 1987).

Regardless of the procedural approach employed, vocal competence
must be improved in relation to the needs of the child in context. A valid
intervention approach must consider the adult–child dyad as the
dynamic unit of vocal competence rather than the child's vocal production alone. The treatment approach should address care givers as critical
to the vocal rehabilitation of their children, under the assumption that
the use of certain interactive and vocal styles allows children to learn
spontaneously from them during habitual conversational exchanges.
Adults can alter linguistic, social and affective aspects of their communicative interactions to help the child actively in vocal rehabilitation. The
critical issue posed by this treatment model is that change generally
occurs when adults and children progress together.

The overriding concern is that the therapeutic goals and activities are developmentally appropriate for the child. Ideally, the clinician helps teachers and family members structure parallel activities and experiences. Therapeutic activities with this age group must be specific and concrete. Therapy sessions should be of short duration and should be supported and expanded by input from parents and other care givers. The clinician should formulate specific, concrete activities using developmentally appropriate linguistic input. Repetition of stimuli is imperative and consistency across care givers is essential. Teachers are helpful consultants in the design and implementation of the therapy programme.

The majority of voice disorders in children are due to abuse and misuse of the voice and result in glottal-margin pathologies. Such pathologies are treated conservatively and the management of choice is voice therapy. In discussing the voice therapy programme for children who engage in vocal hyperfunction with the concomitants of vocal-fold inflammation, oedema and nodules, there is little need to make a clinical distinction in treatment as one is dealing with a common aetiology. The goal of voice therapy for vocal hyperfunction is to reduce vocal-fold trauma through re-education and to modify or eliminate environmental stress.

Voice goals may be organized under the banners of awareness and production. The initial part of the voice therapy programme should concentrate on developing an awareness of the problem and outlining the possible benefits of therapy. Explanation regarding the causative factors of the child's voice problem helps both child and parents to understand the importance of their role in vocal rehabilitation. The role of the parents and significant others in the child's environment cannot be underestimated and it may be that the ultimate success of the voice therapy programme will depend on the success achieved in gaining parental understanding and co-operation at this early stage. During this phase the child learns to isolate appropriate and inappropriate vocal behaviours and to discriminate between them. Successful elimination of faulty vocal habits is predicted on their accurate identification. Substitute vocal behaviours need to be introduced to compensate partly for what the child is relinquishing. The child's use of abusive vocal production is often a reaction to environmental factors. Efficient monitoring and modification of vocal behaviour patterns in the child, therefore, should be extended to include active participation of parents, teachers and significant others. It is inappropriate to engage in vocal modification procedures in the child without focusing on the reciprocal behaviours of both the child and significant others in his environment. The use of a vocal-model therapeutic paradigm, both within and outside the clinical situation, is essential. Such a model obviates the need for verbal and symbolic mediation and instead places emphasis on sensory decoding and encoding (Champley and Andrews 1993).

Carryover and habituation are particularly difficult for children as they are more concerned with day-to-day issues of living than directing their energies towards changing patterns of vocal behaviour. It is difficult for any child to see the value of vocal hygiene. To ignore this reality will result in the clinician's failure to effect change. The amount and nature of responsibility placed on a child will depend on age and on the co-operation of significant others. Unless vocal behaviours are habitually traumatic, time may be more profitably spent in controlling environmental conditions that give rise to vocally abusive patterns. Such control is considerably more certain than control of the child's vocal performance once he is in those conditions.

Following modification of vocally abusive behaviour patterns, techniques such as those recommended by Wilson (1987) and Andrews (1986) to improve vocal production may be undertaken. With many children, progress in the vocal abuse reduction programme results in a definite reduction in glottal-margin pathology and an improvement in vocal quality. Consequently, it is rarely necessary to work directly with the child to influence or modify phonatory behaviour. The use of instrumentation to control the child's vocal behaviour can make voice therapy an interesting and more effective process, as this allows objective assessment of habitual vocal characteristics, awareness of inappropriate vocal parameters by means of auditory and visual feedback, and ease of acquisition of new vocal behaviour patterns. The use of instrumentation in vocal rehabilitation programmes continues to accelerate and professionals will find new and interesting applications for the voice-disordered child.

Ongoing Management

Children undergoing regular voice therapy should have indirect laryngoscopic examination every three months. Laryngeal changes will be apparent at this stage if voice therapy is effective. In addition, to ensure long-term carryover of new vocal behaviours, periodic reviews should be scheduled following completion of the intervention programme. Factors which are influential in determining prognosis include history, duration and severity of the disorder, aetiological correlates, intrinsic and extrinsic motivational factors, and immediate and extended environmental characteristics. The clinician should also consider the question of remission of the presenting symptoms, in the absence of voice therapy. Many childhood voice disorders lessen in degree and frequently resolve with increase in age. This is possibly due to the stabilization of laryngeal size and the acquisition of adult vocal behaviours, during which vocal abuse is less likely to occur.

Effectiveness of Therapy

Speech and language therapists are currently attempting to increase objectivity and accountability in the treatment of communication disorders. Our performance approach to evaluation and treatment and our current emphasis on vocal competence as an aspect of communicative competence is a reflection of such professional emphasis. Although this has produced numerous new rating scales, innovative therapeutic approaches, and technical hardware to enhance our clinical effectiveness, it has also served to re-emphasize the importance of the child/family/clinician relationship in the therapeutic process. Clinicians have a renewed respect for the importance of knowing the child and his family, beyond the objective and accountable data found in the case file.

Communication is a valuable tool in understanding the child's environment and clinicians should foster parental involvement in order to ensure the effectiveness of intervention. Furthermore consideration of vocal function must be made in the light of a child's communicative competence. Therapy has little hope of success if it is not founded on careful and comprehensive assessment and then carried out within the framework of communication.

References

Andrews ML (1986) Voice Therapy for Children. London: Longman.

Aronson AE (1985) Clinical Voice Disorders (2nd ed.). New York: Brian C. Decker Division, Thieme Stratton.

Boone D, McFarlane S (1988) The Voice and Voice Therapy (4th ed.) Englewood Cliffs, NJ: Prentice Hall.

Dobres R, Lee L, Stemple, JC, Kummer, AW, Kretschmer LW (1990) Description of laryngeal pathologies in children evaluated by otorhinolarngologists. Journal of Speech and Hearing Disorders 55: 526–32.

Champley E, Andrews ML (1993) The Elicitation of Vocal Responses from Preschool Children. Language, Speech and Hearing Services in Schools 24: 146–50.

Green G (1989) Psycho-behavioural characterictics of children with vocal nodules; WPBIC ratings. Vocal nodules and aggression. Journal of Speech and Hearing Disorders 54: 306–12.

Leith W, Johnson R (1986) Handbook of Voice Therapy for the School Clinician. London: Taylor and Francis.

Miller SQ, Madison CL (1984) Public school voice clinics, Part 1:A working model. Language Speech and Hearing Services in the Schools 15: 51–7.

Morrison MD, Rammage LA, Belisle GM, Pullan CB, Nichol H (1983) Muscular Tension Dysphonia. Journal of Otolaryngology 12: 302–6.

Ogura JH, Thawley EE (1980) Cysts and tumours of the larynx. In Paparella MM, Shrumick DA (Eds) Otolaryngology. Vol.3. Head & Neck (2nd ed.). Philadelphia, PA: Saunders.

Sloan LP, Montague JE, Buffalo MD (1986) A preliminary survey on the relationship of exogenous factors to laryngeal papilloma. Language, Speech and Hearing Services in Schools 17: 292–9.

Smith RJH, Catlin FL (1984) Congenital anomalies of the larynx. American Journal of Diseases of Children 138: 35–9.

Van Riper C (1939) Speech Correction: Principles and Methods. New York: Prentice Hall.

Wilson DK (1983) Management of voice disorders in children and adolescents. Seminars in Speech and Language 4: 245–58.

Wilson DK (1987) Voice Problems of Children. (3rd ed.) Baltimore: Williams and Wilkins.

Chapter 9
Childhood Stuttering

IRMGARDE A. HORSLEY

Dysfluency, in its various forms such as hesitations, pauses, repetitions, revisions, interjections and prolongations, is a natural aspect of speaking. It reflects various cognitive, affective and linguistic processes that occur when both children and adults are speaking, and, by and large, these dysfluencies are either ignored by the listener or are used as clues to meaning (Brotherton, 1979; Kowal, O'Connell and Sabin, 1975; Sabin et al., 1979). A child's speech is likely to attract the label 'stuttering' when it contains either an excess of these dysfluencies or less common forms of dysfluency, such as part-word repetitions and prolongations and particularly so if there are any signs of facial or physical tension when speaking. It is the type and frequency of speech dysfluencies, rather than their actual duration, that lead listeners to decide that it is stuttering they hear (Zebrowski, 1991). Interestingly, clinicians and untrained lay listeners show good agreement when listening to audio samples regarding the presence of stuttering in young children (Onslow et al., 1992). Clinically, the question is whether or not a child displaying dysfluencies is likely to develop chronic stuttering. The term 'normal non-fluency' is often contrasted with the term 'dysfluency' when describing the speech of young children. Both terms refer to breaks in the continuity of speech, but 'dysfluency' is generally used to describe speech that has more in common with stuttering. Starkweather, Gottwald and Halfond (1990) define stuttering as 'speech that is produced intermittently with excessive effort'.

Stuttering usually appears initially between the ages of 2 and 5 years (Andrews and Harris, 1964; Bloodstein, 1987) at a time when a child's language is in a state of rapid growth. For pre-school children, it has been reported that by 3.5 years of age the risk of stuttering is reduced by 75 per cent (Yairi and Ambrose, 1992b). Early childhood stuttering has been described as being of gradual onset and consisting of easy repetitions in the early stages, with little or no secondary signs such as tension, awareness or negative reactions. However, this traditional concept has been called into question. Recent studies of pre-school children report cases of sudden onset with severe symptoms, including some of the secondary signs (Yairi, Ambrose and Niermann, 1993; Yairie and Ambrose, 1992a, b).

Whether or not delayed speech and language is found more often in children who stutter is unclear (Ryan, 1992; Nippold, 1990). There has been considerable speculation that stutterers have problems with either overall co-ordination of the respiratory, laryngeal and articulatory systems or with one particular system, but the evidence remains equivocal. As Starkweather (1991) points out, it is very possible that some of the aspects of delayed language performance observed in young stuttering children actually represent strategies to avoid using complex utterances and thus reduce the likelihood of stuttering. He also points out that it is not all that uncommon to witness stuttering in a young child whose language performance is advanced. It is more likely, therefore, that only a subset of children who stutter have concomitant speech and language problems.

Fluency breakdown has been reported in some children with developmental language disorders (Hall, Yamashita and Aram, 1993). Boys are more likely to stutter than are girls at an estimated ratio of 3:1 (Bloodstein, 1981). In pre-school children, the male-to-female ratio is 2:1 or even smaller (Yairi and Ambrose, 1992b), whereas with adult stutterers, the male-to-female ratio is 5:1 or even higher (Leske, 1981). The familial risk is also increased if at least one parent ever stuttered and is related to the sex of the relative (Kidd, 1985).

Causative Factors

The current view is that multiple factors, including both genetically disposing factors and environmental contributions, are involved in the aetiology of stuttering (Smith, 1990). The genetically disposing factors which have been proposed are a reduction in central capacity for efficient sensory motor integration (Andrews *et al.*, 1983) or a deficit in the ability to programme and initiate movements (Peters and Hulstijn, 1987), a conclusion mirrored by *some*, but by no means *all*, recent reports on various aspects of sensory motor functioning in stutterers. The environmental or psychosocial factors are those which contribute to and maintain learned aspects of stuttering. These include communicative and general stresses which have been demonstrated to be of importance because their removal or reduction may result in stuttering being removed or reduced. It is important to remember that much of our information about stuttering comes from reports from studies of adult stutterers. As Conture (1991) points out, child and adult stutterers differ in many important ways other than chronological age, which makes extrapolation between them difficult and most likely misleading. It may be that much of the disordered motor and acoustic timing reported in adults is the result of compensatory reactions to long-term stuttering (Molt 1991).

Basically, some children who stutter have a familial history of stuttering and some do not. There are various factors as a child is acquiring speech and language and maturing which may determine whether or not stuttering behaviour emerges. A consideration of environmental factors encompasses aspects of peri- and pre-natal conditions, as well as accidents and illnesses, any of which could have a detrimental effect on a child's capacity for fluent speech organization. Stuttering is also reported to be more prevalent amongst those who have suffered some form of cerebral damage (Bloodstein, 1981; Van Riper, 1982). Whether or not a child without any predisposing factors who was subject to various environmental stresses, would develop a chronic stutter remains a major question.

Assessment Considerations

The speech of any child referred to a clinician because of dysfluency noted by someone in the child's environment needs to be evaluated because, if for no other reason, concern about some aspect of the child's speech development has been expressed. The extent of the evaluation may vary depending on the information gained from the interview with the parents and initial contact with the child. Certainly, assessment should be viewed as an ongoing process. The clinician must satisfy herself about various components of the child's development, which will include more than speech and language. There is evidence that non-speech behaviours, such as facial and body movements that have been described as being associated with stuttering, warrant attention and may be important diagnostic signs (Schwartz, Zebrowski and Conture, 1990; Conture and Kelly, 1991). Finally she needs to decide to what extent environmental factors may be contributing to the difficulty, before deciding on the level of intervention.

The case history, usually through parental interview, is the beginning of the compilation of information and should take place without the child being present. The clinician, through sensitive and informed discussion, will hope to obtain information about familial speech and language development and the stage and course of the child's development of speech and language. Of equal importance is information about general and motor development, behaviour, health, and parental attitudes towards these. The interview should also provide the parent(s) with an opportunity to ask questions and discuss any anxieties. In essence, what is being built up is a picture of the child's communication environment together with a description of the dysfluent behaviours, as well as when and how often they occur. As childhood dysfluency is very often cyclical, one needs to discover the presence and length of such cycles.

The clinician is attempting to discover both overt and covert contributions to the child's dysfluency. However, not every case interview will necessarily be ideal and yield the desired information on the first occasion, and perhaps not even on subsequent ones. Most usually, the informant is one parent who may be unaware of specific aspects of family history and/or who may find it difficult to be informative. In that event even more emphasis will be placed on the second aspect of evaluation. Here, one needs, insofar as possible, an environment that fits the child. This second aspect will include an assessment by the clinician of the child's speech, language and possibly hearing. This should include a recording of the child's spontaneous conversation both with parents and with the clinician, as well as in more structured situations.

Wherever possible, multiple evaluations of the child's speech should be made in naturalistic settings (e.g. in the home, at nursery or school). Traditionally, the age of the child has been a major factor in evaluating stuttering symptoms and deciding on the course of therapy (i.e. the dysfluent pre-school child has usually been treated differently from the school-age child). However, it cannot be overemphasized that each child needs thorough individual evaluation, and so the age of the child can serve only as a rough guide at best. Excellent detailed models of evaluation are provided by Adams (1984a, b), Riley and Riley (1984), Cooper and Cooper (1985), Gregory (1986), Rustin (1987), Starkweather (1987), Starkweather et al. (1990), Costello (1993), Curlee (1993), Gregory and Hill (1993), Wall and Myers (1994) and may also be found in many other current texts. One aim is to attempt to decide to what extent the child's dysfluency is within normal limits, commensurate with both general and speech development and therefore less likely to be a matter of future concern. There is reasonable agreement about what are considered normal and less usual non-fluencies across a number of studies. Overlaps of both types have been found to be present in the speech samples of young children labelled as stutterers and of non-stuttering controls (Hubbard and Yairi, 1988; Yairi and Lewis, 1984; Bloodstein and Grossman, 1981; Wexler and Mysak 1982; Bjerkan, 1980; Floyd and Perkins, 1974; Johnson and Associates, 1959). The important ones to note as abnormal dysfluencies are part-word sound and syllable repetitions (broken words) and sound prolongations. Normal dysfluencies include silent and filled pauses such as interjections of sounds and syllables, revisions and incomplete phrases and whole-word repetition.

Gregory (1986) considers that dysfluencies should be viewed on a continuum from the more usual to the more unusual. Warning signs include the presence of the schwa vowel, airflow disruptions, irregular tempo and/or breathing patterns, and signs of excess tension in articulation. However, dysfluencies of any kind may interact with how frequently they occur in the child's speech. Even so-called normal dysfluencies may lead to a diagnosis of stuttering if they are a substantial portion of the child's speech. Not surprisingly, dysfluent speech often interacts with the acquisition and use of more complex syntactic and semantic structures (Bloodstein, 1981). In a similar way, the pragmatics of a particular situation may affect fluency, e.g. interrupting or directing activities (Myers and Freeman, 1985a, b). A child's awareness of difficulty in speaking takes on different degrees of importance, depending on the extent of this awareness, behavioural reaction to this awareness, and the age of the child. Onslow (1992a, b) presents some of the issues and possible strategies involved in the identification of early stuttering including Adams's (1977) suggestion of an 'at risk' register, which involves regular observations of the child and/or parental telephone contact.

Theoretical Basis of Intervention

Andrews et al. (1983), among others, have pointed out that stuttering onset most often appears at a time when a child is experiencing an explosive growth in language ability, but has an immature speech motor apparatus (usually between 3 and 6 years of age). It is estimated that 60 per cent of children who have stuttered for less than one year will spontaneously recover without direct intervention (Andrews, 1985). Yairi (1993) reports preliminary results of a longitudinal study indicating a recovery rate of 65–75 per cent or even higher. By 16 years of age, the recovery rate is 78 per cent (Andrews et al., 1983). Kent (1976), reviewing acoustic data on various aspects of speech production, concluded that the accuracy of motor control improves with age until about 11-12 years of age, depending upon the child's individual pattern of motor development, until adult-like performance is reached. Also, various aspects of language development continue until adolescence with periods of instability (Palermo and Molfese, 1972). It is possible that cyclical dysfluency in young children is a reflection of periods of linguistic instability combined with variability in motor control. As Curlee (1980) suggests, it is tempting to speculate about the possible relationship between these high recovery rates and maturational processes, i.e. recovery occurs when abilities catch up with linguistic demands.

The Demands and Capacities Model (Starkweather, 1987) states that fluency will falter when demands (either from the environment *or* self-imposed) exceed the speaker's capacity for responding. This capacity for responding includes cognitive, linguistic, motoric and/or emotional factors. Adams (1990) points out that there is no need to think that some deficiencies and/or abnormalities exist. The essential point is that demands exceed capacity. Viewed this way, stuttering can develop when the environment of a child demands more fluent speech than the child is currently capable of producing. The model is presented as a means of organizing our current knowledge about childhood stuttering, *not* as an explanation of the aetiology of stuttering (Starkweather and Gottwald, 1990; Starkweather et al., 1990).

This model explains the rationale behind the most common therapeutic approaches to treatment of young children, particularly for those just beginning to stutter; namely, the indirect approach or prevention.

Main-line Approaches

Preventive therapy encompasses a number of aspects. One is providing the parents with clear and simple information about speech and language development and the variations in fluency that all speakers, particularly young children, experience. Another is the exploration and identification of any environmental factors which are conducive to fluency and those which may be related to increased dysfluency. Through parental counselling and guidance, possible ways of modifying the latter would be arrived at. The assumption and hope of this 'indirect' approach is that a reduction in communicative pressures, environmental stress and parental anxiety will have a positive effect on a child's fluency, i.e. a reduction in demands will mean that the child's communicative capacity is not being challenged. It is also important to establish and maintain contact with the parents over a subsequent period of time and ensure that they will feel comfortable about contacting the clinician should they become concerned at any time about their child's speech.

Irwin (1994), Perkins (1992,) Starkweather et al. (1990), and Van Riper (1973) clearly describe the kinds of difficulties that can arise in the verbal behaviour between parent and child and the importance of introducing positive behaviours and perceptions into the relationship. The type of verbal behaviours identified as potential fluency disrupters include excessive interruptions, finishing the child's statements, filling in words, asking multiple questions at once, constant correction of a child's verbal and non-verbal behaviour, a very rapid speech and conversation rate, and topic switching. More general disruptive communicative behaviours may involve such things as listener loss, competition and time pressure over speaking, display and demand speech. Inconsistent family routines or severe family problems are also potentially emotionally disruptive factors.

However, parental counselling often will need to go beyond that focus. Parents need the opportunity to discuss and understand their own emotional and behavioural responses as well as any other concerns which may arise during the treatment process (Zebrowski and Schum, 1993). There are often subtle aspects of the parent/child relationship, particularly expectations or negative perceptions of the child, which need to be uncovered and discussed. These are often based on ordinary and understandable anxieties caused by comparisons with other children or by negative comments made by other people in the child's environment. Parental expectations about children's speech and general behaviour may be uninformed or unrealistic. Obviously, it is important to avoid imparting a sense of blame and guilt to the parents who are already concerned.

Those individual factors that need to be dealt with will be obtained from both the case history and from observation and analysis of the communicative and general relationship of parents and child. Wherever possible, the counselling process needs to involve all those individuals in the environment likely to have an effect on the child's fluency (e.g. siblings, grandparents and teachers). Adams (1984a) succinctly summarizes the guidelines arising out of differential diagnosis. When a child displays little or infrequent awareness of speech difficulty and therefore no serious reactions, when there are no other developmental problems, behavioural or speech- and-language related, and where the environment presents no apparent difficulties, then the indirect method would be the most likely approach to management.

The use of this indirect approach is widespread, as can be seen in any current text, and its effectiveness is assumed. As Prins (1983) points out, there are many reported clinical observations that manipulating patterns of listening to and responding to the young stuttering child result in fluency changes. Unfortunately, evaluation data are virtually non-existent, and so the real value of this approach remains unsubstantiated. Given the high estimated rate of recovery in childhood, where failure to recover is the exception, plus the absence of the essential matched control groups to evaluate the degree of spontaneous recovery likely to account for positive outcomes, any claims concerning effectiveness of this approach have to be viewed with these reservations in mind.

Direct Therapy

Whether or not some degree of direct therapy with the child is also indicated will depend on the presence and degree of borderline stuttering behaviours previously described, the length of time they have been present, and the child's reactions to his speech disruptions. Direct treatment approaches are therefore employed when the clinician has reason to believe that the child's symptoms indicate the likelihood of a chronic stutter developing and that direct work will not be harmful in the sense of exacerbating the dysfluency or by introducing awareness of speech difficulty where none previously existed. The combination of indirect treatment including parental counselling and environmental manipulation, together with direct modification of the child's speech, is the most common form of treatment which would follow once it was clear that activities geared towards secondary prevention alone were not enough. This approach might be termed 'intermediate'. Descriptions of this combination can be found in Rustin and Cook (1983), Cooper (1984),

Riley and Riley (1984), Wall and Myers (1984, 1994), Gregory (1986), Starkweather et al. (1990) and Gregory and Hill (1993), to name only a few. Some would recommend direct treatment using operant techniques as a first line approach (Ingham, 1983a; Onslow, 1992b; Costello, 1993).

Mainstream Treatment Practices

Despite the fact that the vast majority of childhood dysfluency disorders will, for one reason or another, resolve themselves, we remain desperately short of information as to the course this resolution follows. There have unfortunately been few attempts to follow-up and evaluate therapy with young children which meet the basic requirements for an evaluative study with the notable exception of a report by Onslow, Costa and Rue (1990).

Currently, there are a number of models for treating childhood dysfluency, most of which share similar principles in both differential diagnosis and therapy, but some use different terminology. Consideration will be given to those which have made some effort to assess the effectiveness of their approach or which are considered to represent a significant trend in the management of childhood stuttering. Although they may fail to demonstrate the basic requirements needed to indicate the efficacy of the therapy used (Bloodstein, 1981; Ingham, 1983a), their clarity of approach recommends them as a starting point for the newly qualified clinician.

Differential Diagnosis and Therapy

The first model to be considered is that of Gregory (1973, 1980, 1986) and Gregory and Hill (1980, 1993) because it covers the whole range of possible approaches. By its very nature, it is the least controversial and perhaps the most helpful to the clinician, beginning or experienced. The determination of treatment is systematically explored through the evaluation of the individual child. This model identifies four possible results of differential diagnosis with corresponding treatment approaches. The treatment strategy followed when identifying the 'typically' dysfluent child is preventive parent counselling only. What is important here is that even when the child's non-fluency is clinically considered to be within acceptable ordinary limits, parents who have been concerned about a child's fluency should receive some counselling, usually involving attention to parental concerns and observations about the child.

In the first instance, the 'preventive' counselling process, which has already been described, would be used. Where the child is displaying borderline type dysfluencies, e.g. more unusual dysfluencies, more definite stuttering behaviours but no other difficulties with speech and language development, and the problem has been noted for less than a year, Gregory's approach is again to counsel the parents and see the child for brief therapy. The general principles of preventive counselling are followed, but the parents become more deeply involved in a number of ways. With the child, the clinician models a slower, easier and relaxed speaking method with pauses between shorter phrases. The clinician's modelling behaviour is observed by the parents and is gradually taken over by them.

When the child is showing complicating speech, language, or behavioural problems in addition to dysfluencies *or* when the dysfluencies are largely composed of speech behaviours judged as typical of stuttering behaviours, usually compounded by reports of long-term parental concern, then the approach involves a comprehensive therapy programme. This third strategy obviously includes the elements of the first two approaches, as well as a highly individualized and intensive treatment programme involving both child and parents. The main aim is to enhance fluency by the use of *direct* speech modification procedures, depending on the needs of the individual child. These fluency-enhancing techniques will be mentioned in more detail when considering Cooper's (1978, 1984) approach to treatment, but they are well described in Gregory and Hill (1980, 1993), Costello (1983) and Adams (1984b). Gregory and Hill (1980) reported that, of the children in the comprehensive therapy programme, 70 per cent developed and maintained fluency as evaluated in a follow-up of 9 to 18 months. The remaining 30 per cent were referred to other disciplines after interfering factors were identified. Subsequently, this figure was raised to 75 per cent, and reports about preventive parental counselling, with and without limited treatment for the child, simply state success after four to eight weekly sessions (Gregory, 1986).

Personalized Fluency Control Therapy

Cooper and Cooper (1976, 1985), over an extended period, have developed a programme called Personalized Fluency Control Therapy which integrates cognitive and behaviour therapy for stutterers of all ages. The therapeutic activities are highly individualized and depend on the client's abilities, type of dysfluency problems and environmental factors. There are several useful graphic representations of various aspects of the therapeutic process which would certainly be appealing to the young child. These include the 'stuttering apple' which visually incorporates individual stuttering behaviours. 'My monkeys' help identify negative feelings and attitudes, and the 'FIG' tree aims to identify various fluency-initiating gestures in pictorial form.

Considerable emphasis is placed on the need for a positive relationship between clinician and child. The aim, for any age group, is the feeling of fluency control, which is achieved by working through a well-defined series of stages, with specified short-term and long-term goals. The first stage is identification and structuring, which enables the individual to identify the feelings, attitudes and actual behaviours which are all part of the problem of stuttering and to understand the direction and goals of therapy. It is at this stage that the structure of the therapeutic relationship is established.

The second stage is examination and confrontation. In this stage, the modification of various behaviours related to dysfluency, both within and outside the clinical setting are introduced. Both resistance and success are verbally identified by the clinician and reinforcement of the client's expressions and opinions about the therapeutic process is provided. The emphasis and method in this stage will depend on the individual client's needs. There is, however, a clear marriage between consideration of the stutterer's feelings and attitudes and the modification of stuttering behaviours. The third stage of cognition and behaviour orientation continues the process of reinforcement and facilitation of both self-evaluation and commitment.

The use of fluency-initiating gestures introduces behaviours which promote increased fluency and are methods which form a part of most therapeutic approaches. These are reduction of speech rate, easy voice onset combined with a consciously controlled inhalation. Control of loudness, together with light articulatory contact during speech, as well as manipulation of stress patterns are other concepts introduced to the child, usually together with the parents. Transfer to specific situations outside the clinic is the next procedure followed.

Cooper and Cooper (1985, 1991) believe that the cognitive and affective aspects of stuttering have been neglected because of the focus on what they call the 'frequency fallacy'; i.e. considering the *frequency* of dysfluencies to be the most important factor in assessment, treatment and evaluation of progress. Therapeutic success or failure should be judged on changes in the client's fluency, attitudes, and, in the view of Cooper and Cooper, it is a feeling of fluency control that reflects a successful outcome. They advise that, after therapy is terminated, evaluation follow-ups should continue for at least three years. Assessment and therapy procedures are well described in both the therapy packages (Cooper and Cooper, 1976, 1985). The status report of evaluation insofar as children are concerned is couched in the most general terms, e.g. four out of every five abnormally dysfluent pre-school children can be helped to achieve normal fluency by the time they complete the primary school years (approximately 80 per cent) (Cooper, 1984).

Wall and Myers (1994) present a model for the assessment and treatment of stuttering children which comprises the three factors known to be of interactive importance, namely, psycholinguistic, physiological and psychosocial factors. In their model, variables under each heading are examined and their contribution to the problem evaluated. Basically, theirs is an eclectic and broad-based view which considers the child's overall communicative functioning at every level and so provides the clinician with guidelines which will ensure that no possible contributing factor will be inadvertently ignored.

Operant Conditioning Approaches

The issue of whether the young stutterer should be treated directly has usually been considered in relation to the age of the child, i.e. treatment for the pre-school child should be indirect or preventive and treatment for the school-age child should most likely be a combination of indirect and direct work on stuttering symptoms. Several proponents of direct amelioration of stuttering, even in the very young child, include Ryan (1974, 1986), Costello (1980, 1983, 1984, 1985, 1993), Riley and Riley (1983, 1984) and Shine (1984a, b). These authors take the view that the earlier the direct intervention in any communication disorder, the more likely the chance of success. They reject the idea that calling the young child's attention to stuttering will exacerbate the problem. As has been pointed out, at least some of the spontaneous remission reported may in fact be due to parental intervention of just this type (Ingham, 1983b; Cooper, 1984; Martin and Lindamood, 1986). Assessment aimed at differential diagnosis may range from the simple to complex (Riley and Riley, 1983, 1984) prior to therapeutic intervention. Therapy is based on the principles of operant conditioning which in essence involves the manipulation of consequences to increase or decrease a behaviour; in this case to increase fluency and decrease stuttering. This feedback may be either positive (a reward) or negative (punishment).

Costello (1983, 1985, 1993) succinctly states the rationale for this approach by pointing out several assumptions in the use of the indirect or parental counselling method that may be unwarranted. For one thing, no valid *empirical evidence* exists to indicate that family and environmental variables are functionally related to stuttering. Why then, she asks, should the clinician have the right to ask families to rearrange their lives when it cannot be said with any confidence which, if any, aspects of the child's environment are contributing to and maintaining stuttering?

The second issue she raises is that attempting to change familial behaviour over which one has no control is at best a difficult process and certainly not one amenable to observation or measurement. The clinician is reliant on parental reports of unverifiable accuracy. Instead, her approach is to teach the young child directly how to produce fluent speech, irrespective of environmental aspects. The treatment strategy is simple and structured, moving from short and simple fluent utterances to longer and more complex ones, termed the Extended Length of Utterances (ELU) programme which is similar to the Graduated Increase in Length and Complexity of Utterance (GILCU) of the Monterey

Programme (Ryan, 1974, 1986). During each stage of the treatment programme, the child's behaviour is systematically rewarded or punished and in this way guided to the next stage. Positive reinforcement for non-stuttered utterances is by means of a token system together with social reinforcement, i.e. positive verbal comments of a general nature.

Punishment contingencies for stuttering may take the form of the clinician saying 'stop' (time-out procedure) as soon as a stuttered utterance occurs so that the child does not continue speaking until the next trial begins. Reinforcers are gradually faded out as the programme progresses, so as to prevent the child's becoming dependent on external feedback. In this approach, explanations of the rationale underlying therapy are *not* given to the child nor are they considered advisable.

Other components may be added to the treatment programme if deemed necessary (i.e. if adequate change in fluency is not attained and if evaluation indicates that certain aspects of the child's speech need attention). These are the same fluency-promoting techniques described previously; e.g. rate control, easy voice onset, the reduction of linguistic complexity in utterances, depending again on assessment data. Parents are involved as much as possible, observing every session and being taught to recognize fluent utterances and give *positive* reinforcers, but *not* to use punishment procedures. The latter are avoided because of the danger of inappropriate or excessive use of punishment; this avoidance is considered to be controlled for by not having the parent perform a step in the programme until the child has satisfactorily performed at that level in the clinic.

Several questions arise when considering this approach. For one thing, how does the clinician ensure that parents do not use at home the punishment procedures they have observed in the clinic? In the same vein, how does the clinician ensure that the parent gives positive reinforcers appropriately? The same criticism may be made of this procedure as Costello (1993, 1995) makes about the uncertainty of environmental manipulation, i.e. difficult to verify and ensure. The therapy programme depends on the child performing various speaking tasks of increasing complexity in the clinic. Costello (1993, 1995) states that any child who speaks in connected utterances, and who has been labelled a stutterer, may be a candidate for *direct* work on stuttering. However, some young children who stutter are not easily engaged in verbal activities for a number of reasons. Some may be more interested in play activities which, although capable of eliciting speech, do not invariably lend themselves to the structuring of speech situations. Young children who are engrossed in play situations may not attend to reinforcers. Childhood stuttering is very often cyclical, both in severity and occurrence and there may be too few examples of dysfluency in the clinic.

However, the force and simplicity of the operant approach is obvious.

Ingham (1993) asks why this approach is so little used or advocated in current texts, given earlier reports of its success (Martin, Kuhl and Haroldson, 1972; Reed and Godden, 1977). A possible explanation is that behavioural methods are considered by many to be a mechanistic approach to the problem of stuttering that ignores the individual's feelings and environment. Also, most clinicians are not trained in the use of behavioural methods, do not feel comfortable with them and are apprehensive that they may misapply them. The case for behavioural treatment approaches is not helped by imprecise use of terms and confounding of treatment effects, such as presented in a report by Gagnon and Ladouceur (1992), which gives an account of the 'effectiveness' of a behavioural treatment of child stutterers based on the 'regulated breathing method' (Azrin and Nunn, 1974). In this study, so many different forms of treatment were used that it would be hard to attribute success to any particular one of them, e.g. awareness training, regulated breathing, modification of parental attitudes and beliefs, easy speech and group practice. By contrast, an interesting study by Onslow et al. (1990) trained parents to verbally elicit responses from their children and provide verbal feedback with promising results. Onslow (1992b) admits that the necessary replication studies have not materialized, but in a review of possible treatment procedures, he concludes that operant methodology is conceptually and practically the most justifiable therapeutic approach with young children. With direct approaches to young children, as with indirect approaches, some reservation about the effectiveness of intervention must remain.

Effectiveness of Therapy

For most approaches, published evaluation data in general are at best incomplete and at worst vague and anecdotal. There is little data on recovery as a direct result of treatment available for scrutiny. Consequently, it is not really possible to exclude reported success rates from spontaneous recovery rates estimated at 78 per cent based on the results of several studies. This observation is not meant to suggest that treatment approaches for children are of no or little benefit. Rather it is intended to highlight the need to design one's intervention in such a way as to be able to answer questions about the characteristics of stuttering in young children and how these change over time with and without intervention. Some believe that this can be achieved only by designing and implementing carefully controlled longitudinal studies together with the appropriate control groups (Purser, 1987; St. Louis and Westbrook, 1987). Andrews (1985), puts this view more strongly by saying that no study purporting to benefit pre-school stutterers should be accepted unless it compares a randomized controlled trial of treatment with a placebo condition. However, a good beginning could be made if individual interventions were framed as single case studies. These could supply valuable normative data as well as bringing us nearer to answering the question: why do some things we do work with some children but not others?

Conclusion

Any child who exhibits dysfluent speech behaviours sufficient to cause concern at any level needs to be considered in relation to as many aspects of his/her development and environment as possible. Given the current state of our knowledge, it would seem wise to keep an open mind about the value of different approaches with young children. It is unlikely that there can ever be a blanket approach to the treatment of stuttering in children. What is needed are developmental studies of interventions, both single-case and group, based on objective reliable speech and language data charting the changes in stuttering behaviours that occur and their relation to other aspects of development. With reliable information about the progress from dysfluency to fluency, we can begin to develop a system of soundly based and justifiable differential management.

> Insufficient knowledge of developmental factors of early childhood stuttering appears to be the most serious obstacle for quality research on treatment efficacy for this age group. (Yairi, 1993)

References

Adams MR (1977) The Young Stutterer: Diagnosis, Treatment and Assessment of Progress. Seminars in Speech, Language and Hearing 1: 289–99.

Adams MR (1984a) The differential assessment and direct treatment of stuttering. In Costello J (Ed) Speech Disorders in Children: Recent Advances. San Diego, CA: College Hill.

Adams MR (1984b) The young stutterer: Diagnosis, treatment and assessment of progress. In Perkins WH (Ed) Stuttering Disorders. New York: Thieme Stratton.

Adams M R (1990) The Demands and Capacity Model I: Theoretical Elaborations. Journal of Fluency Disorders 15: 135–41.

Andrews G (1985) Epidemiology of stuttering. In Curlee RF, Perkins WH (Eds) Nature and Treatment of Stuttering: New Directions. London: Taylor and Francis.

Andrews G, Craig S, Feyers AM, Hoddinott S, Howie P, Neilson M (1983) Stuttering: A review of research findings and theories circa 1982. Journal of Speech and Hearing Disorders 48: 22–46.

Andrews G, Harris M (1964) The Syndrome of Stuttering. Clinics in Developmental Medicine (No. 17). London: Heinemann.

Azrin NH, Nunn RG (1974) A rapid method of eliminating stuttering by a regulated breathing approach. Behaviour Research and Therapy 12: 279–86.

Bjerkan B (1980) Word fragmentations and repetitions in the spontaneous speech of

2–6 year-old children. Journal of Fluency Disorders 5: 137–48.

Bloodstein O (1981) A Handbook of Stuttering (3rd ed). Chicago, IL: National Easter Seal Society.

Bloodstein O, Grossman M (1981) Early stutterings; Some aspects of their form and distribution. Journal of Speech and Hearing Research 24: 298–302.

Bloodstein O (1987) A Handbook on Stuttering. Chicago, IL: National Easter Seal Society.

Brotherton P (1979) Speaking and not speaking: processes for translating ideas into speech. In Siegman AW, Feldstein S (Eds) Of Speech and Time. Hillsdale, NJ: Lawrence Erlbaum.

Conture EG (1991) Young Stutterers' Speech Production: A Critical Review in Peters HFM, HulstijnW, Starkweather WC (Eds) Speech Motor Control and Stuttering. Amsterdam: Elsevier.

Conture E, Kelly E (1991) Young stutterers' nonspeech behavior during stuttering. Journal of Speech and Hearing Research 34: 1041-56.

Cooper EB, Cooper CS (1976) Personalized Fluency Control Therapy Kit. Hingham, MA: Teaching Resources.

Cooper EB (1978) Facilitating parental participation in preparing the therapy component of the stutterer's individualised education program. Journal of Fluency Disorders 3: 221-8.

Cooper EB (1984) Personalized fluency control therapy; a status report. In Peins M (Ed) Contemporary Approaches in Stuttering Therapy. Boston: Little Brown.

Cooper EB, Cooper CS (1985) Personalized Fluency Control Therapy. Leicester: (Developmental Learning Materials) Taskmaster Ltd.

Cooper EB, Cooper CS (1991) A fluency disorders prevention program for preschoolers and children in the primary grades. American Journal of Speech-Language Pathology 1(September): 1.

Costello J (1980) Operant conditioning and the treatment of stuttering. In Perkins WH (Ed), Stuttering Disorders. New York: Thieme Stratton.

Costello J (1983) Current behavioral treatments for children. In Prins D, Ingham RJ (Eds) Treatment of Stuttering in Early Childhood: Methods and Issues. San Diego, CA: College-Hill.

Costello J (1984) Operant conditioning and the treatment of stuttering. In Perkins WH (Ed), Stuttering Disorders. New York: Thieme Stratton.

Costello J (1985) Treatment of the young chronic stutterer: Managing fluency. In Curlee RF and Perkins WH (Eds) Nature and Treatment of Stuttering: New Directions. London: Taylor and Francis.

Costello J (1993) Behavioral treatment of stuttering children. In Curlee R (Ed) Stuttering and Related Disorders of Fluency. New York: Thieme Medical

Curlee RF (1980) A case selection strategy for young disfluent children. Seminars in Speech Language and Hearing 1(4): 277–87.

Curlee RF (1984) A case selection strategy for young disfluent children. In Perkins WH (Ed), Stuttering Disorders. New York: Thieme Stratton.

Curlee RF (1993) Identification and Management of Beginning Stuttering. In Curlee R (Ed) Stuttering and Related Disorders of Fluency. New York: Thieme Medical.

Floyd S, Perkins WH (1974) Early syllable dysfluency in stutterers and non-stutterers: A preliminary report. Journal of Communication Disorders 7: 279–82.

Gagnon M, Ladoceur R (1992) Behavioral Treatment of Child Stutterers – Replication and Extension. Behaviour Therapy 23: 113–29.

Gregory H (1973) Stuttering: Differential Evaluation and Therapy. Indianapolis, IN: Bobbs-Merrill.

Gregory H (1980) Prevention of stuttering: Management of early stages. In Curlee RF, Perkins WH (Eds) Nature and Treatment of Stuttering. London: Taylor and Francis.

Gregory H, Hill D (1980) Stuttering therapy for children. In Perkins WH (Ed) Strategies in Stuttering Therapy. New York: Thieme Stratton.

Gregory H (1986) Environmental manipulation and family counselling. In Shames GH, Rubins H (Eds) Stuttering Then and Now. Columbus, OH: Merrill.

Gregory H, Hill D (1993) Differential evaluation—differential therapy for stuttering children. In Curlee R (Ed) Stuttering and Related Disorders of Fluency. New York: Thieme Medical

Hall NE, Yamashita TK, Aram DM. (1993) Relationship between language and fluency in children with developmental language disorders. Journal of Speech and Hearing Research 36(June): 3.

Hubbard C, Yairi E (1988) Clustering of disfluencies in the speech of stuttering and nonstuttering preschool children. Journal of Speech and Hearing Research 31: 228–33.

Ingham RJ (1983a) Stuttering and Behavior Therapy: Current Status and Experimental Foundations. San Diego, CA: College Hill.

Ingham RJ (1983b) Spontaneous remission of stuttering: when will the Emperor realize he has no clothes on? In Prins D, Ingham, RJ (Eds) Treatment of Stuttering in Early Childhood: Methods and Issues. San Diego, CA: College Hill.

Ingham RJ (1993) Current Status of Stuttering and Behavior Modification – II. Principal Issue and Practices in Stuttering Therapy. Journal of Fluency Disorders 18: 57–79.

Irwin A (1994) Stammering in Young Children (2nd ed). Hammersmith: Thorsons.

Johnson W and Associates (1959) The Onset of Stuttering. Minneapolis: University of Minnesota Press.

Kent RD (1976) Anatomical and neuromuscular maturation of the speech mechanism; evidence from acoustic studies. Journal of Speech and Hearing Research 19: 421–47.

Kidd KK (1985) Stuttering as a genetic disorder. In Curlee RF, Perkins WH (Eds) Nature and Treatment of Stuttering: New Directions. San Diego, CA: College Hill.

Kowal S, O'Connell DC, Sabin EJ (1975) Development of temporal patterning and vocal hesitations in spontaneous narratives. Journal of Psycholinguistic Research 4: 195–207.

Leske M (1981) Prevalence estimates of communicative disorders in the U.S.: Speech Disorders, ASHA 23: 217–25

Martin RR, Kuhl P, Haroldson SK (1972) An experimental treatment with two preschool stuttering children. Journal of Speech and Hearing Research 15: 743–52.

Martin RR, Lindamood LP (1986) Stuttering and spontaneous recovery: implications for the speech-language pathologist. Language, Speech and Hearing Services in School 17: 207–18.

Molt LF (1991) Selected acoustic and physiologic measures of speech motor coordination in stuttering and nonstuttering children. In Peters HFM, Hulstijn W, Starkweather, WC (Eds) Speech Motor Control and Stuttering. Amsterdam: Elsevier.

Myers SC, Freeman FJ (1985a) Are mothers of stutters different? an investigation of social-communicative interaction. Journal of Fluency Disorders 10: 193–210.

Myers SC, Freeman FJ (1985b) Interruptions as a variable in stuttering and disfluency. Journal of Speech and Hearing Research 28: 428–35.

Nippold MA (1990) Concomitant speech and language disorders in stuttering children: a critique of the literature. Journal of Speech and Hearing Disorders 55(February): 51–60.

Onslow M (1992a) Identification of early stuttering: issues and suggested strategies. American Journal of Speech and Language Pathology 1(4): 21–7.

Onslow M (1992b) Choosing a treatment procedure for early stuttering: issues and future directions. Journal of Speech and Hearing Research 35: 983–93.

Onslow M, Costa L, Rue S (1990) Direct early intervention with stuttering: some preliminary data. Journal of Speech and Hearing Disorders 55: 405–16.

Onslow M, Gardner K, Bryant KM, Stuckings CL, Knight T (1992) Stuttered and normal speech events in early childhood: the validity of a behavioral data language. Journal of Speech and Hearing Research 35(February): 79–87.

Palermo DS, Molfese DL (1972) Language acquisition from age five onward. Psychological Bulletin 78: 409–28

Perkins W (1992) Stuttering Prevented. San Diego: Singular Publishing Group.

Peters HFM, Hulstijn W (1987) Programming and initiation of speech utterances in stuttering. In Peters HFM, Hulstijn W (Eds) Speech Motor Dynamics in Stuttering. New York: Springer-Verlag.

Prins D (1983) Continuity, fragmentation, and tensions: Hypotheses applied to evaluation and intervention with preschool disfluent children. In Prins D, Ingham RJ (Eds) Treatment of Stuttering in Early Childhood: Methods and Issues. San Diego: College Hill Press.

Purser H (1987) The psychology of treatment evaluation. In Rustin L, Rowley D, Purser H (Eds) Progress in the Treatment of Fluency Disorders. London: Taylor and Francis.

Reed CG, Godden AL (1977) An experimental treatment using verbal punishment with two preschool stutterers. Journal of Fluency Disorders 2: 225–33.

Riley DG, Riley J (1983) Evaluation as a basis for intervention. In Prins D, Ingham RJ (Eds) Treatment of Stuttering in Early Childhood: Methods and Issues. San Diego: College Hill Press.

Riley DG, Riley J (1984) A component model for treating stuttering in children. In Peins M (Ed) Contemporary Approaches in Stuttering Therapy. Boston: Little Brown.

Rustin L (1987) Assessment and Therapy Programme for Dysfluent Children. Windsor: NFER-Nelson.

Rustin L, Cook E (1983) Intervention procedures for the disfluent child. In Dalton P (Ed) Approaches to the Treatment of Stuttering. Beckenham, Kent: Croom Helm.

Ryan B (1974) Programed Therapy for Stuttering in Children and Adults. Springfield, IL: Charles C. Thomas.

Ryan B (1986) Operant procedures applied to stuttering therapy for children. In Shames GH, Rubin H (Eds) Stuttering Then and Now. Columbus, OH: Merrill.

Ryan B (1992) Articulation, language, rate, and fluency characteristics of stuttering and nonstuttering preschool children. Journal of Speech and Hearing Science 35: 333–42.

Sabin EJ, Clemmer EJ, O'Connell DC, Kowal S (1979) A pausological approach to speech development. In Siegman AW, Feldstein S (Eds) Of Speech and Time. Hilsdale, NJ: Lawrence Erlbaum.

St Louis KO, Westbrook J (1987) The effectiveness of treatment for stuttering. In Rustin L, Rowley D, Purser H (Eds) Progress in the Treatment of Fluency Disorders. London: Taylor and Francis.

Schwartz HD, Zebrowski PM, Conture, EG (1990) Behaviors at the onset of stuttering.

Journal of Fluency Disorders 15(2): 77–86.

Shine RE (1984a) Direct management of the beginning stutterer. In. Perkins WH (Ed) Stuttering Disorders. New York: Thieme Stratton.

Shine RE (1984b) Assessment and fluency training with the young stutterer. In Peins M (Ed) Contemporary Approaches in Stuttering Therapy. Boston: Little Brown.

Smith A (1990) Factors in the etiology of stuttering. In Cooper JA (Ed) Research Needs in Stuttering: Roadblocks and Future Directions. ASHA: Rockville, MD. Report No. 18: 39–47.

Starkweather CW (1987) Fluency and Stuttering. Englewood Cliffs, NJ: Prentice Hall.

Starkweather CW (1991) The language-motor interface in stuttering children. In Peters HFM, HulstijnW, Starkweather WC (Eds) Speech Motor Control and Stuttering. Amsterdam: Elsevier.

Starkweather CW, Gottwald SR (1990) The Demands and Capacities Model II: Clinical Applications. Journal of Fluency Disorders 15: 143–57.

Starkweather CW, Gottwald RS, Halfond MM (1990) Stuttering Prevention; A Clinical Method. Englewood Cliffs, NJ: Prentice Hall.

Van Riper C (1973) The Treatment of Stuttering. Englewood Cliffs, NJ: Prentice-Hall.

Van Riper C (1982) The Nature of Stuttering . Englewood Cliffs, NJ: Prentice-Hall.

Wall MJ, Myers FL (1994) Clinical Management of Childhood Stuttering (2nd ed) Austin, TX: PRO-ED.

Wexler K, Mysak E (1982) Disfluency characteristics of 2-, 4-, and 6-year-old males. Journal of Fluency Disorders 7: 37–46.

Yairi E (1993) Epidemiologic and other considerations in treatment efficacy research with preschool age children who stutter. Journal of Fluency Disorders 18: 197–219.

Yairi E, Ambrose N (1992a) A longitudinal study of stuttering in children: A preliminary report. Journal of Speech and Hearing Research 35: 755–60.

Yairi E, Ambrose N (1992b) Onset of stuttering in preschool children: Selected factors. Journal of Speech and Hearing Research 35: 782–8.

Yairi E, Ambrose N, Niermann R (1993) The early months of stuttering: A developmental study. Journal of Speech and Hearing Research 36: 521–8.

Yairi E, Lewis B (1984) Disfluencies at the onset of stuttering. Journal of Speech and Hearing Research 24: 490–5.

Zebrowkski PM (1991) Duration of the speech disfluencies of beginning stutterers. Journal of Speech and Hearing Research 34: 483–91.

Zebrowkski PM, Schum RL. (1993) Counselling parents of children who stutter. American Journal of Speech and Language Pathology (May): 65–73.

Chapter 10
Cleft Palate and Other Craniofacial Anomalies in Children

V. JANE RUSSELL

The speech and language therapist has a recognized and significant role in the management of children born with cleft lip and palate, from the identification of the abnormality and throughout the whole process of medical treatment into adulthood. Because of the physical defect, these children are known to be at risk for factors that adversely influence the development of normal communication skills. Although many will achieve normal speech and language with little or no direct intervention, their progress needs to be carefully monitored by a speech and language therapist so that any potential problems are detected and managed appropriately at an early stage. In addition, following advances in the medical treatment of the rarer and more complex craniofacial anomalies, such cases are now more often encountered in speech and language therapy clinics and may present with communication disorders associated with the physical defect or particular syndrome. These can be further complicated by associated conditions such as hearing loss, learning difficulties and psychosocial factors. These cases, therefore, also require careful assessment, monitoring and treatment by the speech and language therapist.

The aim of this chapter is to describe briefly cleft lip and palate and other craniofacial anomalies and to discuss the potential effects of a physical defect on speech and language development. In addition the ongoing role of the speech and language therapist in the management of such conditions is outlined. In the space available here it is only possible to present an overview of this subject. Reference is made to other texts where more detailed information can be found.

Cleft Lip and Palate

Cleft lip and cleft palate are the most common types of congenital orofacial defects. It is difficult to obtain exact figures but the incidence is estimated to be in the region of one in 750 live births (McWilliams, Morris and Shelton, 1990). This estimate is based on overt clefts which are diagnosed at birth and on a Caucasian population. There are some racial differences, for example, a higher incidence is reported for Chinese/Oriental people and American Indians and the lowest incidence for Afro-Caribbean people (McWilliams et al., 1990). There are two genetically distinct groups, that is cleft lip with or without cleft palate CL(P) and isolated cleft palate (CP). Sparks (1984) describes how clefts can occur with other malformations (see further below) as part of a syndrome. 'Nonsyndromic' clefts (not symptoms of a syndrome) in both CL(P) and CP 'can be caused by familial aetiology or be an isolated event' (Sparks, 1984: 76).

Facial clefts originate in the first three months *in utero* when the anatomical processes which will ultimately form the face, fail to fuse at the appropriate stage in embryological development (Bzoch and Williams, 1979; Watson, 1980, Bzoch, 1989, McWilliams et al., 1990). The resultant defect ranges from slight to severe and can affect the lip, alveolus, hard palate and soft palate. Clefts may be unilateral, bilateral, or median and can occur in different combinations as described by McWilliams et al. (1990). Submucous clefts of the palate, in which there are muscle and bone defects underlying what appears to be an intact palate, often remain undiagnosed unless they give rise to feeding and/or associated speech disorders. Similarly, other congenital defects resulting in 'palatopharyngeal incompetence' and hypernasal speech, in the absence of a cleft palate, are diagnosed from the resulting speech characteristics (McWilliams et al., 1990).

Surgery

In advanced countries, clefts of the lip and palate are routinely repaired surgically, usually in early childhood. There is considerable variation in the timing and type of surgical procedures and a continuing debate concerning the resultant effects on facial growth and speech development (Desai, 1983, Pigott, 1986, Harding and Campbell, 1989, Mars et al., 1991, Harding and Grunwell, 1993). Lip and palate repair in early infancy is thought to facilitate normal speech development, but is reported to lead to a greater number of facial growth deformities which require extensive corrective surgery in adolescence (Harding and Grunwell, 1993).

Craniofacial Anomalies

Craniofacial anomalies are anatomical deviations which may or may not include cleft palate. They are rare but, as McWilliams (1984: 187) comments, they 'constitute a major group of handicaps in children'. Such abnormalities can affect the oral and facial structures, the cranium or both. They are often complex and, as indicated above, may occur with cleft palate as features of a particular syndrome. Although it is possible for similar physical abnormalities to occur as a result of trauma, they are usually congenital and often of genetic origin (Sparks, 1984). McWilliams et al. (1990) describe the patterns of malformation which are associated with clefting and provide a useful overview of this subject. They describe the primary features, incidence, embryology, aetiology, major hazards and communication problems associated with particular syndromes. They include the major syndromes which speech and language therapists may encounter in their clinical practice. These are the Pierre Robin, Apert,[1] Shprintzen and Treacher Collins syndromes and Crouzon disease.[2]

Craniofacial surgery

In the past, congenital craniofacial abnormalities were generally considered to be untreatable. However, technical and technological advances mean that many more patients are receiving corrective surgery (Goldin et al., 1986). Witzel (1983) describes the development of craniofacial surgery and comments that 'the surgery is often drastic, detailed and dangerous'. She describes operative procedures (see also McWilliams et al., 1990) and the effects of craniofacial surgery on articulation and velopharyngeal function. Both Witzel (1983) and McWilliams et al. stress the need for a multi-disciplinary team approach to the management of patients with craniofacial anomalies. The speech and language therapist should be an integral member of such a team in order to document communication difficulties associated with craniofacial anomalies and to record changes in speech patterns following any operative procedures, even when there are no obvious speech problems initially.

Articulation problems associated with orofacial and craniofacial anomalies are described by Peterson-Falzone (1982), Witzel (1983) and McWilliams (1984). Although more severe structural defects are likely to result in greater articulation problems, both Peterson-Falzone and McWilliams comment on the lack of correlation between structure and articulatory function, and the ability of some patients to compensate for severe physical defects. In addition, McWilliams (1984) comments that speech therapy may not be effective in the presence of 'massive oral deformities'. Spontaneous improvement often occurs following surgery, without the need for speech therapy. It should be noted, however, that this does not apply in cases of late cleft palate repair, from about six years upwards, when almost all patients will need some speech therapy (Sell and Grunwell, 1990).

However, it is often the conditions associated with craniofacial anomalies which give rise to the types of speech and language difficulties that require intervention. Language delay, for example, may result from learning difficulties, hearing loss or psychosocial factors (McWilliams, 1984). It is, therefore, important for patients with craniofacial anomalies to receive a comprehensive assessment covering all aspects of communication development. The results of such an assessment must then be carefully evaluated in the context of any associated conditions and with regard to the overall team management of the child.

Cleft Palate and Communication Development

In this section the discussion focuses primarily on the cleft palate anomalies but the reader will appreciate that many of the implications for communication development may also apply to other craniofacial anomalies. From birth the physical defect influences behaviours such as feeding and parent–child interaction, which in turn can subsequently influence normal communication development (Russell, 1989).

Feeding

One of the initial consequences of cleft lip and palate, except the most minor kind, is a disruption of feeding (Campbell and Watson, 1980). Because of the abnormal physical structures the infant is unable to establish normal sucking patterns. Abnormal feeding patterns and the physical defect can also affect oral motor and oro-sensory development (Edwards, 1980; Russell, 1989; Russell and Grunwell, 1993). Bzoch (1979: 73) suggests that abnormal neuromotor patterns may develop because 'auditory decoding and neuromotor encoding skills are learned when the vast majority of infants with a palatal defect have an abnormal mechanism'. Both the abnormal physical structures and neuromotor patterns may result in delayed, or deviant phonetic development.

A further effect of feeding difficulties is the potential disruption of normal mother–child interaction which is vitally important for pragmatic development (Carpenter, Mastergeorge and Coggins, 1983). If feeding is a slow, arduous process and causes anxiety, a pattern of negative interaction may develop. Mother and child may not have the time or inclination to participate in normal communicative interaction because of the pressures of the feeding situation (Russell, 1989).

Hearing

Otitis media is frequently present from birth in children with cleft palate and is though to be due to Eustachian tube malfunction (Heller, 1979; Lencione, 1980; Maw, 1986; McWilliams et al., 1990). This results in a conductive hearing loss which may fluctuate and which can seriously affect auditory skills and communication development (Bamford and Saunders, 1990). Sensori-neural hearing losses may also occur but much less frequently than conductive problems. In craniofacial anomalies there are often associated ear deformities and these can also result in conductive or sensori-neural hearing losses (McWilliams, 1984).

Surgical treatment may be indicated when there is persistent and/or recurrent otitis media (McWilliams et al., 1990). Conductive hearing loss which does not respond to routine surgery is a particular problem in Treacher–Collins syndrome. These children usually require bone conduction hearing aids which may be fitted when they are very young (McWilliams et al., 1990). There is an increasing use of bone-anchored hearing aids which can provide Treacher-Collins patients with near normal hearing.

Parent–child communication

The effect of feeding on mother–child interaction and subsequent pragmatic development is indicated above. It is also possible that the presence of a physical defect will affect the parents' attitude to the child and thus their response to and initiation of communication. As Edwards (1980: 84) points out; 'it has been shown that parents of a child with congenital handicap tend to regard them as being different long after they have in fact moved towards normality'. This may mean that parental expectations of a child's potential are underrated. Attempts by the child to communicate may not be recognized by the parents, particularly because the effects of the cleft on articulation development can cause different vocal output from that which might be expected from the normal child (Russell, 1989). From the start, therefore, the child may experience failure in communication which can result in delayed speech and language development.

Further stress can be placed on the parent–child relationship and communicative interaction by the experience of hospitalization and the trauma of the operation itself (Russell, 1989). In addition, there is also the need to attend out-patient clinics for individual or joint consultations with a number of different professionals, such as the plastic surgeon, orthodontist, otolaryngologist and speech and language therapist. This places an additional strain on the parents, child and other members of the family, which again has the potential to affect family relationships and pragmatic development.

Language development

From the foregoing discussion it will be appreciated that the cleft palate child is at risk for delayed language development. In the many studies of the language development of cleft palate children, there is considerable variation in the aspects of language investigated and the variables taken into account (see McWilliams et al., 1990 for a comprehensive survey). There is, however, general agreement that the language abilities of cleft palate children may be delayed, particularly in expressive language development (Philips and Harrison, 1969; Nation, 1970; Pannbacker, 1971; Fox, Lynch and Brookshire, 1978; Bzoch, 1989; McWilliams et al., 1990). The effect of cleft palate on the phonological aspects of language development is discussed below.

Studies involving younger children have shown that it is possible to detect delay in the pre-linguistic period of development (Fox et al., 1978; Bzoch, 1979; Long and Dalston, 1982). Long and Dalston found that cleft palate children differed significantly from normal children in the development of 'paired gestural and vocal behaviour' at 12 months of age. The combination of gestural and vocal development is a prerequisite for early pragmatic development and is also linked to the origins of grammar (Griffiths, 1979). Fox et al. (1978) found that cleft palate children were performing less well than their normal peers on both linguistic and non-linguistic tasks even below the age of three years. Significant areas of difference were found on both receptive and expressive language subtests. There is, therefore, a need for close monitoring of the linguistic development of cleft palate children commencing in the prelinguistic period of development and continuing into later childhood.

Articulation and phonetic development

Previous studies of the babbling patterns of cleft palate children have confirmed delay and differences from the normal pattern of development (Mousset and Trichet, 1985; O'Gara and Logemann, 1985; Grunwell and Russell, 1987). Grunwell and Russell (1987), and O'Gara and Logemann (1985) report a predominance of glottal and 'back' articulations as well as the frequent occurrence of glides. Mousset and Trichet (1985) report a delay in the development of the voiceless plosives [p] [t] and [k] after palate repair, particularly in the group who had their operation at 18 as opposed to 6 months of age. Dorf and Curtin (1982) report a higher incidence of 'compensatory articulations (mid-dorsum palatal stops, posterior nasal fricatives, velar fricatives, pharyngeal stops, pharyngeal fricatives and glottal stops)' in a group of children who had 'late' (after 12 months) as opposed to 'early' (prior to 12 months) palatal repairs.

Russell and Grunwell (1993) report that following the operation to repair the palate, when there is an improved intra-oral mechanism the children's vocalizations progress towards more normal patterns. However, phonetic deviance characteristic of the cleft palate condition persists for many children. At about two months post operatively, Russell and Grunwell (1993) report an increase in lingual articulations, fewer glottal and pharyngeal articulations and an increased occurrence of plosives. There is, still, however, a lack of labial and lingual plosives. By

18 months of age most children demonstrate further progress, but at this age individual differences indicate that some children are 'at risk' for speech problems. These children continue to evidence extremely delayed and deviant speech patterns (Russell and Grunwell, 1993).

Deviant phonetic patterns have also been reported in the speech of older cleft palate children. Bzoch (1979) and Morris (1979) both describe the predominance of glottal stop articulation, the use of pharyngeal fricatives and the lack of normal plosives and fricatives. Both authorities attribute these characteristics to velopharyngeal insufficiency (see further below) or abnormal learned motor patterns. Bzoch comments that the abnormal learned motor patterns can be identified 'as early as 3 years of age ...'. McWilliams et al. (1990) in an extensive review of the literature, illustrate the high risk of disordered articulation for cleft palate children and the occurrence of improvement with age, especially in the articulation of plosives and fricatives. They also point out the considerable variability between individual cleft palate children in the extent and nature of their speech sound errors and conclude that they are a heterogeneous population in this respect. Russell and Grunwell (1993) also emphasize the heterogeneous nature of speech development in children with cleft palate.

Phonological development

Ingram (1976, 1989) demonstrates by analysing data from previous studies that there are systematic processes in cleft palate speech. Following Ingram's lead, reports employing phonological techniques in the investigation of cleft palate children's speech began to appear in the literature in the 1980s (Hodson et al., 1983; Lynch, Fox and Brookshire, 1983; Broen, Felsenfeld and Bacon, 1986; Grunwell and Russell, 1988). Crystal (1989) highlights the need to investigate the speech of cleft palate children using phonological as well as phonetic analyses in order to determine the extent and nature of any deviance or delay and whether these result primarily from phonetic or phonological bases. McWilliams et al. (1990) also comment on how information about the child's phonological system helps to inform clinical speech therapy management. The relationship between phonetic and phonological development in the speech patterns of cleft palate children is described further in Russell (1989) and Russell and Grunwell (1993). It should be stressed that a child with cleft palate may present with a phonological delay or disorder in the absence of, or in addition to, any phonetic deviance. This may be related to an overall expressive language delay as described above, or to other factors such as hearing problems.

Broen et al. (1986) illustrate how phonological analysis helped to identify, at the age of 2.5 years, children requiring secondary surgery for velopharyngeal insufficiency. Lynch et al. (1983) report differences in the developing phonological systems of two children. For one subject, phonological analysis revealed the characteristics of developmental delay rather than deviation, whereas in the other subject deviant characteristics of 'structural inadequacy' were detected. Grunwell and Russell (1988) also studied two children and report differences in their phonological development. The results for one subject indicate the possibility of spontaneous recovery from phonetic deviance and relatively normal phonological development once palatal surgery has provided an intact intra-oral mechanism. For the second subject, however, there is evidence of persisting phonetic influence on phonological development. Grunwell and Russell (1993) demonstrate that progressively more normal phonetic development leads to normal phonological development but delay in phonetic development causes further delay in the establishment of a child's phonological system.

These studies bear out the observation of McWilliams et al. (1990) mentioned above, that in respect of their articulatory patterns cleft palate children constitute a heterogeneous group. Each individual, therefore, requires a detailed speech assessment including both phonetic and phonological analyses.

Velopharyngeal insufficiency

Inappropriate nasal escape on non-nasal consonants and vowels, and hypernasal resonance during speech may indicate velopharyngeal insufficiency (VPI). VPI occurs when the physical structures which constitute the velopharyngeal sphincter are inadequate or function inadequately. As a result, the child is unable to build up sufficient intra-oral pressure for the articulation of oral phonemes, particularly plosives. The underlying cause may be a residual palatal fistula, poor soft-palate function or a palate which is too short to reach the posterior pharyngeal wall. There may be associated facial movements such as 'nasal or facial grimace' during speech (Sell, Harding and Grunwell, 1994). Patients who are suspected of having VPI need careful investigation including assessment of nasal airflow during speech, radiographic and endoscopic procedures (Huskie, 1989). A comprehensive phonetic and phonological assessment of speech is also required (Russell, 1989). When there is consistent nasal escape and hypernasality as a result of structural inadequacy, rather than abnormal learned motor patterns (see *Articulation and phonetic development* above), secondary surgery is usually indicated. Operative procedures employed in secondary surgery are described by Randall (1980) and McWilliams et al. (1990).

In the space available here it has only been possible to give a brief overview of the influences of cleft palate on communication development. It has been demonstrated that such influences are potentially wide ranging and are not just concerned with the physical nature of the defect. It should also be remembered that, as well as being vulnerable to speech and language problems because of the cleft condition itself, cleft palate children are also subject to the same influences which affect the development of communication in the normal population. For example, a child with a cleft lip only may have a language disorder or delay which is unrelated to the physical condition.

The Role of the Speech and Language Therapist

Once palatal surgery has provided an intact intra-oral mechanism, many cleft palate children will achieve normal speech and language skills with little or no active speech therapy intervention. It is, however, important to monitor closely the communication development of all the children in order to identify as soon as possible those who will require specific help and/or further surgery. In some cases direct intervention may be unnecessary as a result of the ongoing advice and help which the speech and language therapist has given to the parents while monitoring the child's progress.

The therapist's involvement with the cleft palate child should commence at or soon after birth and may continue into the teenage years. The type and frequency of clinical involvement varies, however, according to the age and needs of the child and the counselling needs of the parents. The therapist, therefore, has to adopt a changing role in such cases. Management and treatment of the cleft palate child may be undertaken by the speech and language therapist who is an integral member of the cleft palate team, the therapist in the child's home locality or, in some cases, a combination of both. In the latter situation there should be close liaison between the therapist from the cleft palate team and the child's local therapist, concerning management of the child's communication development. In order to illustrate the changing role of the speech and language therapist, the following discussion describes the clinical management of such children in a developmental chronology.

Before speech

Once the parents have come to terms with the cleft palate condition and have coped with initial problems such as feeding, their next major concern is often associated with speech development. The initial role of the speech and language therapist therefore, is one of counsellor, although there may also be some involvement with regard to feeding. The aim of the therapist is to establish the foundations of a long-term relationship with the parents and to provide them with accurate and comprehensible information regarding speech development. In some cases it is often helpful to supplement verbal with written information but this should be used with care (Russell, 1989).

Excellent guidelines for those undertaking parent counselling are provided by MacDonald (1979). She emphasizes the need to adopt a positive approach and to listen carefully in order to be guided by the parents themselves. In particular the therapist should avoid 'suggesting to the parents what they should be experiencing' by telling them what not to do, for example 'not to feel guilty...' (MacDonald, 1979). The counselling aspect of the speech and language therapist's role is ongoing and should continue throughout childhood and into adolescence and adulthood as required. The family's need for support will change over time and extra help may be required at times of stress, such as when children are in hospital for lip and palate operations, or in adolescence.

At the initial meeting with the parents a brief explanation of the speech and language therapist's involvement with cleft palate children is provided. It is explained that the physical defect may have implications for speech and language development, that many children will develop normal communication skills, but others may need further help from the therapist. This lays the foundation of the therapist's role in monitoring communication development (Russell, 1989), which is usually carried out at subsequent clinic visits in conjunction with the cleft palate team, or with only the speech and language therapist. In some cases it is appropriate for the therapist to visit the child's home.

Most monitoring of early development is carried out through observation and discussion with the parents. Any cause for concern is then investigated in greater detail as appropriate. A knowledge of normal development is obviously essential and it can be useful to refer to developmental checklists such as the REEL scale (Bzoch and League, 1971). The speech and language therapist should monitor all aspects of communication development including parent–child interaction, the development of understanding and expression, and early phonetic development. Appropriate advice can then be offered to the parents who can be shown how to help their child progress on to the next stage of communication development. A home programme for use with children in the pre-speech and early speech stages of development is described in Albery and Russell (1994).

The pre-school child

If there has been no previous concern regarding communication development a routine assessment should be carried out at about the age of 1.5 to 2.0 years, in order to ensure that the child is making satisfactory progress along normal lines. As in the pre-speech stage, all areas of communication development should be screened. The speech and language therapist needs to consider the whole child in relation to his environment. The assessment procedure, therefore, should not differ from that adopted for the speech and language assessment of any young child. Factors relating to the physical defect should obviously be taken into account but these must not prevent the therapist from being open-minded until a differential diagnosis is reached. It should be stressed that a specialist knowledge of cleft palate is not required; the speech and language therapist has the necessary expertise to assess and manage children of all ages. Applicable assessment procedures are outlined in McWilliams et al. (1990), Russell (1989) and Albery and Russell (1994).

In the assessment of a child with a cleft palate or other craniofacial anomaly, there are some additional factors which need to be covered in the case history. Details of early feeding, the nature and extent of the original defect, and information about operations all need to be included. When discussing this with the parents the therapist will be able to gain some insight into their understanding of the problem and their attitudes towards the child (Russell, 1989). In addition, particular attention should be paid to the oro-facial examination (Huskie, 1989) as the child's articulatory ability may be directly related to dentition, occlusion, or the presence of a palatal fistula (residual, usually small, open cleft remaining following palatal surgery). As indicated above, this may in turn influence phonetic and phonological development.

From the results of an initial assessment the therapist is able to identify areas which need further investigation and to implement appropriate action. This may involve reference to other members of the cleft palate team, as in the case of a child who appears to have hearing difficulties, and/or direct or indirect intervention from a speech and language therapist (see below). Cleft palate children should, of course, be receiving regular hearing checks and the routine developmental screening which is carried out on all children.

The school-age child

In an ideal situation the procedures of counselling, monitoring and assessment which have been outlined above will have been ongoing enabling early diagnosis and intervention and, to some extent, the prevention of secondary problems, for example reluctance to communicate because of unintelligible speech. Many cleft palate children will have achieved good communication skills by the time they reach school age, but there will also be those who require continued help. This may be due to the severity of the communication problem, the lack of provision for early intervention and other factors such as poor attendance records for speech therapy.

The speech and language therapist should carry out informal and formal assessment procedures which are appropriate for the age of the child, and assess all areas of communication, including verbal comprehension, vocabulary, syntax, semantics, articulation, phonetic and phonological development and the pragmatic aspects. As highlighted above, factors relating to the physical defect and the child's environment are taken into account in order to construct a profile of the child's communicative abilities. Sell et al. (1994) describe the 'Great Ormond Street Speech Assessment'. This is designed specifically for the assessment of cleft palate speech characteristics and is a comprehensive and practical screening procedure. In addition, it facilitates record keeping and report writing procedures. Appropriate intervention is based on the results of the assessment with referral to other professionals if necessary, for example, when further investigation of velopharyngeal function is indicated. When therapy is not indicated the therapist will continue to monitor the child's communicative abilities at regular intervals in order to record any changes and to identify whether help is needed at some time in the future.

With children of all ages one of the main responsibilities of the speech and language therapist is to document and report to other members of the cleft palate team on the child's communicative development. It is particularly important to include the results of the phonetic and phonological analyses, as well as other speech parameters, in the battery of procedures required to evaluate VPI (Van Demark et al., 1985; Huskie, 1989). Some procedures such as nasal anemometry and radiography may be successfully used with pre-school children, but the more invasive procedure of nasendoscopy requires a higher degree of active co-operation from the child (Pigott, 1980). The likelihood of success with this procedure increases in proportion to the age of the child. With regard to these investigations, the speech and language therapist takes an active role in the recording and interpretation of data with other members of the diagnostic team. Subsequently, the therapist may be involved in counselling the child and parents with regard to secondary surgery. Such surgery may be required to modify the results of the earlier primary lip or palate repair, for example closure of an oronasal fistula or adjustment to the shape of the lip. An operation termed a pharyngoplasty may be needed to provide a competent velopharyngeal sphincter in cases of VPI (Randall, 1980; Pigott, 1986; McWilliams et al., 1990). Further speech assessment and possibly intervention will be required following such surgery.

Mainstream Treatment Practices

The methods of intervention employed by the speech and language therapist will vary according to the age and needs of the child and his family. With the very young child, intervention is usually implemented through the parents who, on a daily basis at home, carry out activities suggested and demonstrated by the therapist (Albery and Russell, 1994). Most intervention with young cleft palate children is carried out on an individual basis with the child and his parents. It may be appropriate, however, to include children, from about three years of age, in groups. These may be made up of cleft palate or non-cleft palate children provided that the needs of the children are similar. Older children may be seen in an individual or group situation and there are considerable advantages when either of these methods is carried out on an intensive basis (Bzoch, 1979; Huskie, 1979; Albery and Enderby, 1984; Grunwell and Dive, 1988; Scanlon, personal communication).

Intervention strategies also vary according to the age of the child and his needs as indicated by the communication assessment. Strategies which can be used with the younger child are described in Hahn (1979), Brookshire, Lynch and Fox (1980), McWilliams et al. (1990), Russell (1989) and Albery and Russell (1994). Brookshire et al. (1980) provide detailed objectives for facilitating speech and language development from birth up to three years of age. These are presented in six monthly stages and this programme is a valuable resource for those lacking experience with younger children. Similarly, Albery and Russell (1994) provide suggestions for activities which can be used during the pre-speech and early speech stages of development. It is important to take advantage of what the child is doing naturally to reinforce and encourage appropriate development so that suitable activities become part of the daily routine (Russell, 1989).

With regard to the treatment of 'cleft palate speech' in older children, a combination of articulatory and phonological strategies versus traditional articulation therapy *per se* may be appropriate (McWilliams et al., 1990; Grunwell and Dive, 1988). Grunwell and Dive studied two children who attended an intensive therapy course and the study demonstrated that a combined articulatory and phonological strategy 'facilitates, the reorganization and expansion of previously static phonological systems, sometimes in spite of persisting articulatory disabilities, sometimes accompanied by improvements in articulatory abilities'. The strategy adopted by the therapist is obviously directly related to the results of the assessment: for example, some children will need help with language and not speech development. In view, however, of the evidence provided by Grunwell and Dive (1988), a phonological approach will enhance and broaden articulation therapy.

Therapy activities for articulation problems are provided by Albery and Russell (1994). They describe techniques for eliciting consonants and suggest ways in which these consonants can be incorporated into words and generalized throughout conversational speech. Some phonological strategies are used, for example minimal pairs to contrast nasal/non-nasal consonants. In addition, Albery and Russell (1994) provide illustrations which can be photocopied and used in therapy.

McWilliams (1984) comments with regard to speech problems associated with craniofacial anomalies, that 'therapy for these patients does not differ in any remarkable way from speech therapy in general'. This is also applicable to children with cleft palate except perhaps in cases where VPI is a significant factor. Even then the therapist can often continue to work on different aspects of speech, such as encouraging appropriate tongue placements, while waiting for investigations of velopharyngeal function to be implemented. Albery (1986) stresses that the therapist 'should always be aware of the possibility of potential competence' of the velopharyngeal sphincter and recommends a period of diagnostic therapy for children with 'a total glottal stop pattern'. The child may therefore learn to produce some consonants, such as bilabial plosives, with the correct articulatory placement, which may improve intelligibility even when there is nasal escape resulting from VPI.

Therapy activities

Therapy activities for articulation problems are provided by Albery and Russell (1994). They describe techniques for eliciting consonants and suggest ways in which these consonants can be incorporated into words and generalized throughout conversational speech. Some phonological strategies are used, for example minimal pairs to contrast nasal/non-nasal consonants. In addition Albery and Russell (1994) provide illustrations which can be photocopied and used in therapy.

When it appears that the VPI is not a result of abnormal physical structures, but is due to the inadequate function of a potentially competent velopharyngeal mechanism, the use of tongue and palate training aids or biofeedback may be indicated (Hardcastle, Morgan-Barry and Nunn, 1989; Stuffins, 1989; McWilliams et al., 1990). Prior to the use of training aids, detailed assessment is required along with close liaison with other professionals such as the orthodontist. It is also important to continue therapy while an aid is being used (Stuffins, 1989). Biofeedback devices, such as the Nasal Anemometer, which visually indicates nasal airflow (Ellis, 1979), and the Electro-palatograph (Hardcastle, 1984), which visually displays tongue contacts against the hard palate, can be used to help the child learn to control the movements of the articulators. A programme for use with the Nasal Anemometer is provided by Albery and Russell (1994). In addition, they describe the Micronose computer program which provides an appealing visual feedback for younger children.

Effectiveness of therapy

It is evident that the effectiveness of therapy with children who have craniofacial anomalies is subject to many variables relating to the nature of the communication difficulty, dentition and occlusion, velopharyngeal adequacy, age and motivation of the child, parent support and other factors. In the author's experience, early intervention of the type described in Albery and Russell (1994) is effective, particularly with regard to preventing secondary problems, for example the use of abnormal plosives and fricatives. For older children, intensive individual or group therapy is often more effective than weekly therapy (Bzoch, 1979; Huskie, 1979; Albery and Enderby, 1984; Grunwell and Dive, 1988). In addition a combined articulatory and phonological approach is effective for articulatory problems (Grunwell and Dive, 1988).

In some cases it may be necessary for the speech and language therapist to compromise over some aspects of speech development. This may occur when accurate articulation is difficult for the child to achieve owing to dental or occlusal abnormalities causing, for example, some lateral escape of air on an /s/. In such instances the decision regarding further therapy depends on the results of the oral examination, the phonetic and phonological analysis, and the motivation of the child. If the problem does not cause the child to be misunderstood and if he is unconcerned, therapy is unlikely to be effective. The therapist should continue to review the child at regular intervals and therapy may be indicated following orthodontic treatment or secondary surgery.

Conclusion

In this chapter the role of the speech and language therapist in the management of children with orofacial defects, in particular cleft palate, has been outlined. The continuing nature of the role from birth and through childhood into adolescence and adulthood has been discussed. It has been demonstrated that the same basic principles of therapeutic practice which are used routinely by the therapist are applicable to the assessment and management of children with cleft palate. The therapist should take into account relevant factors related to the physical defect but a specialist knowledge of cleft palate is not required. When necessary the therapist is able to refer to appropriate texts for further information and to seek the advice of a more experienced colleague who works routinely as a member of a cleft palate or craniofacial team.

Notes

1. *Apert syndrome* (Peterson-Falzone, 1982; McWilliams, 1984; McWilliams et al., 1990). Apert's syndrome is always characterized by craniosynostotis (premature osseous union of bones that are normally distinct) and syndactyly (webbing or union) of the hands and feet. Such children have a high steep forehead, a flattened occiput, hypertelorism and exophthalmos. Thirty per cent of cases have a cleft of the soft palate but a high arched complete palate is more common. Mental retardation may occur in as many as 50 per cent of those affected. Communication skills are affected by factors such as severe malocclusion, an abnormal nasopharyngeal airway, the anomalous shape of the palatal vault, hearing loss and psychosocial problems.

2. *Crouzon syndrome* (Peterson-Falzone, 1982; McWilliams, 1984; McWilliams et al., 1990). Crouzon disease is also known as craniofacial dysostosis. It is less severe than Apert syndrome and is characterized by an abnormally shaped head, maxillary hypoplasia (midfacial deficiency), prognathism (prominent mandible), hypertelorism (wide set eyes), exophthalmus (protruding eyes) and low-set ears. These children are not usually mentally retarded. They may have essentially normal speech but defective speech is usually related to structural abnormalities. Airway problems can restrict respiration and conductive hearing losses are common.

References

Albery EH (1986) Type and assessment of speech problems. In Albery EH, Hathorn IS, Pigott RW (Eds), Cleft Lip and Palate: A Team Approach. Bristol: Wright.

Albery E, Enderby P (1984) Intensive speech therapy for cleft palate children. British Journal of Disorders of Communication 19: 115–24.

Albery E, Russell J (1994) Cleft Palate Source Book. Oxford: Winslow Press.

Bamford J, Saunders E (1990) Hearing Impairment, Auditory Perception and Language Disability (2nd ed). London: Whurr.

Broen PA, Felsenfeld S, Kittleson Bacon C (1986) Predicting from the phonological patterns observed in children wih cleft palate. Paper presented at the symposium on Research in Child Language Disorders, Madison, WI.

Brookshire BL, Lynch JI, Fox DR (1980) A Parent Child Cleft Palate Curriculum: Developing Speech and Language. Oregon: C.C. Publication.

Bzoch KR (1979) Etiological factors related to cleft palate speech. In Bzoch KR (Ed) Communicative Disorders Related to Cleft Lip and Palate (1st ed). Boston: Little, Brown.

Bzoch KR (Ed) 1989 Communicative Disorders Related to Cleft Lip and Palate, 3rd edition. Boston: College Hill Press.

Bzoch KR, League R (1971) Assessing Language Skills in Infancy. Baltimore: University Park Press.

Bzoch KR, Williams WM (1979) Introduction, rationale, principles and related basic embryology and anatomy. In Bzoch KR (Ed) Communicative Disorders Related to Cleft Lip and Palate. Boston: Little Brown.

Campbell ML, Watson ACH (1980) Management of the neonate. In Edwards M, Watson ACH (Eds), Advances in the Management of Cleft Palate. London: Churchill Livingstone.

Carpenter RL, Mastergeorge AM, Coggins TE (1983) The acquisition of communicative intention in infants eight to fifteen months of age. Language and Speech 26: 101–16.

Crystal D (1989) Clinical Linguistics. London: Whurr.

Desai SN (1983) Early cleft palate repair completed before the age of 16 weeks: observations on a personal series of 100 children. British Journal of Plastic Surgery 36: 300–4.

Dorf DS, Curtin JW (1982) Early cleft palate repair and speech outcome. Plastic and Reconstructive Surgery 70: 74–9.

Edwards M (1980) Speech and language disablity. In Edwards M, Watson ACH (Eds), Advances in the Management of Cleft Palate. London: Churchill Livingstone.

Ellis RE (1979) The Exeter nasal anemometry system. In Ellis RE, Flack FC (Eds) Diagnosis and Treatment of Palato Glossal Malfunction. London: The College of Speech Therapists.

Fox D, Lynch J, Brookshire B (1978) Selected developmental factors of cleft palate children between two and thirty-three months of age. Cleft Palate Journal 15: 239–46.

Goldin H, Hockley A, Wake M, Beasley J (1986) Craniofacial surgery. British Journal of Hospital Medicine pp 368–73.

Griffiths P (1979) Speech acts and early sentences. In Fletcher P, Garman M (Eds) Language Acquisition. Cambridge: Cambridge University Press.

Grunwell P, Dive D (1988) Treating cleft palate speech: Combining phonological techniques with traditional articulation therapy. Child Language Teaching and Therapy 4: 193–210.

Grunwell P, Russell J (1987) Vocalisations before and after cleft palate surgery. British Journal of Disorders of Communication 22: 1–17.

Grunwell P, Russell J (1988) Phonological development in children with cleft lip and palate. Clinical Linguistics and Phonetics 2: 75–95.

Hahn E (1979) Directed home training program for infants with cleft lip and palate. In Bzoch KR (Ed) Communicative Disorders Related to Cleft Lip and Palate. Boston: Little Brown.

Hardcastle W (1984) New methods of profiling normal and abnormal lingual palatal contact patterns. Work in Progress, University of Reading Phonetics Laboratory 4: 1–40.

Hardcastle W, Morgan-Barry R, Nunn, M (1989) Instrumental articulatory phonetics in assessment and remediation: case studies with the electropalatograph. In Stengelhofen J (Ed) Cleft Palate, the Nature and Remediation of Communication Problems. Edinburgh: Churchill Livingstone.

Harding A, Campbell RC (1989) A comparison of the speech results after early and delayed hard palate closure: a preliminary report. British Journal of Plastic Surgery 42: 1–6.

Harding A, Grunwell, P (1993) Relationship between speech and timing of hard palate repair. In Grunwell P (Ed) Analysing Cleft Palate Speech. London: Whurr.

Hathorn IS (1986a) Classification. In Albery EH, Hathorn IS, Pigott RW (Eds) Cleft Lip and Palate: A Team Approach. Bristol: Wright.

Hathorn IS (1986b) Dental management. In Albery EH, Hathorn IS, Pigott RW (Eds) Cleft Lip and Palate: A Team Approach. Bristol: Wright.

Heller JC (1979) Hearing loss in patients with cleft palate. In Bzoch KR (Ed) Communicative Disorders Related to Cleft Lip and Palate. Boston: Little Brown.

Hodson BW, Chin L, Redmond B, Simpson R (1983) Phonological evaluation and remediation of speech deviations of a child with a repaired cleft palate: A case study. Journal of Speech and Hearing Disorders 48: 93–8.

Huskie CF (1979) Intensive therapy - Glasgow experience. In Ellis RE, Flack FC (Eds), Diagnosis and Treatment of Palato Glossal Malfunction. London: The College of Speech Therapists.

Huskie CF (1989) Assessment of speech and language status: Subjective and objective approaches to the appraisal of vocal tract structure and function. In Stengelhofen J (Ed) Cleft Palate: The Nature and Remediation of Communication Problems. Edinburgh: Churchill Livingstone.

Ingram D (1976) Phonological Disability in Children. London: Edward Arnold.

Ingram D (1989) Phonological Disability in Children. (2nd ed). London: Whurr.

Lencione RM (1980) Associated conditions. In Edwards M, Watson ACH (Eds) Advances in the Management of Cleft Palate. London: Churchill Livingstone.

Long M, Dalston RM (1982) Paired gestural and vocal behaviour in one-year-old cleft lip and palate children. Journal of Speech and Hearing Research 47: 403–6.

Lynch JL, Fox DR, Brookshire BL (1983) Phonological proficiency of two cleft palate toddlers with school age follow up. Journal of Speech and Hearing Disorders 48: 274–85.

MacDonald SK (1979) Parental needs and professional responses: A parental perspective. Cleft Palate Journal 16: 118–92.

McWilliams BJ (1984) Speech problems associated with craniofacial anomalies In. Perkins WH (Ed) Recent Advances: Speech Disorders. San Diego, CA: College Hill.

McWilliams BJ, Morris HL, Shelton RL (1990) Cleft Palate Speech (2nd ed). Philadelphia: B.C. Decker.

Mars M, Sell D, Houston WJB, Grunwell P, Lamabadusuriya, SP (1991) Lessons to be learned from the Sri Lankan study. Invited presentation at the Fourth European Craniofacial Congress, The Netherlands.

Maw AR (1986) Ear disease. In Albery EH, Hathorn IS, Pigott RW (Eds) Cleft Lip and Palate: A Team Approach. Bristol: Wright.

Morris HL (1979) Evaluation of abnormal articulation patterns. In Bzoch KR (Ed) Communicative Disorders Related to Cleft Lip and Palate. Boston: Little Brown.

Mousset MR, Trichet B (1985) Babbling and phonetic acquisitions after early complete surgical repair of cleft lip and palate. Paper presented at the Fifth International Congress on Cleft Palate and Related Craniofacial Abnormalities, Monte Carlo.

Nation JE (1970) Vocabulary comprehension and usage of preschool cleft palate and normal children. Cleft Palate Journal, 7: 639–44.

O'Gara MM, Logemann JA (1988) Phonetic analyses of the speech development of babies with cleft palate. Cleft Palate Journal 25: 122–34

Pannbacker N (1971) Language skills of cleft palate children: A review. British Journal of Disorders of Communication 6: 37–44.

Peterson-Falzone SJ (1982) Articulation disorders in orofacial anomalies. In Lass N, Northern, J, Yoder D, McReynolds L (Eds) Speech, Language and Hearing. Philadelphia: W. B. Saunders Co.

Phillips BJ, Harrison RJ (1969) Language skills of preschool cleft palate children. Cleft Palate Journal 6: 108–19.

Pigott R (1980) Assessment of velopharngeal function. In M. Edwards, ACH Watson (Eds), Advances in the Management of Cleft Palate. London: Churchill Livingstone.

Pigott R (1986) Primary repair of the cleft lip and palate. In Albery EH, Hathorn IS, Pigott RW (Eds), Cleft Lip and Palate: A Team Approach. Bristol: Wright.

Randall P (1980) Secondary surgery. In Edwards M, Watson ACH (Eds) Advances in the Management of Cleft Palate. London: Churchill Livingstone.

Russell J (1989) Early intervention. In Stengelhofen J (Ed) Cleft Palate: The Nature and Remediation of Communication Problems. Edinburgh: Churchill Livingstone.

Russell J, Grunwell P (1993) Speech development in children with cleft lip and palate. In Grunwell P (Ed) Analysing Cleft Palate Speech. London: Whurr.

Sell DA, Grunwell P (1990) Speech results followng late palatal surgery in previously unoperated Sri Lankan adolescents with cleft palate. Cleft Palate Journal 27: 162–8.

Sell D, Harding A, Grunwell P (1994) A screening assessment of cleft palate speech (Great Ormond Street Speech Assessment) European Journal of Disorders of Communication 29: 1–15.

Sparks SN (1984) Birth Defects and Speech-language Disorders. San Diego: College Hill.

Stuffins G (1989) The use of tongue and palate training aids in the treatment of speech problems. In Stengelhofen J (Ed) Cleft Palate: The Nature and Remediation of Communication Problems. London: Churchill Livingstone.

Van Demark D, Bzoch K, Daly D, Fletcher S, McWilliams BJ, Pannbacker M, Weinberg B (1985) Methods of assessing speech in relation to velopharyngeal function. Cleft Palate Journal 22: 281–5.

Watson ACH (1980) Embryology of cleft lip and palate. In Edwards M, Watson ACH (Eds) Advances in the Management of Cleft Palate. London: Churchill Livingstone.

Witzel MA (1983) Speech problems in craniofacial anomalies. Communicative Disorders 8(4): 45–59.

Part III
Communication Disorders
In Adults

Part II
Communication Disorders
in Adults

Chapter 11
Aphasia: Progress in Theory-based Intervention

RUTH LESSER

As a field dominated by the need to help a continuous flow of sufferers under the constraints of service pressures, rehabilitation is vulnerable to the enthusiasms of changing paradigms. Nowhere is this greater than in the rehabilitation of aphasia (or acquired dysphasia, the language disorder which can follow brain damage from stroke, head injury, surgery or other causes). One reason for this is the multidisciplinary foundations of the study of aphasia, and the aspirations of each discipline to enlighten this study as their interest in it grows. Thus the changing paradigms have been in turn neurological, phonetic, behavioural, linguistic (structural), cognitive-psycholinguistic, sociolinguistic and psychosocial. Yet despite more than a century of probing the nature of this disorder, aphasiology is only just beginning to ask detailed questions about the processes involved in assisting recovery from this condition, and exploring what therapy for aphasia actually does.

The aim of this chapter is to show how each paradigm which has been influential on therapy draws on theoretical foundations for its justification. A thorough review of the current state of aphasia therapy would discuss additional factors, such as service provision in different countries and under different professional conditions with different degrees of technological support. It would include issues such as the efficiency of therapy as assessed through studies of the appropriate time to start therapy, its intensity, its delivery through groups or individual treatment or through volunteers or assistants rather than through professional speech and language therapists. These are factors of considerable relevance to the practising clinician, but they are not directly pertinent to theories which guide the content of therapy as opposed to the means and contexts of its delivery. Neither are questions such as the influence on recovery of different aetiologies, sex, age, cerebral lateralization or site and extent of lesion, though as brain imaging becomes more sophisticated these may well impact on future theories of intervention, as well as their current use as rough guidelines as to the expected pattern of recovery in individuals. The question of effectiveness (in contrast to efficiency), however, has a relevance to theory-based intervention, as effectiveness can provide a preliminary test of how sound the theory is on which the therapy has been based

The present review, therefore, restricts itself to paradigms that have acknowledged the need to relate therapy to theory and which are currently being applied in the practice of aphasia rehabilitation. It is convenient to divide these into three groups: those which focus on the patient as the target of intervention (and are predominantly, though not exclusively, practised in clinical settings), those which focus on communicative interactions in which the patient and others participate together, and those which include elements of both. I shall devote most of the chapter to the first two groups as they are currently the most influential, with a brief acknowledgement of the third group in respect of behaviour therapy and psychosocial intervention.

In what follows assessment and intervention have not been separated. This is not only because theory-based treatment cannot be planned without assessment, but because both are continuing and interactive commitments for the therapist. In our present state of knowledge (and the field is so complex that this is likely to remain valid for many decades to come), assessment is a matter of forming hypotheses which responses to intervention will test and modify. Aphasia therapy is therefore of a very different order from the dominant medical model, in which a patient's symptoms lead to a diagnostic category which has a recommended prescriptive treatment. Speech and language therapists working with aphasic adults have, in fact, for a long time been seeking theories of aphasia which could explain why what they have been doing intuitively with their patients sometimes seems to work and sometimes does not.

Theoretical Bases of Intervention: Focusing on the Patient

I will first discuss those theory-based approaches to aphasia therapy that have focused on the patient's own linguistic and other abilities and deficits and which have generally been applied in a clinical setting, with the direct involvement of the therapist.

Unitary theory and stimulation therapy

Chronologically the first theory to have a significant and lasting impact on clinical practice in aphasia therapy was Schuell's unitary theory of aphasia. This proposed that all aphasic individuals share a common core disorder and emphasized the need to provide patients with repeated stimulation, primarily auditory but supported by other modalities, in order to make the complex events occur in the brain which are needed to support recovery (Schuell, Jenkins and Jiminez-Pabon, 1964). Schuell, a speech pathologist herself, proposed a model of language which required concerted action from the whole of the brain, subcortical structures as well as cortical. She accounted for the superficial differences amongst types of aphasia in terms of different kinds of non-aphasic deficits being added to simple aphasia – for example, sensorimotor deficits adding articulation difficulties, and visual deficits adding particular problems with reading. She advocated and described a range of techniques for coping with essential aphasia and these additional difficulties, which are still widely used in many clinics today.

Unitary theory, as Schuell propounded it, met with its critics because of what seemed in the following decade to have been its undue emphasis on word retrieval rather than grammar. Nevertheless, there are still elements of unitary theory which provide a valuable complement to more modern ideas. We see these in Luria's (1966) theory, which reconciles neurological and unitary theory. Neurologically localizable syndromes are proposed (afferent motor, semantic, sensory, etc.), but as well there is explanation in terms of disruption in neurophysiological activities which concern the whole brain, such as excitation, inhibition, perseveration, retention of traces, and inertia. The current expressions of such a modified unitary theory are in terms of impaired control systems (see Butterworth and Howard, 1987, for an example applied to jargonaphasia), accounts of the disparity between willed and automatic processing (Schacter, McAndrews and Moscovitch, 1988; Berry and Dienes, 1993), and a new 'connectionism' in computer modelling. This last mimics biological networks of neurones in that it employs networks of interconnected processors and engages in interactive parallel activity rather than serial activity referred back to a central memory store (see Schneider, 1987, for an introduction; Allport, 1985 for an application to anomia; and Harley, 1993 for a recent review of its general applicability to aphasia). Though connectionist models can be used to examine what happens when elements are 'lesioned', and thus have been used to test the predictions made by current models of aphasia and alexia, it is too soon to translate such observations into practical implications for therapy. Nevertheless, as Harley has observed, to some extent it has proved possible to re-train lesioned networks, in analogy to recovery of an ability damaged through brain trauma. Conference papers by Plaut and by Martin and her colleagues, which Harley cites, suggest that the retraining which occurs in the networks is faster than the original learning and does indeed parallel what has been observed in recovery from word-retrieval disorders in aphasia. Moreover generalization occurs to semantically associated items, particularly to less prototypical items – an observation which, if sound, could have implications for the selection of materials for therapy for semantic aspects of the disorder in aphasia.

The notion of the need for stimulation still underpins many approaches in aphasia therapy. It has gone beyond the recommendation for intensive drilling in word comprehension and word retrieval, to include drilling in different types of sentence structures (e.g. Helm-Estabrooks, 1981, Helm Elicited Language Program for Syntax Stimulation or HELPSS) and drilling in discourse scripts in a conversational setting (Holland's, 1991, Conversational Coaching). It has also been applied in group settings. Bollinger, Musson and Holland (1993), for example, in an evaluative study compared two types of group therapy that effected improvement on both a formal clinical battery and a measure of functional communication. The therapies comprised Contemporary Group Treatment ('multimodal stimulation with opportunities for listening, reading, speaking, writing-copying and gesturing' (p. 305) supplemented by specific drills and exercises) and Structured TV Viewing Treatment (coaching members of the group in appreciation and recall of storylines from episodes in TV programmes). In updated forms the influence of the unitary theory of aphasia and its recommendation for reactivation through repeated stimulation, therefore, remain significant in clinical practice.

Neurological theory and syndrome-linked therapy

The first elaborated theory of aphasia was a neurological one. Initially proposed in the nineteenth century by Wernicke, it was popularized more recently by Geschwind in the form of connectionist theory (here used in a different sense from that applied to the computer networks described above). This theory proposes that there are zones in the brain that control particular language functions, and tracts which connect them. Damage to these zones and tracts can account for the various phenomena of apraxia, alexia without agraphia and varieties of aphasia. The theory unfortunately brings with it few implications for aphasia therapy. From it an influential battery of tests has been developed, the Boston Diagnostic Examination of Aphasia (Goodglass and Kaplan, 1983), which claims to provide a 'comprehensive assessment of the assets and liabilities of the patient in all language areas as a guide to therapy'. These implications for therapy, however, have not been spelled out in detail. The implications drawn from the test in practice seem to be that, having found that the patient has problems with particular tasks in the examination, the therapist should work on those particular difficulties. For example, if the patient fails on Complex Ideational Material in the Auditory Comprehension Section, the inference is often drawn that the therapist should devise exercises to improve the skill of listening to short paragraphs and attending to their meaning. Thus, such an assessment leads to treatment of a symptom without further exploration of its underlying cause or causes.

Neurological theory classifies aphasia into several syndromes (Broca's aphasia, Wernicke's aphasia, anomia, etc.), and therapists who have been influenced by this neurological approach have devised several therapy programmes which are targeted at such specific syndromes, although the approaches which they apply in therapy have generally been the didactic stimulation one described above: e.g. Helm-Estabrooks's (1981) HELPSS for the agrammatic component of Broca's aphasia, and SLAC (Sentence Level Auditory Comprehension treatment), Naeser et al.'s (1986) programme for comprehension difficulties in Wernicke's aphasia. An addition to the therapist's repertoire, which draws directly on the neuroanatomical model, has been the notion of right hemisphere stimulation to assist the damaged left hemisphere in language recovery or to develop latent language in the right hemisphere as a substitute. The best known application of this is Melodic Intonation Therapy (Sparks and Holland, 1976), which draws on the prosodic abilities of the right hemisphere. A second tentative implication for intervention drawn from the neurological model is pharmacological treatment (Bachman and Albert, 1990). None of these, however, helps us into a deep understanding of the nature of the language deficit in aphasia. The whole notion of syndromes as applied to aphasia has been criticized on the grounds that they are polythetic, with heterogeneous elements combined (see, e.g. Ellis, 1987). For clinical practice, however, these therapy programmes have the considerable advantage of having been published in a structured form, with exact descriptions of their application. They can therefore provide a useful resource from which hard-pressed clinicians can select material, provided that such a selection can be justified on other theoretical grounds. For example, the SLAC programme may be appropriate for a subtype of auditory comprehension disorder, where phonemic discrimination is thought to need to be re-trained. The model of language the neurological approach uses, however, is relatively unsophisticated, and does not offer an insightful theory basis for therapy in itself.

Linguistic theories

Since the two approaches to therapy discussed so far, the unitary and the neurological, use simple concepts of the nature of language, we may ask what the study of language through the discipline of linguistics has been able to contribute to therapy. Linguistics has in fact been extremely helpful to aphasiology, but it has primarily been through providing frameworks for description and analysis (notably the framework which distinguishes the language domains of phonology, morphology, syntax, semantics, discourse and pragmatics). For clinical practice it has provided theory-based notions of rank order of complexity in language, for example in terms of distinctive features in phonology, of phrase structure trees in syntax and of sense relations in semantics. It has also provided empirically derived rank orders associated with order of acquisition by children. As specific linguistic theories have emerged, there have been attempts to apply them to aphasia. Examples are Jakobson's (1964) interpretation of Luria's syndromes, applying the linguistic notion of paradigmatic and syntagmatic dimensions of language, the attempts of Meyerson and Goodglass (1972) to account for aphasic difficulties in terms of transformational complexity, essays of my colleagues and myself at applying Bresnan's lexical functional grammar (Lesser, 1985), and the current interpretations of aphasia by Caplan and his colleagues (Caplan and Hildebrandt, 1988) in terms of government and binding theory. In as much as they make a contribution to aphasia therapy, these efforts have so far added depth to our knowledge of what makes language complex, but they have not yet led to direct applications to remediation.

There are, however, two branches of linguistics which have proved to have more direct implications for the remediation of the aphasic condition; these are, first, the elaboration of psycholinguistics, which forms part of the cognitive neuropsychological study of mental processes after brain damage, and, second, the application of sociolinguistic principles and methodology to the study of naturalistic communicative exchanges in which aphasic people participate, notably through conversation analysis. The implications of the latter approach for therapy are just now being explored, whereas there has recently been a flowering of single case studies of remediation using the psycholinguistic paradigm; this is also much more strongly associated with theoretical propositions. The psycholinguistic approach in aphasia therapy at present falls firmly within therapies which focus on the patient rather than the communicative interaction. In contrast, the sociolinguistic approach lends itself primarily to indirect methods of intervention that involve communicative contexts rather than single impaired individuals. This approach will therefore be addressed later in this chapter.

Psycholinguistic models of single-word processing as applied to therapy

A key notion in this approach is that mental processes are organized in modules. These modules are essentially distinct from each other in their functions although they work interactively and cooperatively. They use essentially abstract notions such as 'logogens', 'buffers', 'phonemes', 'graphemes'. They do, however, seem to be psychologically and neuropsychologically plausible, in that brain damage seems to show that the language system can fractionate in such a way as to disturb these proposed modules selectively. Recent brain imaging studies using positron emission tomography are also suggestive that there may be distinct brain substrates.

The models that have been used as a basis for therapy specify components in the processing of single words and of sentences. Since early psycholinguistic studies focused on single words, it is a single-word model that has so far been most applied in planning remediation for aspects of the aphasic disorder. Brief examples of these therapies will therefore be described first. This will be restricted to the naming of pictures of objects or printed words (i.e. reading them aloud); fuller descriptions of these and other targets of single-word therapy are given in Lesser and Milroy (1993).

A diagram and exposition of a model of single-word processing, which has been highly influential in aphasia therapy, can be found in Ellis and Young (1988). It illustrates the hypothesized processes which operate between seeing and hearing a word and pronouncing or writing it. In reading a word aloud, for example, the stages involved are said to comprise visual analysis, an orthographic input lexicon, the semantic (or meaning) system, a phonological output lexicon, a phonological assembly buffer and other output processes involved in the realization of the word in a spoken form. An additional 'subword' route, direct from visual analysis to the phonological assembly buffer, accounts for the ability to real aloud novel words or non-words. Much of the evidence in support of such a model comes from psychologists' experiments with normal subjects, but the models have been refined from observations of brain-damaged adults. For example, the notion that there may be two lexical routes in writing to dictation, one which bypasses the semantic system as well as one which uses that system, is based on observations from brain-damaged individuals (Patterson, 1986).

For the aphasia therapist to apply such a model to remediation, it is necessary first to be able to identify which of these hypothetical modules or processes may be malfunctioning. If we take reading aloud as an example, the therapist needs to test whether the patient's reading shows the influence of variables which can be linked back to different modules. If the reader is predominantly using the subword route to phonological assembly, rather than the lexical route, there will be effects of whether or not the word has an irregular print-to-sound correspondence. For example, *bear* may be read as 'beer' as if it rhymes with *hear*. Such patients, however, should still be able to read aloud correctly non-words or unfamiliar words, since the subword route is the normal way for coping with such novelties. In other patients, if processing draws on an impaired semantic system there are likely to be effects of the imageability ratings of the words, with high-imagery words producing fewer errors than low-imagery words. There may also be effects which show the influence of other language processes, in that grammatical words result in more errors than nouns, and that inflected and derived words cause more mistakes.

From such measurements, different types of alexia (or dyslexia) syndromes have been described (e.g., surface, phonological, deep and visual dyslexias). In surface dyslexia the lexical route is impaired, and reading shows the effects of use of the subword route. In phonological dyslexia, the subword route is impaired. Deep dyslexia is like phonological dyslexia with added complications implicating the semantic and grammatical systems. Visual dyslexia shows significant effects of word length, and implicates the visual word analysis system. There are many differences of behaviour within these and other dyslexia syndromes, and the same criticism of heterogeneity has been applied to them as to the neurological aphasia syndromes. Nevertheless, as a working framework, they have been applied productively in therapy. For example, de Partz (1986) diagnosed a patient of hers as a deep dyslexic, with malfunctioning subword route, and devised methods of re-establishing this route with such success that the patient then showed signs similar to those of surface dyslexia during his recovery to functional reading.

An extension of the part of this model that relates to the production of names of words in speech attempts to account for different kinds of anomic difficulties on confrontation naming (i.e. looking at a picture of an object and saying what it is). It is proposed that different types of difficulties can be related to the different processes involved, i.e. the semantic system, accessing the item in the phonological lexicon, assembling the accessed item and allophonic, phonetic and motor realization (for a more detailed justification of this model, see Lesser, 1989). All of these can lead to a failure to produce the correct name, although different kinds of behaviours will be observed. For example, a patient with a semantic disorder may produce semantic paraphasias for the target words (such as 'brother' for 'sister'), though this in itself is not definitive of a central semantic disorder, since normal speakers are not immune from such errors. Such a patient is likely, however, to have difficulty on semantic comprehension tests, where fine semantic discriminations have to be made. In order to establish this, the therapist needs to assess the patient using several modalities, and also to test whether the patient accepts cues for semantic associates as correct for the target word.

As a working theory for remediation, such a model has direct implications. Different naming disorders could need different kinds of treatment. The 'semantic' patient may need therapy aimed at clarifying word meaning, and producing sharper distinctions between words and associates. There is essentially no need for the patient to be asked to produce any speech during such therapy, since the assumption is that if the semantic system is improved the rest will follow. The 'phonological lexicon' patient may be assumed to need repeated practice at linking items in the semantic lexicon with those in the phonological lexicon. The rationale for this is that, if such patients show a significant effect of word frequency, as seems typical, then making words more frequently retrieved for this patient should therefore improve the available phonological lexicon. The case for this is somewhat weakened by recent demonstrations that effects which seem to be those of word frequency in the language can in fact be interpreted as related to the age at which the words were acquired (Morrison, Ellis and Quinlan, 1992). It seems likely, however, that some individuals may be influenced by age of acquisition and others by word frequency, suggesting a further differentiation may be needed in planning therapy for 'phonological lexicon' patients (Hirsh and Ellis, 1994). For the 'phonemic assembly' patient the best strategy may be to reduce the complexity of the assembly required by breaking the words down into component syllables, which are processed singly and then combined; classically, seeing the words in written form helps to facilitate this. There are many well known techniques for the other types of patients with more peripheral difficulties in the naming process, which I do not need to rehearse here as they are discussed in Chapters 13 and 14 on dysarthria and apraxia of speech.

This single-word psycholinguistic model, from which such therapy is derived, has been the subject of much criticism for its oversimplifications and, notably from advocates of the connectionist paradigm in lesion modelling, for its dependency on serial and staged processing (Seidenberg, 1988). Consistent with modular theory, it implies that there can be a disorder at any one stage without consequences for other stages, at least for those higher up the system. The model is certainly oversimplified; retrieving items from a phonological lexicon, for example, may well be influenced both by their semantic import for the individual and by their ease of phonemic assembly. But one subsidiary function of therapy is that it can be used to test the validity of such a model. A number of recent studies of therapy have considered this aspect of their results. Nettleton and Lesser (1991), for example, tested the prediction that naming therapy for patients with semantic disorders would be effective without giving the patients any practice themselves in producing names. The study produced equivocal results, in that one patient with a semantic disorder did show significant improvement after such treatment, whereas another did not, although his behaviours changed in that his semantic paraphasias became more related to their targets. The study partially supported the value of assessing patients according to psycholinguistic models in that two patients, whose naming disorder was not related to semantic difficulties, as predicted did not improve from semantic therapy. LeDorze et al. (1994) have looked more closely at the nature of semantic therapy. In a single case study, they controlled not only for the patient's not being asked to produce the names of objects, but also for his not even hearing the name spoken by the therapist. They thus provided two versions of 'semantic therapy': one in which the patient heard only definitions of the object, and had to make decisions about it as a concept; and another, labelled 'formal-semantic therapy', in which the patient did hear the names although was not required himself to produce them. A true semantic disorder, in which semantic concepts had become degraded or unavailable, should respond to the first type of therapy, it was argued. In contrast a disorder which impaired access to the phonological lexicon might respond to formal-semantic therapy through practice in hearing the lexical forms associated with their meaning. The patient, RB, did show a significant, although temporary, improvement after receiving formal-semantic therapy, though not after semantic therapy; this was consistent with other evidence that his impairment was not one of semantics itself, but was in making the desired links between meaning and name at will.

Psycholinguistic models of sentences as applied in therapy

Word retrieval is only one process in the production of speech, and other psycholinguistic models have attempted to explain what happens in between our thinking of what we want to say and uttering this thought as a sentence (this makes the questionable assumption that we do indeed always have sentences in mind when we produce an utterance). The model of sentence production that has been most referred to in aphasia therapy is that proposed by Garrett (1982) and developed by Schwartz (1987; Schwartz et al., 1994). Like the single-word processing model we have just considered, this also is based on studies of normal speakers and therefore has a validity which does not rest on pathological data. In this case the data are from observations of the speech errors made by normal speakers. Prior to the phonetic level of representation, Garrett's model proposes three earlier stages of representation, Message, Functional and Positional. Of these three stages, it is hypothesized disorders at the Functional level which have been proposed as underlying some types of agrammatic speech and which have received most attention in the psycholinguistic approach to therapy for sentence production. At this level functional relations are encoded, according to the model; permitted thematic roles, such as agent, theme, recipient, become mapped on to the predicate argument structure which is specified by predicators such as verbs. This therefore is the interface between meaning and a deep level of grammatical structure. In turn, this predicate argument structure has to be mapped onto a surface structure, through the realization of a syntactic 'tree structure' or constructional frame, which creates positional slots for each word. Thus the Positional Representation is derived, from which phonological processing can be undertaken.

In applying this model to disorders of grammar in aphasia, it seems sensible to see if we can distinguish between disorders which affect the achieving of the different levels of Representation. If the problem lies in moving from the Message to the Functional level, it may be suspected that patients would have difficulty in retrieving the appropriate content words from the semantic lexicon to express their meaning and/or in establishing the thematic roles of the sentence (e.g., who does what to whom, and with what). If the semantic item has been correctly accessed these thematic roles will be specified by the notion which has been retrieved which will form the predicator of the sentence. A transitive verb, for example, will specify that there must be an object for the sentence as well as a subject. Some verbs, such as 'put' and 'set', have arguments which specify location slots which must be filled; others such as 'give' and 'offer' have slots for recipients which generally must be filled. Problems at this level of representation, therefore, have sometimes been considered to be specifically related to difficulty with verbs. Schwartz et al. (1994) argue, however, that the difficulties experienced by patients who have difficulties in 'mapping' between semantics and syntax at the Functional level cannot simply be attributed to verbs. They point out that difficulty with verb arguments as such cannot account for the common finding that it is comprehension only of *moved* arguments (i.e. ones which are not in canonical order) that is difficult for many aphasic people. Nor, since arguments are specific to individual verbs, can such a claim account for therapy results where improvement generalizes to verbs which have not been included in the therapy programme.

Disturbances in the transition from the Functional to the Positional level may also be of different kinds. They may affect the ability to construct a syntactic frame, or they may affect the ability to select and insert the appropriate inflections and grammatical words (indeed, there are linguistically principled reasons, as well as some actual evidence, that subcategories of these may be selectively impaired). The implication of analyses such as these is that the term 'agrammatism' conceals a variety of processing disorders which may be selectively disturbed in different patients, e.g. there may be central verb disorders which affect comprehension as well as production, word-retrieval disorders in production specific to predicators and their arguments, 'mapping' disorders, constructional frame disorders, morphological disorders which affect inflection selection and so on. In fact in this psycholinguistic theory agrammatism and paragrammatism cease to be distinct types of disorders, and even lexical disorders may have secondary effects on grammatical production and comprehension.

Traditional therapy for agrammatism has focused on surface structure or on retraining of function words. Psycholinguistically motivated therapy has to date focused on patients with presumed mapping disorders. Pioneering work on this was first reported in single case studies by Jones (1986) and Byng (1988), with a partial replication by LeDorze, Jacob and Coderre (1991). Schwartz et al.'s (1994) recent study was of eight patients initially considered to have mapping disorders (reduced to six through a further stroke and death). Pre-therapy screening or training ensured that all the patients could identify verbs in sentences and, as in previous mapping studies, the therapy consisted of getting the patients to identify the theme ('What is she doing?') and the agent ('Which one is doing it?), with the different thematic roles colour coded. The sentences used fell into three categories: ones with action verbs (e.g. 'wash'), ones with experiencer verbs (e.g. 'know') and ones with non-canonical order such as passives and cleft sentences. In the event, five out of the six patients improved after therapy as measured through narrative speech or picture description. Two of the patients improved on comprehension tasks (using new sentences). The authors conclude, however, that only one of the cases had been directly suitable for mapping therapy. Despite being four years post stroke, this patient, EW, not only improved on the production of sentences in the narrative task, and showed generalization to the comprehension of new sentences, but also improved on the naming of single words both through reading aloud and naming pictures.

The psycholinguistic approach to the analysis and treatment of aphasia has therefore led to considerable advances in clinical practice. It is not, however, without its critics amongst speech and language therapists. These are not only on the grounds of the underspecification and provisional nature of the models on which it is founded, but primarily because it addresses only fractions of the mental processing of language, leads to language exercises which are not naturalistic, and, most seriously of all, interprets language outside its context of use and without its communicative function. To address this latter aspect, we need to turn to the other branch of linguistics we mentioned earlier, sociolinguistics.

Therapy Focusing on the Interaction

Applications of sociolinguistics through conversational analysis

Of particular concern to sociolinguists is the study of the varieties of spoken language (and a reminder that spoken language is very different from written language). The message has well and truly been got across in aphasia therapy that the therapist is concerned in facilitating restoration of, not some abstract norm of language, but the colloquial spoken language of individual patients in their particular speech communities and social networks. As distinct from central language as a medium for the user's thoughts, spoken language has a dual function. It serves to give and receive information and control the behaviour of others, but it also serves a solidarity function. It establishes the individual in a social context through the style and accent in which he or she speaks and in the content of what is said, including social small talk. The aphasia therapist has to be sensitive to this second dimension of the patient's needs as well as to disruptions in the central use of language and the more obvious information-giving use of language. Hence there is a burgeoning interest for aphasia therapists in conversational analysis.

Detailed work is now being undertaken into the behaviour of aphasic individuals and their partners during conversational exchanges (e.g. de Bleser and Weisman, 1986). To what extent do aphasic speakers retain turn-taking abilities, use cohesive devices for linking sections of discourse, achieve clarifications and repairs, draw on non-verbal communication, for example? Although there are now a number of protocols for measuring this aspect of language (Penn, 1985; Prutting and Kirchner, 1987; Wirz, Skinner and Dean, 1990) they have the limitation of assessing primarily only the aphasic speaker rather than the dynamic exchange between the two partners in the conversational dyad. They also rely on subjective judgements as to what is 'appropriate' and what not. More sensitive protocols are therefore needed which analyse the exchange itself and are data-driven in that they use participants' own reactions rather than applying the analyst's preconceptions. In particular they need to include all the minutiae which can convey conversational signals, and which may be particularly of crucial importance when one of the speakers' language is impaired. Two such protocols which have recently been proposed are those of Gerber and Gurland (1989) and Lesser and Milroy (1993). An increasing number of studies are scrutinizing conversations between aphasic people and their relatives, friends or therapists, and exploring the extent to which the aphasic behaviour affects communication in such settings. The principles which underlie such conversational analysis are reviewed in Lesser and Milroy (1993). Some studies have compared conversations with different interlocutors (Ferguson, 1994; Stimley and Noll, 1994), or focused particularly on how trouble spots in the conversation lead to collaborative repairs and who initiates such repairs (Milroy and Perkins, 1992; Ferguson, 1994). Collaborative repairs are characteristic of many such conversations, and point to the shared role of the participants in achieving communication.

For the therapist, the question is how to turn such observations into ideas for helping the aphasic patients and their partners. Since communication is a two-way process, it would appear that aphasic people's condition could be improved, not only by direct help with their defective language system, but by changing the environment which surrounds them. There are different levels of detail at which this can be done. The most obvious way is for the aphasia therapist to think of the patient not as an isolated individual but as a member of a community. Since many patients are initially referred in a hospital setting and are treated in clinical settings, this is not always as obvious as is assumed. Very often the patient's community may be a shrunken community as a result of the physical and communication handicaps. The therapist may seek to extend this where possible, for example by introducing the patient to a Speech after Stroke Club or by arranging for visiting volunteers where this is appropriate. At a second level of detail, the therapist's efforts will be directed at improving the patient's spouse's role in the communicative exchange through a better understanding of the nature of aphasia, with advice on how to improve communication through such strategies as repeating statements, simplifying language, speaking clearly and pausing (Green, 1984). The application of conversational analysis in aphasiology has recently permitted a third level of detail in how communication difficulties in aphasia may be ameliorated. This parallels the development of the psycholinguistic approach in that it provides individualized recommendations based on a detailed analysis of the individual's behaviour, though in this case it is the behaviour of individual carers and aphasic people interacting together. This allows the strategies which the therapist recommends to the carer and patient to be tailor-made for the particular dyad. For example, from a detailed analysis of recorded conversations between patient and carer at home, samples of successful or not-so successful repairs can be selected, and used as illustrations as to how future difficulties can be overcome (Lesser and Algar, 1995). If this goes in harness with a greater understanding in the carer and the patient of the psycholinguistic nature of that individual's disorder, the therapist has a further powerful potential tool for assisting remediation which combines the differing strengths of the psycholinguistic and the pragmatic approaches.

Other therapies

Other theory-related therapies do not fall so neatly into a dichotomy between patient-focused and interaction-focused. Only brief mention of them will be made here, as they have less current impact on clinical practice in this field.

The first is behaviour therapy. A strong influence on intervention for other speech and behavioural disorders in the 1960s and 1970s, it seemed on the surface less applicable to the overtly organic disorder of aphasia. It has well-developed theoretical principles underlying its practice, however, and there is no prima facie reason to assume that aphasic people are less prone to 'non-organic' behavioural disturbances than others. Indeed, given the circumstances they face, it could be argued that they might well experience more. The implication is that patients may not be using to the full the residual resources they have retained, perhaps due to emotional reactions or the development of maladaptive habits. There are a few examples reported in the literature of behaviour therapy successfully using token reward, modelling or desensitization procedures with aphasic patients and/or their carers (see, for example, Goodkin, Diller and Shah, 1973; Smith, 1974; Damon, Lesser and Woods, 1979), and this paradigm may well be underacknowledged in current clinical practice in aphasia therapy.

If the behaviour therapy paradigm in intervention for aphasia is currently experiencing a lull, another is poised for development. This is the psychosocial approach. This also straddles the grouping between patient-focused and interaction-focused. In some ways it is an extension of the behavioural paradigm in that it attempts an explanation for some behavioural difficulties. One facet emphasizes the repercussions on the patient of loss of 'self', drawing an analogy between the aphasia-producing stroke and sudden bereavement (Brumfitt, 1993). If such an analogy is accepted as uncontroversial, Holland and Beeson (1993) make some suggestions as to how the therapist may adjust her behaviour and the pattern of intervention in order to ameliorate the distress. Brumfitt and Clarke (1989) describe the therapeutic techniques of counselling, which they feel can be used with aphasic people in order to help to contain the distress and confusion. The model of psychotherapy they advocate, however, is that of 'good parenting' or 'making things manageable the way a parent does for an upset child' (p. 100), and some therapists may question how appropriate this would be in working with adults whose independence needs to be sustained. Mackenzie (1993) raises another issue, and that is the extent to which the speech and language therapist's role extends into psychosocial intervention and such specialized counselling.

Others acknowledge that the distress is likely to extend to the whole family, and therefore advocate family therapy (Wahrborg, 1989). It is argued that there is a relationship between active family support and successful stroke rehabilitation; it is spouses' interpretation of the aphasic member's impairment rather than the actual degree of impairment itself which is more important for social isolation. Families (and the aphasic member) may therefore benefit from help to overcome anxiety, guilt feelings, their own self-perceptions and rejection. Many aphasia clinics have set up support groups for relatives in an attempt to meet this need, but the detailed analysis of family reactions to aphasia has still to be undertaken, and this aspect of aphasia rehabilitation has yet to develop a sound theoretical basis.

Effectiveness of Intervention

A final aspect of this discussion of the relationship between theory and practice in aphasia therapy is the question of evaluation of the effectiveness of therapy. This is important in any kind of intervention and applies to pragmatic intervention with spouses, using a sociolinguistic, behavioural or psychosocial perspective, as much as to psycholinguistic or other intervention directly with the patient. With any theory-based approach there is an additional value in that the results of therapy (i.e. whether it was effective or not) can feed back into the theoretical model and justify it or show how it needs modification. This in turn feeds back into clinical practice. Evaluation requires accurate and replicable measurement. The means for achieving this in terms of the psycholinguistic models described are available (see, for example, Kay, Lesser and Coltheart, 1992), as are replicable procedures in analysing conversations (see, for example, Gerber and Gurland, 1989). There have been several expositions in the literature recently of designs which can be used in single case studies of the effectiveness of therapy; in particular, AB designs which contrast treatment and non-treatment periods of two different tasks, multiple-baseline designs where treatment is expected to be item-specific and extended-baseline designs. The latter can be used where the treatment might be expected to have generalized effects but where the effects of a non-treatment period can be subtracted from the effects of treatment (for reviews see McReynolds and Thompson, 1986; Pring, 1986; Howard and Hatfield, 1987).

All these are beginning to make evaluation of therapy a practical proposition in the working clinic, given that reliable and practical instruments are available to measure changes in the processes or situations which are being treated. Great advances have been made in linking theory and the practice of aphasia therapy over the last few years; students are now graduating from their degree courses better equipped than ever before to push both theory and practice forward together, and an increasing number of clinicians are recognizing that making time to apply the newer theories to therapy and evaluate their effectiveness promises to benefit their patients and the families who share the consequences of their condition.

References

Allport DA (1985) Distributed memory, modular subsystems and dysphasia. In Newman S, Epstein R (Eds) Current Perspectives in Dysphasia. Edinburgh: Churchill Livingstone.

Bachman DL, Albert ML (1990) The pharmacotherapy of aphasia: historical perspective and directions for future research. Aphasiology 4: 407–13.

Berry DC, Dienes Z (1993) Implicit Learning. Hove: Lawrence Erlbaum.

Bleser R de, Weisman H (1986) The communicative impact of non-fluent aphasia on the dialogue behavior of linguistically impaired partners. In Lowenthal F, Vandamme F (Eds) Pragmatics and Education. New York: Plenum Press.

Bollinger RL, Musson ND, Holland AL (1993) A study of group communication and intervention with chronically aphasic persons. Aphasiology 7: 301–13.

Brumfitt S (1993) Losing your sense of self: what aphasia can do. Aphasiology 7: 569–75.

Brumfitt S, Clarke P (1989) An application of psychotherapeutic techniques to the management of aphasia. In Code C, Muller D (Eds) Aphasia Therapy (2nd ed). London: Whurr.

Butterworth B, Howard D (1987) Paragrammatisms. Cognition 26: 1–37.

Byng S (1988) Sentence processing deficits: theory and therapy. Cognitive Neuropsychology 5: 629–76.

Caplan D, Hildebrandt N (1988) Disorders of Syntactic Comprehension. Cambridge, MA: MIT Press.

Damon S, Lesser R, Woods RT (1979) Behavioural treatment of social difficulties in an aphasic woman and a dysarthric man. British Journal of Disorders of Communication 14: 31–8.

Ellis AW (1987) Intimations of modularity, or, the modelarity of mind: Doing cognitive neuropsychology without syndromes. In Coltheart M, Sartori G, Job R (Eds) The Cognitive Neuropsychology of Language. London: Lawrence Erlbaum.

Ellis AW, Young AW (1988) Human Cognitive Neuropsychology. Hove: Lawrence Erlbaum.

Ferguson A (1994) The influence of aphasia, familiarity and activity on conversational repair. Aphasiology 8: 143–57.

Garrett MA (1982) Production of speech: Observations from normal and pathological language use. In Ellis AW (Ed) Normality and Pathology in Cognitive Functions. London: Academic Press.

Gerber S, Gurland GB (1989) Applied pragmatics in the assessment of aphasia. Seminars in Speech and Language 10: 263–81.

Goodglass H, Kaplan E (1983) Assessment of Aphasia and Related Disorders. Philadelphia: Lea and Febiger.

Goodkin, R, Diller L, Shah N (1973) Training spouses to improve the functional speech of aphasic patients. In Lahey B (Ed.) The Modification of Language Behavior. Springfield, Illinois: C.C. Thomas.

Green G (1984) Communication in aphasia therapy: Some of the procedures and issues involved. British Journal of Disorders of Communication 20: 35–6.

Harley TA (1993) Connectionist approaches to language disorders. Aphasiology 7: 221–49.

Helm-Estabrooks N (1981) Helm Elicited Language Program for Syntax Stimulation. Austin, TX: Exceptional Resources Inc.

Hirsh KW, Ellis AW (1994) Age of acquisition and lexical processing in aphasia: a case study. Cognitive Neuropsychology 11: 435–58.

Holland A (1991) Pragmatic aspects of intervention in aphasia. Journal of Neurolinguistics 6: 197–211.

Holland A, Beeson PM (1993) Finding a new sense of self: what the clinician can do to help. Aphasiology 7: 581–4.

Howard D, Hatfield FM (1987) Aphasia Therapy: Historical and Contemporary Issues. London: Lawrence Erlbaum.

Jakobson R (1964) Towards a linguistic typology of aphasic impairments. In de Reuck AVS, O'Connor M (Eds) Disorders of Language. Edinburgh: Churchill.

Jones EV (1986) Building the foundations for sentence production in a non-fluent aphasic. British Journal of Disorders of Communication 21: 63–82.

Kay J, Lesser R, Coltheart M (1992) Psycholinguistic Assessments of Language Processing in Aphasia. London: Lawrence Erlbaum.

LeDorze G, Boulay N, Gaudreau J, Brassard C (1994) The contrasting effects of a semantic versus a formal-semantic technique for the facilitation of naming in a case of anomia. Aphasiology 8: 127–41

LeDorze G, Jacob A, Coderre L (1991) Aphasia rehabilitation with a case of agrammatism: a partial replication. Aphasiology 5: 63–85.

Lesser R (1985) Sentence comprehension and production: an application of lexical grammar. In Rose FC (Ed) Recent Advances in Neurology, 42: Progress in Aphasiology. New York: Raven.

Lesser R (1989) Some issues in the neuropsychological rehabilitation of anomia. In:

Seron X, Deloche G (Eds) Cognitive Approaches in Neuropsychological Rehabilitation. London: Lawrence Erlbaum.

Lesser R, Algar L (1995) Towards combining the cognitive neuropsychological and the pragmatic in aphasia theory. Neuropsychological Rehabilitation 5: 67–92.

Lesser R, Milroy L (1993) Linguistics and Aphasia: Psycholinguistic and Pragmatic Aspects of Intervention. London: Longman.

Luria AR (1966) Higher Cortical Functions in Man. London: Tavistock.

Mackenzie C (1993) Concern for the aphasic persons sense of self: why, who and how. Aphasiology 7: 564–9

McReynolds LV, Thompson CK (1986) Flexibility of single-subject experimental designs. Part 1: Review of the basics of single-subject designs. Journal of Speech and Hearing Disorders 51: l94–203

Meyerson R, Goodglass H (1972) Transformational grammars of three agrammatic patients. Language and Speech 15: 40–50

Milroy L, Perkins L (1992) Repair strategies in aphasic discourse: towards a collaborative model. Clinical Linguistics and Phonetics 6: 27–40.

Morrison CM, Ellis AW, Quinlan PT (1992) Age of acquisition, not word frequency, affects object naming, not object recognition. Memory and Cognition 20: 705–14.

Naeser MA, Haas G, Mazurski P, Laughlin S (1986) Sentence level auditory comprehension treatment program for aphasic adults. Archives of Physical Medicine and Rehabilitation 67: 393–6.

Nettleton J, Lesser R (1991) Application of a cognitive neuropsychological model to therapy for naming difficulties. Journal of Neurolinguistics 6: 139–57.

Partz MP (1986) Reeducation of a deep dyslexic patient: rationale of the method and the results. Cognitive Neuropsychology 3: 149–77.

Patterson KE (1986) Lexical but non-semantic spelling? Cognitive Neuropsychology 3: 341–67.

Penn C (1985) The profile of communicative appropriateness: a clinical tool for the assessment of pragmatics. The South African Journal of Communication Disorders 32: 18–23.

Pring T (1986) Evaluating the effects of speech therapy for aphasics: developing the single case methodology. British Journal of Disorders of Communication 21: 103–15.

Prutting CA, Kirchner DM (1987) A clinical appraisal of the pragmatic aspects of language. Journal of Speech and Hearing Disorders 52: 105–19.

Schacter DL, McAndrews MP, Moscovitch M (1988) Access to consciousness: dissociations between implicit and explicit knowledge in neuropsychological syndromes. In Weiskrantz L (Ed) Thought Without Language. London: Oxford University Press.

Schneider W (1987) Connectionism: Is it a paradigm shift for psychology? Behavior Research and Methods 19: 73–83.

Schuell HM, Jenkins JJ, Jiminez-Pabon E (1964) Aphasia in Adults: Diagnosis, Prognosis and Treatment. New York: Harper and Row.

Schwartz MF (1987) Patterns of speech production deficit within and across aphasia syndromes: application of a psycholinguistic model. In Coltheart M, Sartori G, Job R (Eds) The Cognitive Neuropsychology of Language. London: Lawrence Erlbaum.

Schwartz MF, Saffran E, Fink RB, Myers JL, Martin N (1994) Mapping therapy: a treatment programme for agrammatism. Aphasiology 8: 19–54.

Seidenberg M (1988) Cognitive neuropsychology and language: the state of the art. Cognitive Neuropsychology 5: 403–26.

Smith MD (1974) Operant conditioning of syntax in aphasia. Neuropsychologia 12: 403–5.

Sparks R, Holland A (1976) Method: melodic intonation therapy for aphasia. Journal of Speech and Hearing Disorders 41: 287–97.

Stimley MA, Noll JD (1994) The effects of communication partner on the verbal abilities of aphasic adults. Aphasiology 8: 173–80.

Wahrborg P (1989) Aphasia and family therapy. Aphasiology 3: 479–82.

Wirz S, Skinner C, Dean E (1990) Revised Edinburgh Functional Communication Profile. Tucson, Arizona: Communication Skill Builders.

Chapter 12
Acquired Speech Dyspraxia

NIKLAS MILLER

In an outline chapter on speech dyspraxia it is impractical to cover even a fraction of what is known and argued about in the field. Questions facing clinicians include: what is (speech) dyspraxia; how do I recognise it; what bearing do theoretical issues have on my approach to assessment and rehabilitation; how do I work scientifically towards a firmer knowledge of how to treat speech dyspraxia? The aim here is to sketch out a framework of facts and issues considered relevant to the subtitle of the book, *The Science of Intervention*, with readers left to fill in the detail from references given and their clinical experience.

What is Dyspraxia? First Sightings

The apraxias are a group of disorders (Miller, 1986; Roy and Square-Storer, 1990) which have in common problems in the selection, organization and execution of appropriate motor responses for the volitional control of learned action. This may involve limb movements, eye movements, oral non-verbal movements, or movements concerned with speech production. The latter disorder is discussed under numerous labels, including speech dyspraxia, apraxia of speech, verbal dyspraxia, efferent motor dysphasia, cortical dysarthria, and many more. This broad definition, imperfect though it might be (see below), already contains some pointers to the recognition of dyspraxia just from observing a person and carrying out routine clinical examinations.

The disruption of voluntary action control at the stage of selection, organization and execution of movements, rather than at the stage of conduction of neural impulses from the motor cortex to the periphery, or at the stage of actual muscle contractions, leads to several characteristics that typify dyspraxic behaviour, including dyspraxic speech production. There is no loss of power or change in tone; reflexes are normal, as are the range and speed of movements that the person can be capable of. Sensory functions are also normal, with no change in auditory, visual and tactile perception. Furthermore, dyspraxic breakdown does not stem from non-cooperation, low motivation, non-comprehension, attentional deficits, nor any generalized intellectual deficit. Of course, dyspraxia may co-occur with any one or more of these problems. For example, the speech dyspraxic person often has a (right) facial weakness; the limb dyspraxic person may have a hemiparesis, loss of sensation, or underutilization of a limb due to neglect. In such cases the clinician's task is to unravel which impairment is contributing in what way and to what degree to the person's disability. The presence of a marked dysphasia may render differential diagnosis and the treatment approach even more difficult.

Since the disorder affects volitional, conscious action control, the person may be apparently unable to accomplish a task when trying to do it to some purposeful end, or when directly requested to carry out a command. However, when not actually thinking about it, or responding reflexively, they may succeed without error. So, the limb dyspraxic person may not be able to demonstrate how to put their hand on their head when asked, but seconds later do it while nonchalantly scratching their head. The person with buccofacial dyspraxia may not succeed in moving their tongue round their lips in an oral physical assessment, but execute it perfectly having just eaten a jam doughnut. The clinician may struggle in vain with the dyspraxic speaker to elicit the syllable /mi/ only to hear the person say it perfectly when someone calls 'who does this £10 note belong to?'.

This variation between volitional and more 'automatic' actions is better seen as a continuum rather than a neat dissociation. In speech dyspraxia, for instance, there is not an invariant boundary for all speakers that divides so-called automatic speech from volitional speech. The dividing line varies according to level of severity and situational factors. In cases of severe speech dyspraxia utterances deemed automatic for less severely affected speakers, such as proverbs, idioms, cliches, or rote learned lists like the days of the week, may be inaccessible, with only the most highly reflexive utterances heard, such as um's and er's or expletives. The more habitual the situation is for the performance of a particular action, the more predictable an action is from the context, the more likely it is to succeed automatically. Something deemed automatic, reflexive, or overlearned, such as counting, or saying a 'Hail Mary', is not necessarily still 'automatic' if one tries to elicit it in atypical circumstances.

Two other features are attributable to the types of breakdown believed to underlie dyspraxic behaviour. Stemming from variable success at accessing or organizing appropriate movement patterns, responses can be highly inconsistent. This can be apparent even on immediately succeeding repetitions of the same word. Because sensory, receptive processes are intact, dyspraxics are aware of their inaccuracies and typically try to correct them. This leads to characteristic trial and error struggle, with repeated attempts at a target or compensatory, slow 'tip-toe' homing in on the desired response.

These are general behavioural traits of dyspraxic performance. In the individual dyspraxia types (limb, constructional, buccofacial, etc.) there are also characteristic derailments to performance that divide them from other disorders and may be the targets of treatment. Since this chapter is on speech the focus now will be on this. Those wishing to follow up other dyspraxias might consult Miller (1986), Kimura and Watson (1989), Square Storer (1989), Roy and Square Storer (1990), and Rothi, Ochipa and Heilman (1991).

What is Speech Dyspraxia? A Closer Look

The manifestations of speech dyspraxia naturally vary according to the severity of the disorder. In mild cases speech may sound slow, deliberate, hesitant, with minor apparent dysfluencies and dysprosody. Speakers may sound as if they are talking with a foreign accent (Ingram, McCormack and Kennedy, 1992). Despite this, intelligibility is functionally intact, with only articulatorily complex strings of sound provoking breakdowns in intelligibility that require repetition for clarification. As severity increases, dysfluency and dysprosody grow. Unexpected pauses appear between, and even within, words. These silences may be filled with visible oral-facial struggle or audible struggle to reach the target sound. The impression of foreign accent gives way to definite distortions. Atypical allophones are heard, e.g. unaspirated [t] or nasalized vowel in *two*. Distortion might be so marked as to suggest another sound has been substituted – *two* is heard as [du]. At other times unwanted sounds seem to be added, or expected ones omitted – [tfu], [u:], again for *two*. This pattern of distortion, apparent substitution, addition and omission is, as intimated above, characteristically inconsistent, so that in the same phonetic context on repeated occasions, a quite different production ensues, e.g. *Two teas please* could be realised as [ˈtuˈtiz pliz], [ˈtsi ˈtaɪs ˈfliz], or [a ˈdʉt ˈʔeɪz pf.pɹ..pleɪ.plis].

In more severe cases shorter and less intelligible utterances predominate. Even on single words success may be seldom, especially if they have a complex syllable structure or are less frequent words in the person's vocabulary. In the severest cases there may not even be any utterances. Patients may be aphonic. Attempts at spontaneous conversation or even imitating single syllables end after effortful struggle in frustrated silence.

The pattern of perceived segmental errors was earlier claimed to differentiate speech dyspraxia from other speech disorders. However, more recent work has been unable to confirm this (Zyski and Weisiger,

1987; Odell et al., 1990; 1991; Miller, 1993). This does not mean that different underlying neurological conditions do not cause differing disruptions to speech production. Rather, multiple types of disturbance result in similar perceived surface derailments, and perceptual features that might lead clinicians to the underlying impairment are too difficult to hear sufficiently reliably with the naked ear to provide interjudge agreement regarding their presence or severity. On the one hand this has stimulated attempts to uncover differential diagnostic traits and treatment targets for different disruptions to speech production via acoustic and physiological investigations. On the other hand it has strengthened searches for alternative ways of relating perceived, physiological and acoustic features to the posited underlying neurolinguistic disruption(s) to the demands of therapy for the communication breakdown. These two directions will be briefly examined before proceeding to the 'science of intervention'.

Acoustic and Physiological Investigations of Speech Dyspraxia

Workers have used a variety of acoustic and physiological measures to describe dyspraxic speech and contrast it with other speech disorders – most notably dysarthria. Whether the approach has been to use fibre-optics (Itoh and Sasanuma, 1984), sound spectrography (Kent and Rosenbek, 1983), electropalatography (Edwards and Miller, 1989) or electromagnetic articulography (Katz et al., 1990), there is general concurrence about the kinds of features that characterize dyspraxic speech. In some way the spatial and/or temporal coherence of movements for speech is disrupted – in contrast to (certain) dysarthrias where instrumental indications point to a decrease in absolute velocity and range of movements in association with degraded speech. McNeil, Caliguiri and Rosenbek (1990) investigated acceleration and velocity times for apraxics. They too emphasized that in apraxia it is relative and not absolute values that are disturbed. They found, despite delayed initiation and intra-individual variation, that apraxics and normals behaved similarly regarding speed and range of movements. Dysarthrics were characterized by failure to reach peak velocities and to attain the desired range of movement (Ziegler and von Cramon, 1986).

A detailed review of all the above studies is not possible here. An essential point to note, however, concerns the nature of the relationship between movement and sound. Speech sounds issue from movements. One may read in some introductory phonetics textbooks descriptions of sounds that look like descriptions of static postures, but the essence of articulation is movement, simultaneously, of the many parts of the vocal tract. These multiple movements are not independent of each other. Onset and termination of movements, the range and speed of movements relative to each other of distant (e.g. diaphragm, larynx, lips) and neighbouring (e.g. upper and lower lip; intrinsic and extrinsic tongue muscles) articulators are tightly organized and constrained. Movements are intricately interweaved, such that at any point in time one may discern elements of previous, current and upcoming movements and their corresponding sounds. Alteration of the fine spatial–temporal tuning of the characteristic co-articulatory pattern for a given language gives rise to changes in a person's speech perceived as distortions, substitutions, omissions, and so on. This is what appears to be happening in speech dyspraxia. There is impairment of the spatial–temporal tuning of movements needed to produce sounds and move from one sound to the next. It is not absolute timing and placement that seems to be affected but the relative timing between articulators necessary for fluent, coherently co-articulated speech.

In mild cases listeners may only perceive the disruption as an idiosyncratic way a speaker has of producing certain sounds or sound combinations. In less mild circumstances the gradual uncoupling of the co-articulatory features may lead to the impression of a foreign or strange accent. As dissolution deteriorates definite distortions to sounds may be heard. It can be seen how the dissolution of normal timing and co-articulation leads to perceived errors. For instance, problems with voice onset time distinctions lead to the impression of 'substitutions' (they are not substitutions in the sense that the person 'selected' the wrong target, rather the target has been so distorted as to be perceived as having crossed a categorical boundary) of voiceless for voiced sounds in word initial position (in English). Mistiming of velar movements (Itoh and Sasanuma, 1984) can lead to intermittent, inappropriate hyper- or hyponasality or in more extreme cases to the impression of 'substitution' of oral for nasal sounds or vice versa. What are heard as stopping and affricatization difficulties tie in with problems of controlling contact force and time/duration.

Two significant findings, not apparent to the naked ear, are that even during 'silent' pauses considerable abortive articulatory activity may be taking place, and that many sounds that appear correct to the listener are actually produced with abnormal articulatory postures (Edwards and Miller, 1989; Hoole, Schroeter-Morasch and Ziegler,1989; Gentil, 1992).

Of course, saying that the difficulty seems to lie with mis-specification of spatial and/or temporal parameters is no real answer to what the underlying disorder is in dyspraxia. It simply begs a new set of questions. Some of the problems hiding behind such statements are now turned to.

Models of Speech Production and Problems of Pronunciation

No comprehensive definition of speech dyspraxia has been offered – not without reason. The main problem is that there is no agreed definition of speech dyspraxia that is not loaded with debatable terms and open to alternative theoretical interpretations. The chapter opened with a broad statement that (speech) dyspraxia represents a disorder in the selection, organization and execution of movements for learned volitional actions. Even this endeavour to remain neutral contains contentious terms. Does this mean that selection, organization and execution are three separate processes? Do they run independently of each other, in the order given here? If not, what is their order or state of interdependence? How do they relate to other aspects of movement control? Even if the choice of words is supportable from experimental, theoretical and/or clinical evidence, *what* is selected; in what form; where is it selected from; how is the appropriate selection targeted in the first place? What is organized, in what way and by what means? What is executed, what form do the 'instructions' for execution take, and what are they addressed to? The list of unanswered questions is endless.

Some accounts of the speech production process (e.g. Abbs, 1988) have tried to give body to these general notions. A suggestion has been that after choice of a semantic target, a second lexical look-up identifies the abstract phonological string for the word; this is converted at some stage into phonemes, which are slotted in the correct sequence for subsequent real-time production, before being converted into motor commands which are addressed to the necessary muscles. This is close to earlier hierarchical models, such as that of Garrett (1984). This scholarship sharply divided a pre-motor, language (phonological), planning stage from a later, phonetic, motor, execution stage. The latter was linked to speech dyspraxia, while the former was designated a dysphasia. Dysarthria was considered to be associated with a stage after the phonetic one, involving disruption to conduction of the nerve impulses to the muscles to realize the preassembled blueprint.This sketch, though, raises more questions than it answers. Are there really independent semantic and phonological 'stores'? What form does the abstract phonological specification take? What is a phoneme? Do they really exist as anything more than a convenient descriptive device for psycholinguists, and if so in what form and where? Do, and if so how do, abstract phonological forms turn into the physical form required for actual movement? What form do the 'commands' to muscles take? Are they in terms of spatial targets, acoustic targets, (spatial) temporal linkages across muscle(s) groups?

The instrumental investigations mentioned above lure one to talk of timing specifications, since on the surface that is what seems to be disrupted in speech dyspraxia. But, even should that be true, what is timed? Is it muscle contraction duration, interarticulator phasing, or what? Where does the timing come from? Is it intrinsic or extrinsically determined? Or, is the timing disruption only secondary to another factor? For instance, mis-specification of spatial targets would also lead to apparent changes in timing of movements, relative onsets and offsets and so forth.

The failure to solve these questions within a hierarchical framework has stimulated other ways of conceptualizing the entire speech production process. Alternative arguments, both theoretical (Fowler, 1985; K. Stevens, 1989; Saltzman and Munhall, 1989), linguistic (Browman and Goldstein, 1992; Dell, 1988) and clinical (Folkins and Bleile, 1990; Weismer and Liss, 1991) have challenged rigid compartmentalization of underlying processes in production and their posited associated pronunciation breakdowns. From a theoretical standpoint interactive accounts of speech production have been argued for which de-emphasize the independence, or even existence, of separate stages (Harley, 1993). Motor-control perspectives have offered alternative physical, mechanical accounts of action which try to solve the problems of the mental–physical leap involved in hierarchical accounts of speech programming. These have been complemented by developments in linguistics seeking physical, articulatory accounts of all aspects of speech production (Hawkins, 1992) which view the notion of 'phoneme' and the control units of production in a quite different light to, say, traditional segmental phonology. Still others have sought to clarify the control conundrums by starting not from the notions of what neurolinguistic processes and organization might lie behind speech, but what are the movement characteristics of the vocal tract, how do these relate to the properties of real and perceived sounds, and what kind of control processes are compatible with the empirical data (K. Stevens, 1989; Lindblom, 1990).

Reductionist accounts tried to explain speech production and its disorders by tracing perceptual features back to their assumed constituent acoustic elements, these in turn to their presumed physiological constituents, and so on. However, the thrust of heterarchical arguments is that the secret of speech and its control does not reside in any one structure or process. Rather, speech emerges out of an interaction among all the processes and actions involved in speaking – both internal and external to the speaker. In this perspective there is no central, fixed programme that unfolds in some invariant fashion with subsequent levels of control simply unfolding or translating codes prepared at an earlier phase. There is no one-to-one correspondence between neurophysiological, kinematic, acoustic and perceived 'units'.

Each of these angles can provide a valid description of speech, but the intricacies of speech as communication can only be appreciated by viewing the interaction of speaker and listener, language (semantics and syntax) and speech, segmental and suprasegmental parameters of speech, and the complex (i.e. not simple translation one-to-one) relationship of movement, sound as spoken and sound as perceived.

At the least this has resulted in the admission of interactive and bottom-up as well as top-down notions into hierarchical models (e.g. Levelt, 1989); in extreme departures from hierarchical perspectives the development has been to a complete coalescence of all productive and perceptive parameters (e.g. in the direct realist approach of Fowler, 1985).

This is not all idle ivory tower speculative debate which has no bearing on clinical work. On the contrary, resolution of theoretical questions, or, pending resolution, choice of a particular theoretical view, determines what one believes one is differentially diagnosing from what; which criteria diagnosis is based on; what the targets of therapy should be; which aspects of speech represent core symptoms of a disorder, which are the result of compensatory readjustment throughout the system; and what methods there might be of manipulating the variables to effect communicative change. These points are picked up below in the discussion on intervention. The next section considers some implications for assessment.

Assessment Considerations

There are two general paths on which to approach assessment. They are not mutually exclusive, but adopt a different attitude to the speaker and can bear on the later path through therapy. One could be labelled the functional approach, the other a medical-model, syndrome approach.

The functional approach starts from the perspective of the person who feels in some way dissatisfied with their intelligibility and seeks to answer the question, *why* is their communication impaired? Evaluation may then start with investigations of the overall communicative environment to see how far the problem is in the ear of the listener and not the performance of the speaker. To gauge the loss of communicative power of the person's speech a diagnostic intelligibility test would be administered (Kent, 1992). This should indicate which aspects of speech appear to undermine intelligibility. Analyses might cover:

- the relative effects of the loss of particular contrasts, e.g. ± voice, ± nasal, stop vs. fricative, velar vs. alveolar;

- differences according to the position of derailments in words, e.g. initial vs. final, consonant vs. vowels;
- the influence of syllable and/or sentence length and complexity;
- the effects of prosodic disturbance;
- the effect on listener judgements of trial-and-error struggle behaviour;
- the relative interference with message transmission of, for example, displacement (anticipation; perseveration; transposition) vs. substitution derailments.

In speech dyspraxia and phonemic paraphasia a relevant variable to examine might also be the consequences for intelligibility of the variable nature of pronunciation breakdown.

From these alternatives, the choice of therapy targets would be decided with the speaker on the basis of: what level of intelligibility he wishes or needs to reach, and which variables constitute the main barrier to this desired level of intelligibility. The functional path meets the syndrome-based path when it comes to deciding which of these features is open to therapeutic influence and in what way they can be influenced. It is helpful for the clinician to know not only what features of impaired pronunciation affect intelligibility, but also why those features arise – be it problems with ± voice; loss or blurring of particular articulatory position(s), or manner(s), or whatever. This helps clarify which therapeutic techniques and strategies will be appropriate for influencing the underlying impairment(s) leading to the aspects of performance that affect intelligibility.

Of course, for differential diagnosis it is assumed that the criteria for separating underlying impairments exist and that the links between one aspect of performance (e.g. strength and speed of articulator movement and intelligibility – Dworkin and Aronson, 1986) or analysis (e.g. spectrographic printout and articulatory configuration – Weismer and Liss, 1991; Gentil 1992) are transparent. It was suggested above that clinicians and researchers are not on firm ground in this respect. It is also apparent, as mentioned earlier, that theoretical issues are not irrelevancies removed from clinical concerns. How one believes speech is produced, and what consequences different disruptions have for the speech production process overall, radically influence what one looks for in differential diagnosis, how one looks for it, and what one does about it in intervention. Issues in diagnosis are detailed elsewhere (Wertz, LaPointe and Rosenbek, 1984; Square Storer, 1989; Kearns and Simmons, 1990) and cannot be dissected here. The next paragraphs offer a sketch of these issues with some rules of thumb for differential diagnosis.

Whatever the procedure and theoretical standpoint adopted, the aim will be to apply it with systematic, objective, and testable rigour. The aim, through testing the various routes and /or interactions hypothesized to exist between different inputs (auditory; reading; picture naming; spontaneous speech), different outputs (spoken; written), different tasks (real vs. nonsense words; single words vs. sentences; closed vs. open class words etc.) is to isolate those processes which appear to account for why a particular speech picture exists and which variables therefore should be the targets of therapy. As intimated above, no definitive model or procedure exists. Even within relatively narrow areas of hypothesized models dealing with relatively small aspects of speech production there remains divers and often conflicting evidence. Compare for instance the review of the functional localization of conduction dysphasia (Buckingham, 1992) and the views of Dell (1988) and Levelt (1989) on related questions.

As methods of approaching individual cases the approaches in the references mentioned above provide a good framework. However, how much they have to say on the totality of questions in speech production (consider the flavour of possible questions given above) and the persistence of disagreements about *the* solution limit their scope for answering all clinical decisions at present. In the absence of final answers one has to make do with general directions, especially as people one meets in day-to-day clinical routine so seldom seem to present as such neatly delineable cases as those selected for publication and hypothesis testing. This is not to underestimate or understate the importance of the clinician's role in refining and confirming or refuting the soundness of such rules of thumb through a systematic and objective attitude to assessment. What disruptions, dissociations, interactions, and so forth, to investigate brings us back to the question of theoretical perspective and what to look for. Solutions differ between, for instance cognitive psycholinguistic approaches and connectionist views. Despite this there are some general areas where relative agreement exists about areas it may be fruitful to look in.

Assessment Areas

Does the person know what word he is trying to target in the first place? Tests of semantics will be needed here (e.g. feeling of knowing, tip of the tongue, semantic association tasks). Observation of the person can also help – despite inability to speak a word, is he nevertheless able to gesture, draw, or write it. The specific speech error type does not allow one to distinguish specific underlying neurophonological or motor disorders, but general trends can point in certain directions to explore further. Do attempts at words bear any resemblance to the target – in terms not only of the sounds in the utterance, but also of the number and structure of the syllables. The lower the scores on the semantic tests, the less the evidence from other expressive media that the person 'knows' the target, and the greater the utterance departs from the target in content and structure, the more likely one is dealing with a non-speech problem. This does not preclude the possibility of semantic disorders having an effect on sound patterning, or vice versa (Caramazza and Hillis, 1990; Caramazza and Miceli, 1990).

If there is evidence for semantic intactness, does the speaker know the sound pattern he is aiming for? Can he identify targets from amongst foils which are controlled for minimal paradigmatic and syntagmatic pairs? Here one is examining the ability to monitor that the correct sound is about to be or has been produced, and in the correct position in a string. Again, observation of speech attempts may complement more formal tests. Can fragments of the target be discerned in the output? Do attempts at least match the target in syllable number and stress assignment? Are the 'errors' largely of ordering, with a predominance of anticipations, perseverations or transpositions? Can apparent substitutions be related to derailment triggers in the general word or phrase environment? Do repeated tries at a target bring widely (in terms of place-manner features) varying realizations (e.g. Valdois, Joanette and Nespoulous, 1989) in contrast to homing in which displays close-to-target deviations with a gradual progression towards the right sound? How fluent, how effortful or effortless are the run-ups; how accommodated to native language phonology do the 'errors' appear; how far are derailments restricted to particular word classes (e.g. form vs. content)? Can the person endeavour to write the word, even if mis-spelled, or gesture correctly, despite the pronunciation problem?

It is unlikely that there will be a clear-cut picture. However, if the trend is towards fluently articulated displacement or far-from-target perceived errors that are accommodated to the person's native phonology, with matching syllable number and stress and restricted to content words, then the greater the likelihood that the central problem lies in the specification of the correct sound in the correct position. In traditional terms this is labelled phonemic, or literal, paraphasia. Buckingham (1983) terms it apraxia of language.Classically it is the disorder associated with reproduction conduction dysphasia. Of course, *why* such a breakdown occurs and *what* is being mis-specified depends on your theoretical standpoint.

This contrasts with, or in interactive perspectives blends through to, a picture where perceived target order is essentially intact, but a problem emerges of fine tuning for targets, especially transitions between neighbouring sounds. The person performs well on semantic tasks, is able to write the word correctly and pick it out from amongst foils closely matched on sound and meaning (in so far as no dysphasia coexists with the dyspraxia). Perceptually there are fewer if any displacements. Speech 'errors' are discernibly closer to the target (predominantly one place–manner feature) with a predominance of distortions, additions and substitutions. The latter two, together with apparent omissions, are arguably variations of the distortions that arise as the person effortfully struggles to achieve target sounds and smooth transitions from one sound to the next. This is supported by instrumental findings, where even in perceptually intact sounds, distortions and homing in on targets are shown (Kent and Rosenbek, 1983; Edwards and Miller, 1989; Weismer and Liss, 1991).

Prosody can be disrupted, though it remains disputed whether this constitutes a primary feature of this speech dyspraxic disorder (Square Storer and Appeldoorn, 1991; Kent and Rosenbek, 1982), or whether it is secondary to the audible and visible struggle to get the articulators to where the person knows they should be, but they just will not obey. Flow of speech is also typically disrupted by between- and in-syllable pauses, usually filled with struggle behaviour. Prosody too might be characterized by recurrent restricted patterns and/or syllabification (Kent and Rosenbek, 1982). Again it is unclear whether this represents a core behaviour or is a compensatory tactic people adopt to lighten the control load. Despite apparent laborious slow movements instrumental and straightforward oral physical examinations demonstrate no primary sensory motor impairment, and, even if there is a facial hemiparesis, the nature and degree of this are far from adequate to explain the speech picture.

This is classical speech dyspraxia. As a dyspraxia it is not surprising to find performance influenced by the degree of propositionality, or the familiarity of the word and sound sequence. Compare *you* with *ewe*, and *him*, *he's fair* with *hemisphere*, where the first of each pair proves easier. Inconsistency (Miller, 1992) of error pattern across and within elicitation modes and matched sound contexts is also relatively prominent here.

In contrast to the above constellations of behaviours, in dysarthria the predominance of perceived errors moves towards distortions and omissions, indicated by instrumental assessments as arising from failure to reach target velocities or full range of movement excursions. Oral physical examination uncovers a close coupling between site and severity of weakness and the speech picture. Furthermore, unlike in speech dyspraxia and phonemic paraphasia the error pattern and severity remain constant across elicitation modes, real and nonsense words and closed vs. open class words. Struggle, if present, is commensurate with the degree and severity of weakness and can be seen or heard as attempts to reach target velocity and position, not to correct mis-selection or ordering of articulatory features. Also the neuromuscular symptoms link to the overall neuromuscular (ataxic, hypokinetic etc.) picture. Relative consistency of (un)successful realization of a given sound in a given context is the rule rather than the exception, especially in spastic and flaccid dysarthrias.

Assessment of the person's language can also help give pointers to diagnosis and therapy. The greater the comprehension deficit, at least as regards stroke aetiology, the more likely one is looking at a dysphasic problem, with the sound pattern difficulty linked to problems in fixing the appropriate target word, not syllable structure and sounds. Even if the pronunciation breakdown stems from a disruption to speech production, low comprehension is likely to receive priority in treatment over speech output. The presence of language difficulties should also alert the clinician to possible speech-language interaction in 'error' genesis. For instance [lãĩgəɹ] might be suspected of originating in competition between lion and tiger, or [fɹɔkɪnnaɪf] from fork and knife vs. carving knife. Sorting out which dysfluencies and dysprosody arise from word finding, sentence structuring or speech production factors is another task the clinician may face.

A further consideration in diagnosis, is that differentiation is not simply between dysphasia, dysarthria and dyspraxia. They each have subtypes with their own characteristics. Teasing out speech dyspraxic features from ataxic dysarthria (Kent and Rosenbek, 1983) presents a different task to separating it from upper motor neuron lesion dysarthria (Hartman and Abbs, 1992). Different criteria pertain to dividing apraxia of language, as opposed to speech dyspraxia behaviours, from dysphasic elements, and within the latter will change according to whether it is a Broca's or Wernicke's type. Coexisting limb and/or constructional dyspraxia may be important to uncover (Miller, 1986) as potential factors influencing the person's ability to gesture, write or draw a word they cannot say.

The message remains that, despite claims in the literature for 'pure' forms of hypothesized underlying disorders and dissociations, the majority of people met in clinic will show a mixture of behaviours and only approximate posited 'pure' pictures. This underlines the advantages of a case-by-case approach to diagnosis, avoiding the temptation to label a person as manifesting disorder x and proceeding to make all the diagnostic and intervention assumptions derived from a blanket term, heedless of the specific profile with which the individual presents. Thus in the first instance diagnosis should proceed from the speaker, his insights, needs and wishes; followed by the diagnostic intelligibility evaluation and a search for why the surface intelligibility situation has arisen. This will detail the strengths and weaknesses in the *individual's* pattern of dissociations and the variables that influence success at speaking and communicating overall. Intervention in this way can be much better tailored to the speaker's needs. If labels are going to be helpful, they are better couched in terms of the maximum likelihood formulae (Bates *et al.*, 1991), or similar. Such data do not yet exist for speech disorders.

Treatment: Some General Principles

The *science* of intervention has been longer in reaching the therapy front than the theory and assessment field. Careful and systematic identification and control of variables are no less important in the clinic than in the laboratory for establishing which therapies do or do not work, which ones are the optimum approaches for particular goals and/or symptom pictures, and which are the best times and methods for implementation, and so forth.

There are several prerequisites to a fruitful path through therapy. A reliable differential diagnosis goes without saying. Knowing the underlying motor problem will point towards what therapeutic techniques are appropriate. Contrary to previous claims, off-the-peg programmes linked to particular medical-model syndromes will not necessarily address the needs of the individual client, other than by default. Content comes first from asking and negotiating with the person what his priorities in communication are, and what he wants to achieve through therapy. Second, it comes from an examination of the speech signal in the communicative context to focus therapist, speaker and listener on those elements of the signal that should be targets for change and give constructive and purposeful direction to therapy. Third, pinpointing nodes of breakdown within a speech-production model framework indicates which processes in speech production are leading to the identified breakdowns in intelligibility and in turn shape the content and form of therapeutic tasks.

Following this the therapist needs to construct therapy tasks and recruit techniques and strategies that:

1. involve processes in the production area where breakdown occurs;
2. will effect change in those areas; or,
3. if needs be, provide routes round a breakdown by alternative and/or augmentive means.

Therapy needs to be designed and monitored such that the clinician can verify:

1. whether change is taking place or not;
2. if it is taking place, is it in the targeted variables;
3. can change be attributed to therapy elements, if so which; or
4. whether change is coincidental to therapy content and methods.

If therapy proves not to be working, the clinician needs to determine which variables, altered in which way, seem to change the situation.

Several works deal in a general way with the objective design of intervention (McReynolds and Kearns, 1983; Dworkin, 1991). There are also several exemplary approaches to speech dyspraxia and other motor speech treatment which illustrate the systematic construction and monitoring of therapeutic tasks and change (Wertz et al., 1984; articles in Square Storer 1989; Dworkin, Abkarian and Johns, 1988). Dworkin et al.

stress the importance of describing the specific nature of tasks to be used; delineation of the type and sequence of steps to be followed; establishment of criteria used for progressing within and between steps; quantification of the time and trials required to achieve (sub)goals; indication of which steps proved easy or difficult; consideration of which modifications to methodology may have produced more efficient/ quicker outcomes. To these one can add the importance of incorporating measures of generalization – how far are changes restricted to directly targeted items, how far does change generalize to similar/same classes of behaviour. It is also necessary to design and measure therapy in a way that permits calculation of whether changes within a behaviour, or of the behaviour compared to another (±treated), are statistically significant. Dworkin et al. (1988) employed a multiple baseline design and used multiple retrospective and prospective probes to ascertain data on effectiveness. Dworkin (1991) espouses a model approach to treatment and nothing said here can currently add to that. Other carefully designed routine clinic-based studies of speech dyspraxia therapy include Lambier et al. (1989), Rau and Golper (1989), Square-Storer and Hayden (1989), and E. Stevens (1989).

The importance of such care in design cannot be overstated. It is not a clinical luxury nor an obsession with particularness. It is the *sine qua non* of advancement in clinical science that every clinician can and must participate in daily. Results do not have to be publishable, but if the therapist wishes objectively to demonstrate the efficacy of her treatment to herself, to the client, and to administrators and to refine her knowledge of what works with whom, when and what for, then such an approach is indispensable.

Apart from these organizational principles, there are other guiding considerations for the content and context of therapy. Management naturally varies with both the degree of speech impairment and the extent to which other dysfunction either impinges on communication or might influence therapeutic methods. Treatment of the speech disorder may not be the prime priority. Progress in spoken language may be dependent on comprehension, syntax, word finding, monitoring skills, limb dyspraxia, or other concurrent impairment. Judicial balancing of prerequisites and priorities is part of the skill of the clinician, and informed and properly monitored passage through such an obstacle path will speed recovery for the speaker, save morale-sapping months of input with no change, and thereby cut down the time needed for one person and increase time available for other people.

In addition to the principled approach to assessment and case design, the principled structure that can be lent to therapy from lessons in psychology and linguistics enters the ring here. This assures that overall goals are meaningful and worthwhile ends; subgoals along the way are manageable steps; and generally the principles of learning psychology are observed. Linguistic principles (Miller and Docherty, 1995) guide the construction and succession of tasks from subphonemic features to suprasegmental dimensions, as well as give insight into variables that can be manipulated to arrive at direct or compensatory goals. Thoughtful and informed therapy also knows when to stop. If monitoring shows that progress has halted and that alternative routes have been exhausted, preparation for discharge and counselling for other approaches to communication must prevail.

Focus on the minutiae of voice onset time or formant transitions should not blind (or deafen?) the clinician to the communicative aims of therapy, i.e. incorporation of (re)acquired skills into the communication context. The whole person and overall context must not be forgotten. So, from the start one must remember that an informed and trained listener (Miller, 1989; Vogel and Miller 1992; Dongilli, 1994) is as important as a good speaker. Mystery about the nature of the disorder, the direction of therapy, and the role of the listener should not be added hurdles on the road through therapy. Nevertheless, experience has shown that successful speakers are those able to take over their own therapy. Therapy which is ever dependent on the clinician is of limited or no value. Therapy must teach the person not only what to do, but how to do it. If a technique, content or goal has no use in its own right, or as a stepping stone to communicative independence, it is redundant.

Some Treatment Practices

Fashions in therapy are continually evolving. Today's clinical spring collection is tomorrow's old hat. Therapy content is shaped by clinicians' views on what they believe to be the cause and course of the disorder, what has seemed to work in the past, and the organization of their rehabilitation service. Clinicians should not close their eyes to methods not mentioned here, nor to novel combinations of those mentioned. If careful monitoring is built into therapy, it should soon become clear whether a particular path is the treatment of choice.

Intervention varies with severity of the disorder. In very severe cases the person may be mute and efforts will be directed towards eliciting any sound and establishing some (alternative) communication channel (Coelho and Duffy, 1990; Fawcus, 1990). Methods include stimulation via so-called automatic actions (singing, humming, over-learned material and series); via paralinguistic and non-verbal gestures (tut-tut, yawning, blowing a kiss); by physical placement of the articulators by the therapist; through imitation (±verbal); and by following static or moving pictograms/articulograms. Emphasis will be on looking, feeling, and listening as much as on speaking. The why and how of following pictograms, copying clinicians and using mirrors all need to be trained. They are not magic wands. As soon as a sound is possible it should be given a use. Elicitation and control techniques must also be taught to the family.

Less severe cases may manage approximations to sounds. The above techniques can be used to stabilize and extend the repertoire. Once a sound is stable it can be used to derive other positions/sounds, and to stand in contrast with another element. Except in extreme instances when problems arise even in producing isolated sounds, speech dyspraxia manifests itself more when concatenation of sounds and syllables commences. Sounds/syllables in isolation tend to be relatively preserved.

Which sound do you start with? Group data suggest a gradient of difficulty rising through vowels, plosives, nasals, laterals and fricatives to affricates. Individual people do not necessarily conform. Hence the need to establish each individual's pattern. Order of teaching will depend on this and factors such as visibility, feelability, direct manipulability, frequency of occurrence in familiar words and phrases (family names, pets, over-learned and social words), and, importantly, usability in terms of the expansion to a person's communication afforded by the (re)acquisition of a given contrast. For instance, /ð/ in English is visible, feelable, manipulable, and occurs frequently – but it is limited in the number of other sounds it stands in minimal contrast with. Consequently choosing /ð/ in favour of say /s/ or /t/ would not normally be a recommendation. Debate continues on whether it is better to proceed through meaningful or nonsense syllables. Programmes employing nonsense syllables (e.g. Deal and Florance, 1978) aim to tackle the actual motor speech dysfunction more directly, with the justification that, because meaningful syllables are tied to linguistic and situational variables, there may be less generalizability. There are no hard data to support either way. Functionally, for the speaker, it is hard to wait months before meaningful stimuli are introduced, and many would say that if a technique works (meaningful syllables), then why ignore it? Either way, therapy progresses through increasing syllabic complexity, moving from familiar single-syllable words in predictable, habitual circumstances to uncommon (for the person) polysyllabic words in simple, and then complex, grammatical utterances, in situations of increasing propositionality and decreasing external (visual, tactile, contextual, etc.) support.

With the attainment of stable syllables progressing to multisyllables, several more important ways of extending communicative competence are available. Tonal variation offers scope for saying the same utterance with an imperative, questioning, or doubting tone. Different nuances can be expressed by contrasting stress on different syllables. Contrastive stress drills take a phrase and practise it with alternative stress and intonational patterns, e.g. '*buy* him a red shirt', 'buy *him* a red shirt', 'buy him a *red* shirt', 'buy him a red *shirt*', uttered as statements, commands, or questions. However, there is evidence that contrastive stress exercises may not (Liss and Weismer, 1994) be equally successful with all speaker groups. In some cases intelligibility may be improved simply by concentration on suprasegmental features. Hargrove and McGarr (1994) give, in their Prosodic Teaching Model, methods of training tempo, intonation, stress and rhythm, directed to pragmatic, syntactic, lexical, attitudinal, and other roles of prosody. They also present a rationale for choosing and prioritizing treatment targets and methods within the sphere. Thus, in mild cases, depending on the wishes and needs of the speaker (do they need to talk over the phone, to a hearing impaired spouse, in a noisy background, etc.?) emphasis may be on prosodic variables or techniques to manage unfamiliar, complex words.

The gap can be bridged between single and polysyllabic words by first introducing longer words composed of well rehearsed single syllable elements; toe-ma-toe for *tomato*; pan-D-mow-knee-M for *pandemonium*; car-ten for *carton* and *curtain*. This last strategy points to a way of settling for non-'perfect' articulation, which is nevertheless unambiguous in context. By the same token one can exploit the perceptual equivalence of sounds not necessarily produced with 'standard' articulatory settings, e.g. /m/ as ɱ; /f/ as ɸ; /t/ with the tongue body, not the tip. As an especial difficulty in speech dyspraxia is smooth transition from syllable to syllable, techniques are useful which ease this by teaching with co-articulations incorporated, e.g./hæmbæg/ for *handbag*; modifying transitional complexity – /bəlæk/ for *black*; or permitting a degree of distortion, e.g. the carton/curtain and /ɱ/ for /m/ examples above. These strategies are dealt with more by Miller and Docherty (1995). In using such methods dyspraxic speaker and therapist are seeking the best trade-off between articulatory precision and functional intelligibility.

Another method of deriving connected speech is by movement towards propositional language from less volitional. An often cited example is *fried egg* from *Friday*. Others would be *want to* from *1, 2*; *deaf* from *D.E.F.* Relearned or intact 'chunks' can serve as carrier phrases for these or other words. Gonna, wanna, /ɪsa/ (it's a. . .) /wezə/ (where's the . . .), especially if combined with other (approximations to) familiar utterances (/ta/ – thanks; /næŋks/ – no thanks, etc.) can boost communicative morale.

Mention has been made of direct therapy, various ways of reorganizing intact skills to replace lost skills and gaining access to utterances through alternative channels. For some patients speech will always remain elusive or inadequate and substitution or augmentation through other media will be necessary.

Replacement Therapies

Some dyspraxic speakers are fortunate enough to have (relatively) intact writing. Others will be able to utilize alphabet charts or mechanical equivalents to these. Concurrent language problems, alas, often mean that use of such equipment is as limited as spoken communication. Machines that employ pictographic, prerecorded messages associated with a single button, or synthesized speech as alternative or augmentative expression may be more suitable here.

Gestural systems from *ad hoc* personal choices to complete systems provide another avenue of expression. The presence of limb dyspraxia and severe dysphasia may inhibit learning in some subjects (Rothi and Heilman, 1985). Also, as Coelho and Duffy (1987) point out, there are people who acquire manual gestures but who just do not or cannot use them.

This has been a very fleeting skim over some central principles in therapy for speech dyspraxia. One is aware that as much has been left out as included, especially regarding treatment of fluent apraxia of language (Kohn, Smith and Arsenault, 1990; Bruce and Howard, 1987; Nickels, 1992) and the potential of instrumental techniques (EPG, laryngograph, see, for example, MorganBarry, 1989; Goldstein et al., 1994). The concerned clinician must consult the more detailed references for closer guidance.

Effectiveness of Treatment

There are no large-scale studies on the efficacy of apraxia therapy equivalent to reviews attempted on dysphasia intervention. LaPointe (1984) conducted a single case multiple-baseline study and Wertz (1984) reported the performance of dyspraxic–dysphasic people in a larger survey of people with dysphasia. Investigations exist into the usefulness or not of various components of overall apraxia treatment, e.g.melodic intonation therapy (Tonkovich and Marquardt, 1977); fading of integral stimulation (Holtzapple and Marshall, 1977); a hierarchical continuum of integrated stimulation (Deal and Florance, 1978); the pairing of vibrotactile stimulation with speech production (Rubow et al., 1982); and the works cited above.

The work of LaPointe and Dworkin demonstrated improvement and the patients in the report by Wertz improved if they received motor speech training, but not as a result of general language therapy. Given the controlled conditions stipulated in the studies (as opposed to diluted, haphazard application, which is always a danger in clinic), it is clear that speech dyspraxia can respond to therapy. All approaches involved an intensive pattern of therapy. Even if not seen daily by a therapist, patients carried out daily practice. The studies also re-emphasize the need for objective, principled structuring of therapy steps and the assessments that monitor them – establishing baselines and controls, systematically manipulating variables (input, response demands, etc.) and monitoring which mode and combination of therapies are proving most effective for the individual. Only in this way will unproductive practice be eliminated and speakers reap maximum benefit from intervention.

Conclusion

The centre ground of a definition and description of speech dyspraxia is relatively uncontroversial. But, despite the fact that instrumental techniques have added greatly to our descriptive knowledge, many issues of explanation remain undecided. Evidence has been cited supporting the notion that the central disruption in what is traditionally considered to be speech dyspraxia lies in a breakdown in the temporal and spatial cohesion of speech action. But how do these actions originate, how are they organized and carried out within the central nervous system and what exactly is disrupted? What should be the units of analysis? Are there different types of speech dyspraxia according to which aspects in the assembly and unfolding of actions are disordered?

Suggestions for solutions point towards an interplay between an ideational, conceptual, cognitive–linguistic planning disorder (traditionally termed phonemic paraphasia), an ideomotor executive production breakdown (traditional speech dyspraxia) and a so-called limb-kinetic dyspraxic-dysarthria. These arise from different disruptions to a heterarchically organized speech motor system.

It has further been emphasized that speech dyspraxia may be a motor disorder, but it exists within a linguistic framework, which in turn exists within social interaction. Elements of planning and execution may be higher cortical, but this activity interacts and is in turn dependent on subcortical organization. Hence dyspraxia may be influenced by, and simultaneously itself influence, co-existing language and dysarthric disorders. Therapy may be via direct attention to (assumed) underlying dyspraxic breakdown, but manipulation of other aspects of planning and communication can also be used to influence speech output. A philosophy of intervention was introduced that was aware of and exploited all these interdependencies.

Accordingly, therapy, at different times or through different approaches, concentrates on direct, so-called intrasystemic, attempts to restore malfunctioning areas; indirect, so-called intersystemic reorganization of intact functions to compensate for or circumvent deficits; and creation of an optimal communication environment. This chapter has suggested first steps in these directions.

References

Abbs J (1988) Neurophysiologic processes of speech movement control. In Lass N, McReynolds L, Northern J, Yoder D (Eds) Handbook of Speech Language Pathology and Audiology. Toronto: Decker.

Bates E, MacDonald J, MacWhinney B, Appelbaum M (1991) Maximum likelihood procedure for the analysis of group and individual data in aphasia research. Brain Language 40: 231–63.

Browman C, Goldstein L (1992) Articulatory phonology: an overview. Phonetica 49: 155–80.

Bruce C, Howard D (1987) Computer generated phonemic cues. British Journal of Disorders of Communication 22: 191–201.

Buckingham H (1983) Apraxia of language vs. apraxia of speech. In Magill R (Ed) Memory and Control of Actions. Amsterdam: Elsevier.

Buckingham H (1992) Phonological production deficits in conduction aphasia. In Kohn S (Ed) Conduction Aphasia. Hillsdale: LEA.

Caramazza A, Hillis A (1990) Where do semantic errors come from? Cortex 26: 95–122.

Caramazza A, Miceli G (1990) Structure of the lexicon. In Nespoulous J-L et al. (Eds) Morphology, Phonology and Aphasia. New York: Springer.

Coelho C, Duffy R (1987) Relationship of the acquisition of manual signs to the severity of aphasia, Brain Language 31: 328–45.

Coelho C, Duffy R (1990) Sign acquisition in two aphasic subjects with limb apraxia. Aphasiology 4: 1–8.

Deal J, Florance C (1978) Modification of the eightstep continuum for treatment of apraxia of speech in adults. Journal of Speech and Hearing Disorders 43: 89–95.

Dell G (1988) Retrieval of phonological forms in production. Journal of Memory and Language 27: 124–42.

Dongilli P (1994) Semantic context and speech intelligibility. In Till J, Yorkston K, Beukelman D (Eds) Motor Speech Disorders. Baltimore, MD: Brookes.

Dworkin J (1991) Motor Speech Disorders. St Louis, MI: Mosby.

Dworkin J, Abkarian G, Johns D (1988) Apraxia of speech: the effectiveness of a treatment regimen. Journal of Speech and Hearing Disorders 53: 280–94.

Dworkin J, Aronson A (1986) Tongue strength and alternate motion rates in normal and dysarthric subjects. Journal of Communication Disorders 19: 115–32.

Edwards S, Miller N (1989) Using EPG to investigate speech errors and motor agility in a dyspraxic patient. Journal of Clinical Linguistics and Phonetics 3: 111–26.

Fawcus M (1990) Information transfer in four cases of articulatory dyspraxia. Aphasiology 4: 207–12.

Folkins J, Bleile K (1990) Taxonomies in biology, phonetics, phonology, speech motor control. Journal of Speech and Hearing Disorders 55: 596–611.

Fowler C (1985) Current perspectives on language and speech production. In Daniloff R (Ed) Speech Science London: Taylor & Francis.

Garrett M (1984) Organisation of processing structure for language production. In Caplan D (Ed) Biological Perspectives of Language. Cambridge. MA: MIT Press.

Gentil M (1992) Variability of motor strategies. Brain Language 42: 30–7.

Goldstein P, Ziegler W, Vogel M, Hoole P (1994) Combined palatal lift and EPG feedback therapy in dysarthria: a case study. Clinical Linguistics and Phonetics 8: 201–18.

Hargrove P, McGarr N (1994) Prosody Management of Communication Disorders. London: Whurr.

Harley T (1993) Connectionist approaches to language disorders. Aphasiology 7: 221–49.

Hartman D, Abbs J (1992) Dysarthria associated with focal unilateral upper motor neuron lesions. European Journal of Disorders of Communication 27: 187–96.

Hawkins S (1992) Introduction to task dynamics. In Docherty G, Ladd D (Eds) Papers in Laboratory Phonology II. Cambridge: Cambridge University Press.

Holtzapple P, Marshall N (1977) Application of multiphonemic articulation therapy with apraxia patients. In Brookshire R (Ed) Clinical Aphasiology Conference Proceedings. Minneapolis, MN: BRK.

Hoole P, Schroeter-Morasch H, Ziegler W (1989) Disturbed laryngeal control in apraxia of speech. Proceedings XXI IALP Conference, Prague, August.

Ingram J, McCormack P, Kennedy M (1992) Phonetic study of a case of foreign accent syndrome. Journal of Phonetics 20: 457–74.

Itoh M, Sasanuma S (1984) Articulatory movements in apraxia of speech. In Rosenbek J, McNeil M, Aranson A (Eds) Apraxia of Speech. San Diego: College Hill.

Katz R, Machetanz J, Orth U, Schoenle P (1990) Kinematic analysis of anticipatory coarticulation in the speech of anterior aphasic subjects using electromagnetic articulography. Brain Language 38: 555–75.

Kearns K, Simmons N (1990) Efficacy of speech language pathology intervention: Motor speech disorders. Seminars in Speech and Language 11: 273–95.

Kent R (Ed) (1992) Intelligibility in Speech Disorders. Amsterdam: Benjamins

Kent R, Rosenbek J (1982) Prosodic disturbance and neurologic lesion. Brain Language 15: 259–91.

Kent R, Rosenbek J (1983) Acoustic patterns of apraxia of speech. Journal of Speech Hearing Research 26: 231–49.

Kimura D, Watson N (1989) Relation between oral movement control and speech. Brain Language 37: 565–90.

Kohn S, Smith K, Arsenault J (1990) Remediation of conduction aphasia via sentence repetition. British Journal of Disorders of Communication 25: 45–60.

Lambier J, Andrews F, Atwell D, Couper M (1989) Comparison of two treatment techniques for the remediation of acquired dyspraxia. Australian Journal of Human Communication Disorders 17: 3–19.

LaPointe L (1984) Sequential treatment of split lists: a case report. In Rosenbek J, McNeil M, Aranson A (Eds) Apraxia of Speech. San Diego: College Hill.

Levelt W (1989) Speaking: From Intention to Articulation. Cambridge, MA: MIT Press.

Lindblom B (1990) On the notion of possible speech sounds. Journal of Phonetics 18: 135–52.

Liss J, Weismer G (1994) Selected acoustic characteristics of contrastive stress production in control geriatric, apraxic and ataxic dysarthric speakers. Clinical Linguistics and Phonetics 8: 45–66.

McNeil M, Caliguiri M, Rosenbek J (1990) Comparison of labiomandibular kinematic durations, displacements, velocities and dysmetrias in apraxic and normal adults. In Prescott T (Ed) Clinical Aphasiology. Boston, MA: College Hill.

McReynolds L, Kearns K (1983) Single Subject Experimental Designs in Communicative Disorders. Baltimore, MD: University Park.

Miller N (1986) Dyspraxia and its Management. Beckenham, Kent: Croom Helm.

Miller N (1989) Strategies of language use in assessment and therapy for acquired dysphasia. In Grunwell P, James A (Eds) Functional Evaluation of Language Disorders. Beckenham, Kent: Croom Helm.

Miller N (1992) Variability in speech dyspraxia. Clinical Linguistics and Phonetics 6: 77–85.

Miller N (1993) Perceptual errors in acquired speech disorders. Presentation, British Aphasiology Society Conference, September, Warwick.

Miller N, Docherty G (1995) Acquired speech disorders: applying linguistics to treatment. In Grundy K (Ed) Linguistics in Clinical Practice. London: Whurr. In preparation.

MorganBarry R (1989) EPG from square one. Clinical Linguistics and Phonetics 3: 81–91.

Nickels L (1992) The autocue? Self generated phonemic cues in the treatment of a disorder of reading and naming. Cognitive Neuropsychology 9: 155–82.

Odell K, McNeil M, Hunter L, Rosenbek J (1990) Perceptual characteristics of consonant production by apraxic speakers. Journal of Speech and Hearing Disorders 55: 345–59.

Odell K, McNeil M, Rosenbek J, Hunter L (1991) Perceptual characteristics of vowel and prosody production in apraxia, aphasic and dysarthric speakers. Journal of Speech and Hearing Research 34: 67–80.

Rau M, Golper L-A (1989) Cueing strategies. In Square Storer P (Ed) Acquired Apraxia of Speech in Aphasic Adults. London: Taylor and Francis.

Rothi L, Ochipa C, Heilman K (1991) Cognitive neuropsychological model of limb praxis. Cognitive Neuropsychology 6: 443–58.

Rothi L, Heilman K (1985) Ideomotor apraxia: gestural discrimination. Comprehension and memory. In Roy E (Ed) Neuropsychological Studies of Apraxia and Related Disorders. Amsterdam: Elsevier.

Roy E, Square Storer P (1990) Evidence for common expressions of apraxia. In Hammond G (Ed) Cerebral Control of Speech and Limb Movements. Amsterdam: Elsevier North Holland.

Rubow R, Rosenbek J, Collins M, Longstreth D (1982) Vibrotactile stimulation for intersystemic reorganization in the treatment of apraxia of speech. Archives of Physical Medicine and Rehabilitation 63: 150–3.

Saltzman E, Munhall K (1989) Dynamical approach to gestural patterning in speech production. Ecological Psychology 1: 333–82.

Square Storer P (Ed) (1989) Acquired Apraxia of Speech in Aphasic Adults. London: Taylor & Francis.

Square Storer P, Apeldorn S (1991) Acoustic study of apraxia of speech in patients with different lesion loci. In Moore C, Yorkston K, Beukelman D (Eds) Dysarthria and Apraxia of Speech. Baltimore: Brookes.

Square Storer P, Hayden D (1989) PROMPT treatment. In Square Storer P (Ed) Acquired Apraxia of Speech in Aphasic Adults. London: Taylor & Francis.

Stevens E (1989) Multiple input phoneme therapy. In Square Storer P (Ed) Acquired Apraxia of Speech in Aphasic Adults. London: Taylor & Francis.

Stevens K (1989) On the quantal nature of speech. Journal of Phonetics 17: 4–45.

Tonkovich J, Marquardt T (1977) Effects of stress and melodic intonation on apraxia of Speech. In Brookshire R (Ed) Clinical Aphasiology Conference Proceedings Minneapolis, MN: BRK.

Valdois S, Joanette Y, Nespoulous J-L (1989) Intrinsic organisation of sequences of phonemic approximations. Aphasiology 3: 55–73.

Vogel D, Miller L (1992) A top down approach to the treatment of dysarthric speech. In Vogel D, Cannito M (Eds) Treating Disordered Speech Motor Control. Austin, TX: Pro Ed.

Weismer G, Liss J (1991) Acoustic/perceptual taxonomies of speech production deficits in Motor Speech Disorders. In Moore C, Yorkston K, Beukelman D (Eds) Dysarthria and Apraxia of Speech. Baltimore, MD: Brookes.

Wertz R (1984) Response to treatment in patients with apraxia of speech. In Rosenbek J, McNeil M, Aranson A (Eds) Apraxia of Speech. San Diego, CA: College Hill.

Wertz R, LaPointe L, Rosenbek J (1984) Apraxia of Speech in Adults: The Disorder and its Management. New York: Grune Stratton.

Ziegler W, von Cramon D (1986) Spastic dysarthria after acquired brain injury: an acoustic study. British Journal of Disorders of Communication 21: 173–87.

Zyski B, Weisiger B (1987) Identification of dysarthria types based on perceptual analysis. Journal of Communication Disorders 20: 367–78.

Chapter 13
Dysarthria Assessment: Some Perspectives for Treatment

ROXANNE DEPAUL AND JAMES H. ABBS

The last two decades have been witness to an unprecedented increase in clinical research on the disorders of speech associated with brain impairments. A new era of theory, description, and diagnosis of dysarthria was begun with the pioneering efforts of James Hardy at the University of Iowa and Ronald Netsell, then at the University of Wisconsin, in describing these disorders using techniques previously reserved for physiology studies. In parallel and of equal significance were the extensive and landmark nosological analyses of Frederick Darley and his colleagues at Mayo Clinic, including a comprehensive attempt at providing a complete set of categories of these inflictions. In this context, the present chapter is an attempt to update and extend that earlier work, as well as correct some misconceptions that appear to reflect over-interpretation or misunderstandings in its subsequent application.

The quality of clinical treatment is generally related to the degree of knowledge of the pathophysiology and the extent to which reliable assessment procedures can be devised to exploit that knowledge. Dysarthria treatment is not an exception to this principle. Based upon a recent orientation towards the assessment of the underlying pathophysiology, treatment of dysarthria increasingly has involved focused physical intervention, including biofeedback, palatal lifts, posturing, abdominal binding, respiratory exercise, bite-block prostheses, etc. (Hixon, 1975; Rosenbek and LaPointe, 1978; Netsell and Daniel, 1979; Rubow, 1981; Lybolt, Netsell and Farrage, 1982; Bless, Rubow and Braun, 1983; DePaul-McNamara, 1983; Rubow and Netsell, 1979; Yorkston, Beukelman and Bell, 1988; Dworkin, 1991). In contrast to more global approaches (e.g. behavioural modification techniques aimed at general behavioural variables such as 'correct articulation') the prescription of such focused, physically oriented intervention, requires detailed information concerning the speech-mechanism pathophysiology (Netsell and Daniel, 1979; Netsell, Lotz and Barlow, 1989; Netsell, 1994). For example, it would not be justified to undertake biofeedback as a means to reduce muscle tone if information was not available on (a) the severity and distribution of that increased muscle activity and (b) whether or not it causes problems in speech performance. It is obvious that the long-term advancement of intervention in dysarthria depends upon the reliability and validity of assessment in revealing the underlying motor pathophysiology. New rehabilitation techniques are difficult to develop, apply or refine without concrete information concerning these characteristics. Unfortunately, the effectiveness and validity of current dysarthria assessment procedures have not been evaluated quantitatively in their relative sensitivity to the underlying pathophysiology. As noted by Netsell (1994), a recent study of speech clinicians in the Department of Veterans Affairs suggested that 'the clinician's reluctance to use instrumentation may result from a lack of knowledge and a lack of evidence to support the contributions of instrumentation in dysarthria management' (Gerratt et al., 1991: 86–7). Indeed, many assessments for dysarthria have been developed in isolation and hence are idiosyncratic to particular clinicians or particular clinics, making global evaluation difficult. Despite these problems it is worthwhile to examine dysarthria assessment with a view towards the strengths and weaknesses of the different approaches currently being utilized.

Effectiveness of Current Dysarthria Assessment

Generally, there appear to be two general avenues in dysarthria assessment: (1) the listener judgement–inferential approach and (2) the multiple component approach (see Abbs, Hunker and Barlow, 1983, for a further description of these two approaches). Within a broader perspective, these two avenues have increasingly merged in the last fifteen years (as reflected in Rosenbek and LaPointe, 1978), although this may not be uniformly manifest in most clinical settings. In any case, at present there is not a widely accepted or standardized set of approaches to this problem. These issues not withstanding, a brief review of these two major assessments highlights a number of key issues in clinical management of dysarthria.

Evaluation of Assumptions Underlying Assessment

The listener judgment–inferential approach, as it was originally advocated for use in many clinical settings, involves several serial steps in determining the speech system neuropathophysiology. Initially, a speech pathologist listens to and evaluates the dysarthric speech with attempts, via speech task manipulations, to identify the nature of impairments in the three 'major' components of the speech production system (i.e. respiratory, phonatory, and articulatory). In most clinical settings this evaluation is augmented by a routine, but usually unstandardized, examination (the oral peripheral exam) and sometimes a test of articulation (Logemann et al., 1978). The second stage of this particular assessment process involves differential categorization of the apparent dysarthric subgroup based upon the auditory-perceptual classification of the speech patterns (Darley, Aronson and Brown, 1969a, b; 1975). The final step in 'determining' the underlying pathophysiology is based upon inferences from the dysarthric subgroup categorization. These critical inferences commonly are drawn from (1) parallel neurological examinations of limb impairments, and (2) classical profiles of the non-speech symptoms and signs as provided in traditional neurological descriptions. For example, if the differential diagnosis (step 2) results in the categorization of hypokinetic dysarthria (namely, dysarthria associated with Parkinson's disease), the speech motor problem has been suggested to be due to hypo- or bradykinesia, rigidity, and tremor in the muscles and movements of the speech production system. This profile of signs and symptoms is, of course, the classical one found in descriptions of limb impairments in this population (DeLong and Georgopoulos, 1981; Marsden, 1982).

There is no question that a number of experienced speech and language clinicians can categorize a given speech motor disorder by listening to the associated speech patterns. However, the question is whether such identification provides optimal or useful directions for treatment. In particular, it is apparent that there is not a common profile of symptoms and signs for all patients with a given neurological disease. The further presumption that inferences from limb signs and symptoms to orofacial motor impairments are clinically valid is also unsupported. In evaluating the viability of these inferences, interestingly, one must in turn address the multiple speech component approach, as reflected in the physiological perspectives of Hardy (1967) and the representation of the speech production system offered by Netsell and Daniel (1979). Table 13.1 delineates this multicomponent orientation, which evolved from the concept that assessment of individual speech motor subsystems (e.g. lips, jaw, tongue, velum, larynx, etc.) is necessary to develop optimal programmes of focused, physically-oriented rehabilitation. This approach is particularly appealing in evaluating potential lower motoneuron disorders where differences in subsystem impairments might be present due to select damage in some cranial nerves.

However, it also appears valuable to conduct multiple subsystem assessment in dysarthrias of suprabulbar origin. Earlier data from articulation tests in patients with dysarthrias due to supranuclear lesions indicate non-uniform patterns of impairment (Logemann et al., 1978). Further, most neurologists and speech and language clinicians are acutely aware of the fact that individuals with Parkinson's disease, congenital or acquired spasticity, etc. do not have equivalent degrees of

Table 13.1 Functional vocal tract components as a framework for focused assessment and treatment in dysarthria

Speech system component	Structures
Respiration	Rib cage
	Abdomen
	Diaphragm
Phonation	Larynx
Articulation	Pharynx
	Velum
	Tongue: anterior
	posterior
	Jaw
	Lips

impairment across all orofacial or limb motor systems. Obviously, if supranuclear lesions yield differential impairments among orofacial and limb muscle groups, it would be difficult to make inferences from limb motor impairments to determine the pathophysiology in the orofacial system (Darley et al., 1975).

By way of direct physiological measures, several recent observations in hypokinetic, ataxic, spastic, and flaccid dysarthrics indicate that differential impairment among the motor subsystems of the speech production mechanism is the rule rather than the exception. These studies indicate differential degrees of:

1. rigidity and hypokinesia in the upper vs. lower lips of Parkinson subjects (Hunker, Abbs and Barlow, 1982);
2. hypertonicity, fine force control, fine position control impairment in the lips, tongue, jaw and upper limbs of congenital spastic subjects (Barlow and Abbs, 1984; 1986);
3. multimovement decomposition in the orofacial vs. respiratory motor systems in ataxic patients (Abbs et al., 1983; Abbs, 1985);
4. variations in bradykinesia of speech movements of the upper lip, lower lip, and jaw of Parkinson patients (Connor et al., 1987);
5. motoneuron loss for the tongue, lip, jaw and laryngeal muscles in patients with amyotrophic lateral sclerosis (DePaul et al., 1988; DePaul and Brooks, 1993);
6. fine force control impairment among the lips, tongue, and jaw of Parkinson patients (Abbs, Hartman and Vishwanat, 1987); and
7. weakness and dysdiadochokinesis associated with focal unilateral upper motoneuron patients (Hartman and Abbs, 1992; Duffy and Folger, 1986; Ropper, 1987).

Given these data, one major issue concerns the nature of impairment differences among different orofacial and limb motor systems. If these differential impairment profiles are systematic, one would be able to utilize that information clinically. For example, it appears that there are subgroups of patients within the Parkinsonian population with different sub-clusters of motor signs and deficits (Hunker and Abbs, 1984; Mortimer et al., 1982). Different treatments for these two groups of Parkinson patients might be indicated.

A second major issue is related to the underlying reason for a differential distribution of impairment manifestations across orofacial, laryngeal, respiratory, and limb muscle groups. Obviously, multiple factors are involved, at least in some disorders. Focal dysfunctions of portions of the primary motor or premotor cortex, the basal ganglia or the cerebellum could selectively impair parts of the orofacial system, or the upper or lower limbs, especially given the consistent somatotopy manifest throughout the nervous system. Variation due to differential loss of neural tissue is most probable with lacunar insults such as those associated with cerebral vascular accident or trauma. However, it appears that consistent patterns of differential impairment are manifest in systemic diseases as well, including amyotrophic lateral sclerosis and Parkinson's disease. In individual patients, progressive neuromotor diseases are commonly first observed in a single part of the body and then in other parts over the time course of the disease. Studies with differential impairment profiles associated with amyotrophic lateral sclerosis (ALS) and Parkinson's disease address this point quite well.

Differential Impairment

Retrospective clinical studies of ALS support differential orofacial muscle group impairment. For example, Carpenter, McDonald and Howard (1978), studying 123 bulbar ALS patients, observed that weakness and fasciculations were most common in the tongue (66 per cent, 54 per cent respectively) and much less prominent in the facial (23 per cent, 8 per cent), velopharyngeal (8 per cent, 2 per cent) or jaw muscles (10 per cent). Predictably, these patients also reported greater difficulties in tongue muscles (68 per cent) than in laryngeal (14 per cent), pharyngeal (13 per cent) or jaw muscles (1 per cent). These kinds of differential impairments have important implications for the progression of functional deterioration, especially with regard to manifestations of dysphagia, aspiration and dysarthria.

More recent quantitative work with ALS patients, along with neuropathological data further addressed the consistency of this differential pattern and the neuropathological origins. In one study, maximum strength was measured for the lips, tongue, and jaw of ALS patients using special force transducers (DePaul et al., 1988). Figure 13.1 shows force signals for multiple MVC (Maximum Voluntary Contraction) trials. As shown, tongue MVC signals in the ALS patient are substantially more reduced (in relation to the normal subject) and the lip or jaw MVC signals. Quantitatively, the normal MVC values of the tongue, lips and jaw vary substantially from one another (reflected in the calibration bars in Figure 13.1); as such it is not meaningful to compare absolute ALS decrements in lip, jaw and tongue strength directly. To permit such comparisons, MVC values for ALS patients were expressed as a percentage of normal (i.e. one-half normal equals a 50 per cent decrement). Figure 13.2 illustrates the percentage of strength loss for the lip, jaw and tongue of two subgroups of these ALS patients – (1) bulbar ALS patients, and (2) those manifesting the earliest signs of ALS in the extremities (non-bulbar[1]).

Clearly, in both subgroups, the tongue is significantly weaker than either the lips or the jaw. However, it also is worthy to note (Figure 13.2) that the non-bulbar subgroup does not have normal lip, jaw or tongue strength. These data thus not only support the clinical observations of Carpenter et al., (1978), indicating a disproportionate degree of tongue muscle group involvement in ALS, but are consistent with Gubbay et al. (1985) finding that even patients with initial ALS symptoms in the extremities manifest bulbar signs. Obviously separating ALS patients into bulbar and non-bulbar subgroups is tenuous.

Obtaining instrumental measures of this kind is difficult in most clinical settings. Of additional concern is whether maximum strength measures lack sensitivity in some stages of ALS during which motoneuron (MN) collateral reinnervation minimizes actual muscle strength

MAXIMUM VOLUNTARY CONTRACTIONS

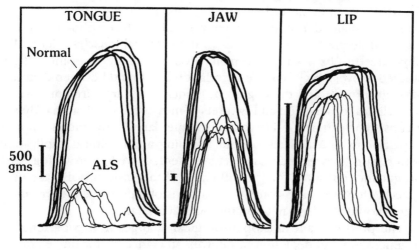

One Second

Figure 13.1 MVC signals showing differential involvement of facial, trigeminal and hypoglossal motoneurons for one ALS subject relative to a normal control.

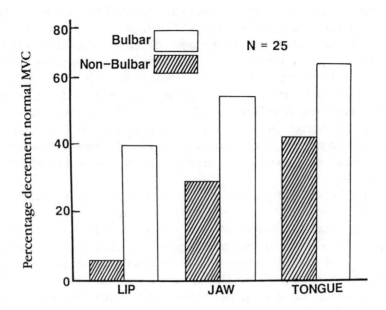

Figure 13.2 Differential involvement of facial, trigeminal and hypoglossal motoneurons for bulbar and non-bulbar ALS subjects relative to normal controls.

changes. As such, it is useful to consider other techniques which reflect other manifestations of motor neuron disease, including fasciculations, muscle wasting and mobility. Such data, while largely unpublished (see, however, DePaul and Abbs, 1987), were obtained using a standardized dysarthria examination, the Frenchay Test (Enderby, 1980, 1983a, b). The data obtained from the Frenchay examination corroborate the findings of differential ALS symptoms in the orofacial muscles. Figure 13.3 illustrates results from the Frenchay evaluations for 15 of the patients studied above; a high positive correlation was found between degree of MVC decrement and the degree of Frenchay test impairment. Overall, with clinical observation and two sets of measures, it is clear that there is a consistent pattern of differential tongue, larynx, lip, and jaw muscle impairments in ALS. These results have important clinical implications with regard to assessment and management, as well as providing better prognostic indicators for the influence of this insidious disease upon speech. However, such consistent patterns of differential motor impairment should also have neuropathological correlates.

The predominant neuropathological changes in ALS patients are degeneration and depletion of neurons in cranial motor nuclei, degeneration of the corticospinal pathways (Hughes, 1982; Hirano, 1982), and primary loss of motor cortex pyramidal cells. While limited data are available, neuropathological studies in ALS patients support the MVC and Frenchay profiles shown in Figures 13.1 to 13.3. Specifically, all available

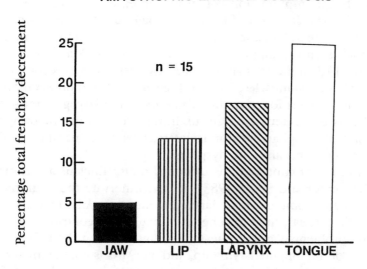

Figure 13.3 Differential orofacial impairment of mandibular, labial, laryngeal and lingual subsystems for ALS subjects using the Frenchay dysarthria assessment (Enderby, 1983b). Percentage decrement relative to normal controls.

studies indicate differential degrees of involvement in cranial motor nuclei V, VII, X and XII. For example, Lawyer and Netsky (1953) reported hypoglossal nucleus alterations in 50 of 53 patients, with only four of the 50 brains manifesting trigeminal motor nucleus changes; facial nucleus involvement was not mentioned. These observations directly support the data reported above. Notably, only 14 of Lawyer and Netsky's 53 patients initially manifested cranial motor signs. Comparable observations have been made by other authors (Bonduelle, 1975; Brain, Croft and Wilkinson, 1969; Shiraki and Yase, 1975). Specifically, Bonduelle (1975) noted common alterations of motoneuron cells in the hypoglossal nucleus, while motor trigeminal nucleus was much less impaired and there was only limited isolated groups of MN loss in the facial nucleus. Shawker and Sonies (1984) also argued for differential impairment of extrinsic and intrinsic tongue muscles; however, a paucity of information on the organization of the hypoglossal nucleus makes evaluation of potential neuropathological correlates difficult.

In addition to XIIth and Vth cranial MN changes, Lawyer and Netsky (1953) also observed changes in the nucleus ambiguous in 43 of their 53 patients and in the dorsal motor nucleus of 35 of these patients. Although frequencies of MN alteration were not given, Bonduelle (1975) made comparable observations regarding nucleus ambiguous and dorsal motor nucleus involvement. Some authors assert that the intrinsic laryngeal muscles do not manifest involvement in ALS (Kushner et al., 1984). However, change in phonation is typically an early ALS symptom and, given the obvious alteration of nucleus ambiguous MNs, this assertion may simply be due to limitations in objective measures of these muscles in ALS patients. Interestingly, the observations of the Frenchay evaluation (Figure 13.3) indicate that laryngeal involvement was second only to that of the tongue muscles. Further, the very common observation of ALS aspiration argues for some impairments in the laryngeal muscles. Potential loss of nucleus ambiguous innervation to the pharyngeal constrictor and velopharyngeal muscles may relate to 'nasality' in the speech of ALS patients and with dysphagia.

While the motor contributions of dorsal motor nucleus are controversial (Carpenter and Sutin, 1983), if MNs innervate the pharyngeal constrictors and some extrinsic laryngeal muscles (Alba et al., 1976; Davis and Nail, 1984), their degeneration could also contribute to ALS swallowing problems. Overall, these data illustrate that the differential impairment of the tongue, larynx, lip, and jaw MNs is consistent across the ALS population and because this is a systemic disease, these differences must be due to variation in susceptibility of different cranial motoneuron pools to the underlying disease process.

In the same way, one could argue that differences in Parkinson upper lip, lower lip, tongue and jaw impairments relate to differences in the way that these muscle groups are influenced by this systemic metabolic disease. The work by Abbs et al. (1987) indicates that with an isometric fine force control task the tongue was much more impaired than the lips or jaw. Clinical profiles from 18 individuals with idiopathic Parkinson disease support these instrumental measures. Using the Frenchay (Figure 13.4) we found that the tongue (28.7 per cent) and larynx (27.95 per cent) were the most impaired orofacial muscle groups, with the lips (17.92 per cent) and the mandible (5.56 per cent) being much less impaired (DePaul, Turner and Backonja, 1988). The addition of laryngeal measures demonstrate further that the degraded speech characteristics associated with Parkinsonian dysarthria also are likely associated with decrements in laryngeal parameters (Darley et al., 1975; Logemann et al., 1978; Ramig et al., 1988).

In terms of underlying pathophysiology, it would appear that the movement impairments associated with Parkinson's disease (PD) are related to aberrant basal ganglia (BG) inputs to the motor or somatic sensory cortices (Mortimer and Webster, 1978; Tatton and Lee, 1975). That is, the tongue muscles, without spindle afferent projections to MNs or the cerebellum (Bowman and Combs, 1969), should be particularly reliant upon sensorimotor actions at the motor cortex (Neilson et al., 1979) and hence, as observed, would be disproportionately impaired in PD. Interestingly, however, the lip muscles, devoid of muscle spindles, manifest PD rigidity similar to that observed in the extremities (Hunker et al., 1982).

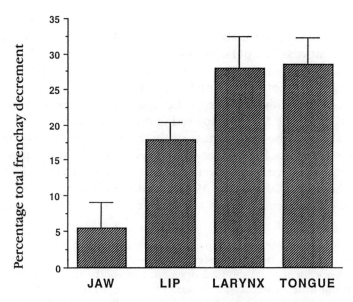

Figure 13.4 Differential orofacial impairment of mandibular, labial, laryngeal and lingual subsystems for 18 Parkinson subjects using the Frenchay dysarthria assessment (Enderby, 1983b). Percentage decrement relative to normal controls.

The disproportionate tongue impairment observed in Parkinson's disease is also subject to an alternative interpretation. While major BG outputs project to cortical sites (DeLong and Georgopoulos, 1981), there are also descending pathways directly to the brain stem. Several studies (Lidsky et al., 1978; Labuszewski and Lidsky, 1979; Weitzel, Schwarting and Huston, 1984) indicate that BG lesions yield particular orofacial dysfunctions consistent with swallowing in Parkinson's disease (Palmer, 1974; Logemann, Blonsky and Boshes, 1975; Robbins, Logemann and Kirshner, 1986), and upper airway respiratory (Vincken et al., 1984) problems. Inasmuch as the motor cortex is not primarily involved in the functions of swallowing or respiration, these latter disorders are difficult to reconcile with the concept that PD impairments are due to aberrant BG influences upon the motor cortex. However, reported orofacial reflex aberrations in PD (Gracco and Abbs, 1984; Kimura, 1973) are consistent with swallowing and upper airway breathing problems and with the Abbs et al. (1987) data.

In view of the special anatomical and physiological characteristics of the orofacial system, and apparently unique interrelationship with the basal ganglia, orofacial motor impairments in PD are likely to be different from those manifest in the extremities. As such, orofacial movement disorders with PD may not respond to drug manipulation in the same way as the muscle groups of the extremities. Thus, the Abbs et al. (1987) data in PD suggest that efficacy of treatment in the limb and the orofacial muscles should be evaluated separately. These considerations in Parkinson's disease also indicate that the possible basis for differential impairments may be due not only to variable susceptibility of different neural centres to a disease process, but possibly also to the particular central representation of a given muscle group. Apparently the somatic sensory aspects of the tongue are not represented at the levels of the cerebellum and cerebrum in the same manner as the lips and jaw, which provides a possible basis for their being impaired to differing degrees.

While a comprehensive review of the multiple neurophysiological and neuroanatomical factors that might predict differential impairments would be prohibitive in the present chapter, other reviews in earlier papers (Abbs, 1985; Abbs et al., 1983) provide sufficient documentation that these differences are commonplace. Indeed, in an earlier paper it was noted that

> the major and unquestionable neurophysiological and neuroanatomical differences among different speech system muscle groups was almost irrefutable evidence that the CNS does not control the spinal and cranial systems nor their respective subsystems in the same manner ... and hence, if there is damage to the nervous system at a suprabulbar/supraspinal level, the result will be impairments in movements and muscle contractions that are different among the speech production systems and the limbs. For example, hypo- and hyper- gamma drive to muscle spindles, loss or aberrations in recurrent inhibition, and impairment of selective influences on motoneuron recruitment patterns all have enjoyed some popularity as partial pathogenic explanations for spasticity, rigidity, tremor, ataxia, hypotonia, dysmetria, and asthenia. If some of these explanations are even partially correct, and the implicated physiological processes (e.g. presence of spindles, operation of recurrent inhibition) differ from one motor system to another, then the pathophysiology must vary as well (Abbs et al., 1983: 30).

The implications of this non-uniformity of speech motor subsystem impairments are several. Initially, because global measures of the speech motor system are generally unlikely to reveal such impairments, determination of speech motor subsystem pathophysiology may need to be enhanced by use of direct observations using voluntary, non-speech tasks. In this manner, it may be possible to identify those speech motor subsystems manifesting the greatest degree of impairment and focus treatment for maximum effectiveness.

Improvements in speech motor function also could possibly be enhanced by initial emphasis upon those subsystems that either are most severely impaired or allow for the most direct and effective intervention.

Diagnostic Signs, Neural Control Aberrations and Performance Deficits

Table 13.2 provides an overview of the signs and movement aberrations classically associated with different classes of movement disorders. This is a catalogue of some value in distinguishing among these disorders. However, it has become increasingly apparent in the last decade that it is not satisfactory to describe or list the various speech motor system aberrations associated with a given neuromotor disorder. That is, describing the presence or absence of particular pathophysiological signs across the speech motor subsystems and the limbs is of limited value unless it is possible to determine whether the salient aberrations are primary or causal factors in the speech motor performance deficit, or simply tertiary manifestations that accompany the syndrome. More specifically as shown in Table 13.2, the relations among the major and minor signs and the movement aberrations are uncertain. As such, the effort must be made to ensure that each particular aberration has a causal relation to the performance deficits prior to the expenditure of energy, time and money on treatment programmes to eliminate or minimize it. Neurological signs or motor manifestations that are simply different from normal do not necessarily play a causal or important role in a patient's clinical disability.

Aberrant manifestations that are tertiary were recognized by Hughlings Jackson over 100 years ago, and labelled positive signs (e.g. due to 'release' of certain nervous system functions or simply irritations to nervous system tissue). Negative signs, according to Jackson, are aberrant disease characteristics that are causally associated with the performance deficit or the clinical disability, *per se*. Clearly the white lock of hair (a positive sign) associated with Waardenberg's syndrome is not a causal factor in the hearing disability (a negative sign) also manifest in this population. In this vein, one also must be very careful in interpreting abnormal patterns that might be compensatory in nature. For example, the ubiquitous slowing of speech in many dysarthric subjects may be primarily a compensation for certain general aberrations of control that are deleterious at a more rapid rate. No one would undertake to treat the Waardenberg white hair lock with an expectation of improving the patient's hearing. Attempting to treat such compensatory patterns as speech slowing also could be counterproductive unless the complex factors associated with this behaviour are also understood.

In this context, it is enlightening to consider some of the assessment procedures utilized in dysarthria and evaluate the extent to which it is possible to discriminate positive signs and compensations from factors causally intertwined with actual performance deficits. By using customary diagnostic procedures, it has been common to distinguish the different neuromotor pathologies of speech via contrastive profiles of descriptive behaviours. As highlighted above, a common assumption has been that diagnostic indicators of a particular neuropathological syndrome are coincident with or underlie the debilitating performance deficits associated with the disease. An assumption of this kind is found with the so-called spastic dysarthric. In this group, it has been indicated

Table 13.2 Neurological signs and movement aberrations associated with different movement disorders

	Major signs	*Other signs*	*Movement aberrations*
Flaccid cluster	Hypotonia Weakness Muscle atrophy	Reduced or absent reflexes Fasciculations	Reduced velocity and extent of movement Restricted or weak movement Loss of fine adjustments
Spastic cluster	Spastic hypertonicity Clasp-knife reflex (lengthening reaction) Clonus	Hyper-brisk stretch reflexes Babinski sign	Restricted or weak movement Loss of fine adjustments
Cerebellar cluster	Ataxia Tremor: postural and intention Hypotonia	Reduced stretch reflex Pendular reflexes Rebound phenomenon	Asynergia Decomposition of multi-joint movement Dysmetria
Hypokinetic cluster	Rigidity: plastic/ lead-pipe and cogwheel	Shortening reaction Reflex reinforcement absent	Hypo-, brady- and akinesia Kinesia paradoxica
Hyperkinetic cluster	Fluctuating tone Shortening reaction	Reflex reinforcement absent Stretch reflexes variable	Athetosis Chorea Dystonia Ballismus

that several of the distinct speech motor symptoms can be related to increased muscle tone or muscle spasms. Such a phenomenon as the feature of strain-strangled voice observed in these patients has been argued to be caused by co-contraction of antagonistic intrinsic laryngeal muscles or spasms in the same. This example presents several problems clinically. Firstly, the term spasticity is ill-defined, even in neurology. Secondly, assumptions have been made that (1) the antagonistic co-contraction thought to be manifest in the limbs is also operating in the larynx, and (2) this spastic hypertonicity is a causative factor underlying the speech motor disability.

Unfortunately, muscle activity in the intrinsic laryngeal muscles is difficult to record and thus has not been evaluated in a patient with spastic dysarthria; as such, the argument for antagonistic co-contraction or laryngeal muscle hypertonicity is without documentation. Further, the clinical neurology literature is ambiguous as to the definition of spasticity or its quantification (Lance, 1980; Landau, 1980). Controversy continues as to whether spasticity is primarily a velocity of stretch-related activation of stretch reflexes yielding a pathological resistance to a clinical examiner's passive displacement, or rather is descriptive of an entire syndrome which includes increased reflex excitability, muscle weakness, clumsiness, greater than normal stiffness, and flexion reflexes that are hyperactive. Aside from this controversy, obviously spasticity is not unidimensional. Of greatest importance is the fact that clinical neurologists realize that spasticity (narrowly defined) is primarily a clear diagnostic sign, but largely unrelated to the actual motor performance deficits manifest in this population. Perhaps no author has been more clear in stating these points than Landau (1980), who in reviewing several sets of corroborative studies of evidence (Denny-Brown, 1980; Duncan, Shahani and Young, 1976; Landau, 1974, 1980; Sahrman and North, 1977) commented directly regarding the hypertonicity and motor disability in individuals with spasticity:

> However useful to clinical diagnosis may be the increase of excitability at anterior horn cells and to some extent muscle spindles, these phenomena have little more relation to the patient's disability than does the insertion of the rectal thermometer in pneumonia (Landau, 1980: 20).

Obviously in this context, one must seriously question the assertion that so-called strain-strangled voice is the result of antagonistic muscle/spastic hypertonus in the larynx.

These observations point very clearly to the need for distinguishing between diagnosis and assessment! That is, while it often appears logical to infer that diagnostic signs are a major underlying cause of motor disabilities in individuals with neuromuscular disease, even the most 'apparent' of these inferences need to be tested empirically. That is, it is likely that some of the most striking distinguishing features for differential dysarthria classification may not be related causally to the speech deficits. One must examine the extent to which certain features of speech abnormality are related causally to deficits in functional communication or speech movement co-ordination and control. In the example of spasticity discussed above, reducing or eliminating flexor spasms or hyperactive stretch reflexes through various treatments is not of particular benefit in improving motor function. Treating certain superficial speech aberrations may be similarly futile unless such aberrations have been demonstrated to be related to deficits of speech performance. Apparent compelling causal relations among symptoms and signs one might observe in clinical populations may not be valid; the nervous system usually functions in ways not intuitively obvious, and the requirement for testing of unquantified assertions, no matter how appealing they may be, cannot be compromised.

Can Motor Speech Impairment be Predicted from Non-speech Measures?

If one accepts the arguments that (1) the various speech motor subsystems are differentially impaired and (2) many aberrations or signs accompanying a particular disorder do not have a causal relation to deficits in speech movement performance, then measures obtained during ongoing speech behaviour may be very difficult to interpret as a basis for determining the critical elements of the underlying pathophysiology. For example, if one observes alterations in the temporal properties of speech, it may be very difficult to discern whether those aberrations are due to a uniform impairment in all speech system muscle groups, or primarily disproportionate aberrations in one or two components. For example, analyses of the influence of disproportionate aberrations in jaw control (DePaul and Abbs, 1984) suggested that such aberrations were manifest during speech in structures that are mechanically isolated from the jaw (e.g. the upper lip), possibly reflecting attempts at compensation for the jaw control aberrations. These and other related data indicate that experimental and clinical assessment of motor speech disorders could be enhanced through the utilization of measures obtained during non-speech tasks.

Many measures currently utilized either experimentally or in clinical settings with instrumental capabilities indicate that measures of speech motor subsystem performance simplify assessment substantially by dealing with one subsystem at a time. Differential impairment is clearly manifest as in the work described previously with cases of amyotrophic lateral sclerosis (DePaul et al., 1988) and Parkinson's disease (Abbs et al., 1987; Connor et al., 1987). Presumably with such information one can consider focusing rehabilitation or clinical management at those more specific, less global motor malfunctions. In general, this seemingly logical approach is dependent upon the assumption that non-speech motor impairments are of value in assessing and managing motor speech disorders. This assumption raises the classical issue of whether speech and non-speech motor functions are dependent upon a sufficiently common neural substrate so that impairments in speech can be predicted from non-speech measures and further that enhancements in non-speech performance will lead to parallel improvements for speech tasks.

It has been a long-standing question in the assessment and treatment of motor speech disorders as to whether (1) impairments in the motor control of non-speech activities such as chewing and swallowing, or volitional non-speech manoeuvres (as observed in the oral peripheral examination) correlate with or are indicative of parallel impairments in speech motor function, and further, whether (2) rehabilitation focused upon either feeding or non-speech voluntary control of speech motor systems will effectively carry over to speech control. This issue has been debated most intensely regarding speech motor problems resulting from supranuclear damage, of either a congenital or an acquired nature.

There are several lines of evidence that appear particularly relevant. It is, however, important that speech and non-speech motor tasks be defined from a current neurophysiological perspective. Chewing, swallowing and other orofacial vegetative functions are known to be neurophysiologically distinct from non-speech tasks performed voluntarily. That is, these vegetative functions appear, to a large extent, to be controlled via certain subcortical pattern generators and/or networks of brainstem reflexes (Dubner, Sessle and Storey, 1978; Wyke, 1974). For example, Hoffman and Luschei (1980) demonstrated that primary motor cortex activity was not related to movements during chewing in rhesus monkeys. However, operantly conditioned biting (a 'more voluntary' task using the same jaw muscles) was clearly under motor cortex influence. Hoffman and Luschei (1980: 345) noted that, 'a likely explanation for this observation is that the reciprocal action of the jaw-closing and opening muscles during chewing is patterned elsewhere in the brain'. Other work suggests a parallel dichotomy for the muscles of the respiratory system (Phillips and Porter, 1977) and the facial muscles (Denny-Brown, 1960). As noted by Evarts (1981: 1113):

> It might at first seem odd that corticospinal neurons controlling precise skilled movements terminate on motoneurons controlling intercostal muscles that participate in an act as automatic and primitive as respiration, but Phillips and Porter point out that these terminations are probably related to the use of respiratory muscles in speech and song rather than in breathing ... Destroying the corticospinal projection to thoracic motoneurons does not impair the use of respiratory muscles for respiration, though these same muscles may be useless for speech.

These considerations offer a different perspective on the long-standing speech–non-speech controversy. That is, these recent neurophysiological observations indicate that this issue is not one of speech versus non-speech motor control. The critical distinction may be whether the non-speech movements are controlled in a conscious, voluntary manner as in speech, or, by contrast, represent vegetative movements that are more automatic. This interpretation is compatible with earlier and more recent data that address this issue. As was noted recently in a re-evaluation of this issue:

> These data and the previously considered neurophysiological/neuroanatomical findings suggest that non-speech control of precise, voluntary activities is likely to be impaired in the same manner and to the same degree as speech motor behaviour (Abbs and Rosenbek, 1985: 39).

The implications for assessment and for rehabilitation based upon this working hypothesis are several. Recent data indicate that assessment of impairments solely on the basis of spontaneous speech behaviour, whether one uses movement observations, acoustic analyses or simply a sage clinical ear, may not permit discrimination of a jaw control impairment from a lip or tongue impairment. Spastic and hypokinetic dysarthric data in particular address an important point made previously regarding the relative insensitivity of more global indices provided by acoustic or aerodynamic analyses. For example, changes in the speech of a congenital spastic subject by inserting a bite-block was not discernible from such measures as perceptual judgements (DePaul and Abbs, 1984). Similarly, conventional global measures are not likely to be sensitive to the differential degree of upper and lower lip rigidity in the Parkinsonian dysarthrics. Hence, observations of voluntary non-speech control tasks apparently are useful for disambiguating potential subsystem motor impairments. This line of reasoning applies to treatment as well. If impairments in voluntary non-speech control are parallel to those for speech, improvements on selected, voluntary non-speech tasks should enhance speech control as well, depending on the site of the lesion and neural tissue remaining to support less automatic behaviours.

These interpretations have interesting implications for other forms of rehabilitation as well. For example, some schools of cerebral palsy treatment have emphasized that facilitation of chewing and swallowing is a means for improving speech function. Despite the enthusiasm for these particular programmes, direct evidence to support their value for speech improvement is lacking. Indeed, difference in neural control between chewing and speech–non-speech voluntary behaviour argues against the utility of these therapies for speech. This argument is supported by the observations of Love, Hagerman and Taimi (1980) who found no consistent relation between severity of speech impairment in 60 cerebral palsied children and the presence of dysphagia. Other data to this point are those of Schliesser (1982), who reported that in the cerebral palsy population certain non-speech alternate motion rate tasks predicted dysarthria severity quite well.

While these considerations offer a supporting basis for assessment and treatment of dysarthria via non-speech voluntary control tasks, the details of this approach need to be considered in light of current state-of-the-art assessment procedures and their underlying neurophysiological rationale. Obviously, it is of particular value to test the above distinctions empirically in studies designed to offer more direct evidence for predicting speech motor impairment from non-speech measures.

What are the Implications for Treatment?

At the outset of this chapter it was noted that the most promising new approaches for treatment of speech motor disorders lay with physically-oriented techniques such as prostheses, biofeedback to reduce increased muscle tone, muscle strengthening exercises, and so on. Obviously, the ultimate objective of dysarthria assessment in this context must be to provide empirical indications of the pathophysiology in each of the speech motor subsystems (Abbs et al., 1983; Netsell and Daniel, 1979; Netsell et al., 1989; Netsell, 1994). However, to date many of these efforts have involved instrumentally based techniques; one is faced with the question as to the practical clinical utility of measures that largely have been confined to research laboratories. Based upon some efforts in the last 15 years, we have been increasingly convinced that some measures of this kind provide information of potential clinical value to the patient's physicians and speech and language clinicians. However, the issue is whether technically complex and instrumentally intensive procedures can be readily adopted for routine clinical evaluation. Certainly, most speech and language clinics will not be able to exploit these measures in the foreseeable future without some assistance from engineering and computer experts as well as an influx of moneys with which to purchase electronic and computer systems. To this end however, one may be able to rely upon non-instrumental measures. In two circumstances, we have been able to replicate the results of instrumental analyses utilizing non-instrumental measures. Specifically, as described, utilizing the Frenchay dysarthria test it has been possible to replicate the results of Abbs et al. (1987) with Parkinson patients and the findings of DePaul et al. (1988) with ALS patients. Given the relatively high reliability of this examination (Enderby, 1980; 1983a,b), it would appear reasonable to include a standardized orofacial examination in clinical assessment procedures to assist in identifying differential impairment profiles. From the foregoing considerations it appears that the optimal success of treatment is conditioned not only by the degree to which the distribution of motor impairments across muscle groups is identified, but also by whether determinations are made as to which of the identified aberrations are contributing factors to the patient's speech motor disability. Treatment of so-called positive signs is unlikely to be useful. However, even if these important conditions are satisfied, the directions of treatment must also be conditioned by other factors.

One of these factors is the careful consideration of the disease process and awareness of what influences treatment might have on that process. For example, in diseases influencing motoneurons (e.g. ALS), strengthening exercises appear to be of questionable value and may even be contraindicated. Specifically, it appears, based upon preliminary evidence in the limb musculature, that exercise may stress motoneurons and accelerate their death and exacerbate consequent muscle weakness (DePaul and Abbs, 1987). The data on post-polio syndrome clearly point in this direction. Additionally, such exercise does not appear to provide even transient plateaux of muscle strength in those patients so tested. In such cases, where say, for example, one wishes to minimize the influence of substantially weakened ALS tongue muscle group function, the alternative approach may be to begin working towards enhancing a patient's ability to use compensatory jaw or extrinsic tongue muscles in anticipation of failure of primary muscles. This approach to treatment thus implies that all differential impairment profiles must be individually evaluated with an understanding of disease prognosis and pathophysiology to determine the optimal course.

Conclusion

As reflected in this chapter, irrespective of the specific treatment or management programme undertaken, the current emphasis in motor speech disorders is on improved objective measures of system performance. With such measures subtle alterations in performances can be documented in relation to various therapeutic endeavours, or to the progression of the disease condition. Improved measures limit speculation and assumptions; medical colleagues can be provided with clearly defined observations rather than subjective impressions of symptoms and signs. In this manner, handling of patients with motor speech disorders is certain to improve.

Note

1. Pre-bulbar is used interchangeably with non-bulbar to denote the absence of clinical bulbar signs. Pre-bulbar is preferable because considerable MN death occurs prior to the appearance of clinical signs and symptoms, and bulbar signs will manifest in sporadic ALS (DePaul et al., 1990).

References

Abbs JH (1985) Motor impairment differences in orofacial and respiratory speech control with cerebellar disorders: A response to Hixon and Holt. Journal of Speech and Hearing Disorders 50(3): 306–12.

Abbs JH, Hartman DE, Vishwanat B (1987) Orofacial motor control impairment in Parkinsons disease. Neurology 37: 394–8.

Abbs JH, Hunker CJ, Barlow SM (1983) Differential speech motor subsystem impairments with suprabulbar lesions: Neurophysiological framework and supporting data. In Berry WR (Ed) Clinical Dysarthria. San Diego: College Hill.

Abbs JH, Rosenbek JC (1985) Some motor control perspectives on apraxia of speech and dysarthria. In Costello JM (Ed) Recent Advances Speech Disorders in Adults. California: College Hill.

Alba A, Pilkington LA, Kaplan E, Baum J, Schultheiss M, Ruggieri A, Lee MHM (1976) Long-term pulmonary care in amyotrophic lateral sclerosis. Respiratory Therapy, Nov-Dec, pp 1–11.

Barlow SM, Abbs JH (1984) Orofacial fine motor control impairment in congenital spastics: Evidence against muscle spindle-related performance deficits. Neurology 34: 145–50.

Barlow SM, Abbs JH (1986) Fine force and position control of select orofacial structures in the upper motor neuron syndrome. Experimental Neurology 94: 699–713.

Bless DM, Rubow RT, Braun S (1983) Speech breathing patterns in cerebral palsied adults. Folia Phoniatrica 24: 107.

Bonduelle M (1975) Amyotrophic lateral sclerosis. In Vincken PJ, Bruyn GW and DeJong JM (Eds) Handbook of Clinical Neurology. New York: Elsevier.

Bowman J, Combs CM (1969) Discharge patterns of lingual spindle afferent fibers in the hypoglossal nerve of the Rhesus monkey. Experimental Neurology 21: 105–19.

Brain, Lord, Croft P, Wilkinson M (1969) The course and outcome of motor neuron disease. In Norris FH, Kurland LT (Eds) Motor Neuron Disease: Research on ALS and Related Disorders. New York: Grune and Stratton.

Carpenter RJ, McDonald TJ, Howard FM (1978) The otolaryngologic presentation of amyotrophic lateral sclerosis. Otolaryngology 36: 479–84.

Carpenter RJ, Sutin J (1983) Human Neuroanatomy. Baltimore, MD: Williams and Wilkins.

Connor NP, Forrest K, Cole KJ, Gracco VL, Abbs JH (1987) Kinematic analyses of Parkinsonian dysarthria. Paper presented at the American Speech-Language-Hearing Association Convention, New Orleans, Louisiana.

Darley FL, Aronson AE, Brown JR (1969a) Differential diagnostic patterns of dysarthria. Journal of Speech and Hearing Research 12: 246–69.

Darley FL, Aronson AE, Brown JR (1969b) Clusters of deviant speech dimensions in the dysarthrias. Journal of Speech and Hearing Research 12: 462–69.

Darley FL, Aronson AE, Brown JR (1975) Motor Speech Disorders. Philadelphia, PA: W.B Saunders.

Davis PJ, Nail BS (1984) On the location and size of laryngeal motoneurons in the cat and rabbit. Journal of Comparative Neurology 230: 13–32.

DeLong M, Georgopoulos AO (1981) Motor functions of the basal ganglia. In Brooks VB (Ed) Handbook of Physiology, Section 1, Vol 2: Motor Control, Part 2. Maryland: American Physiological Society.

Denny-Brown D (1960) Motor mechanisms – introduction: The general principles of motor integration. In Magoun HW (Ed) Handbook of Physiology. Washington, DC: American Physiological Society.

Denny-Brown D (1980) Preface: Historical aspects of the relation of spasticity to movement. In Feldman RG, Young RR, Koella WP (Eds) Spasticity: Disordered Motor Control. Chicago: Year Book Medical Publishers.

DePaul-McNamara R (1983) A conceptual holistic approach to dysarthria treatment. In Berry WR (Ed) Clinical Dysarthria. California: College Hill.

DePaul R, Turner G, Backonja M (1988) Differential impairment in Parkinsons disease. Paper presented at the American Speech, Language and Hearing Association, Boston, Massachusetts.

DePaul R, Abbs JH (1984) Physiologic and acoustic analyses of the effect of a bite-block prosthesis in a spastic dysarthric. Paper presented at the Clinical Dysarthria Conference, Tucson, Arizona.

DePaul R, Abbs JH (1987) Manifestations of ALS in the cranial motor nerves: dynametric, neuropathologic, and speech motor data. In Brooks BR (Ed) Neurologic Clinics of North America: Amyotrophic Lateral Sclerosis, Vol 5. Philadelphia: W.B Saunders.

DePaul R, Abbs JH, Caligiuri MP, Gracco VL, Brooks BR (1988) Hypoglossal, trigeminal and facial motoneuron involvement in amyotrophic lateral sclerosis.

Neurology 38: 2, 281–3.

DePaul R, Brooks BR (1993) Multiple Orofacial Indices in ALS Journal of Speech and Hearing Research 36(6): 1158–67.

DePaul R, Brooks BR, Wang M, Sanjak M (1990) Quantitative natural history of amyotrophic lateral sclerosis (ALS): Early rapid linear loss of tongue isometric muscle strength in pre-bulbar patients. Annals of Neurology 28: 46.

Dubner R, Sessle BJ, Storey AT (1978) The Neural Basis of Oral and Facial Function. New York: Plenum.

Duffy JR, Folger NW (1986) Dysarthria in unilateral central nervous system lesions. Paper presented at the Annual Meeting of the American Speech-Language Association, Detroit, Michigan.

Duncan GW, Shahani BT, Young RR (1976) An evaluation of baclofen treatment for certain symptoms in patients with spinal cord lesions. A double cross-over study. Neurology 26: 441–6.

Dworkin JP (1991) Motor speech disorders: A treatment guide. St Louis, MO: Mosby Year Book.

Enderby PM (1980) Frenchay dysarthria assessment. British Journal of Disorders of Communication 15: 165–73.

Enderby PM (1983a) The standardized assessment of dysarthria is possible. In Berry WR (Ed) Clinical Dysarthria. San Diego, CA: College Hill.

Enderby PM (1983b) Frenchay Dysarthria Assessment. San Diego, CA: College Hill.

Evarts EV (1981) Role of motor cortex in voluntary movements in primates. In Brooks VB (Ed) Handbook of Physiology, Section 1, Vol II: Motor Control, Part 2. Maryland: American Physiological Society.

Gerratt BR, Till JA, Rosenbek JC, Wertz RT, Boysen AE (1991) Use and perceived value of perceptual and instrumental measures in dysarthria management. In Moore CA, Yorkston KM, Beukelman DR (Eds.) Dysarthria and Apraxia of Speech: Perspective on Management. Baltimore, Md: Brookes Publishing Co. pp 77–93.

Gracco VL, Abbs JH (1984) Sensorimotor dysfunction in Parkinsons disease: observations from a multiarticulate speech task. Society for Neuroscience Abstract.

Gubbay SS, Kahana E, Zilber, J, Cooper G, Pintov S, Leibowitz Y (1985) Amyotrophic lateral sclerosis: A study of its presentation and prognosis. Journal of Neurology 232: 295–300.

Hardy JC (1967) Suggestions for physiological research in dysarthria. Cortex 3: 128–56.

Hartman DE, Abbs JH (1992) Dysarthria associated with focal unilateral upper motor neuron lesion. European Journal of Disorders of Communication 27: 187–196.

Hirano A (1982) Aspects of the ultrastructure of ALS. In Rowland LP (Ed) Human Neuron Diseases. New York: Raven Press.

Hixon TJ (1975) Respiratory-laryngeal evaluation. Paper presented at the Veterans Administration Workshop in Motor Speech Disorders, Madison, Wisconsin.

Hoffman DS, Luschei ES (1980) Responses of monkey precentral cortical cells during a controlled jaw bite task. Journal of Neurophysiology 44: 333–48.

Hughes JT (1982) Pathology of ALS. In Rowland LP (Ed) Human Motor Neuron Diseases. New York: Raven Press.

Hunker C, Abbs JH (1984) Physiological analyses of Parkinsonian tremors in the orofacial system. In McNeil MR, Rosenbek JC, Aronson A (Eds) The Dysarthrias: Physiology-Acoustics-Perception-Management. San Diego, CA: College Hill.

Hunker CJ, Abbs JH, Barlow SM (1982) The relationship between Parkinsonian rigidity and hypokinesia in the orofacial system: A quantitative analysis. Neurology 32(7): 740–54.

Kimura J (1973) The blink reflex as a test for brain-stem and higher central nervous system function. In Desmedt JE (Ed) New Developments in Electromyography and Clinical Neurophysiology, Vol. 3. Basel: Karger.

Kushner MJ, Parrish M, Burke A, Behrens M, Hays AP, Frame B, Rowland LP (1984) Nystagmus in motor neuron disease. Clinicopathological study of two cases. Annals of Neurology 16: 71–7.

Labuszewski T, Lidsky TI (1979) Basal ganglia influences on brain stem trigeminal neurons. Experimental Neurology 65: 471–7.

Lance JW (1980) Pathophysiology of spasticity and clinical experience with baclofen. In Feldman RG, Young RR, Koella WP (Eds) Spasticity: Disordered Motor Control. Chicago: Year Book Medical Publishers.

Landau WM (1974) Spasticity: The fable of a neurological demon and the emperors new therapy. Archives of Neurology 31: 217–9.

Landau WM (1980) Spasticity: What is it? What is it not? In Feldman RG, Young RR, Koella WP (Eds) Spasticity: Disordered Motor Control. Chicago: Year Book Medical Publishers.

Lawyer T, Netsky MG (1953) Amyotrophic lateral sclerosis: A clinicoanatomic study of fifty-three cases. Archives of Neurology and Psychiatry 69: 171–92.

Lidsky TL, Robinson JA, Denaro FJ, Weinhold PM (1978) Trigeminal influences on entopeduncular units. Brain Research 141: 227–34.

Logemann JA, Blonsky ER, Boshes B (1975) Dysphagia in Parkinsonism. Journal of the American Medical Association 231: 1, 69–70.

Logemann JA, Fisher HB, Boses B, Blonsky E (1978) Frequency and co-occurrence of vocal tract dysfunctions in the speech of a large sample of Parkinson patients. Journal of Speech and Hearing Disorders 43: 47–57.

Love RJ, Hagerman EL, Taimi EG (1980) Speech performance, dysphagia and oral reflexes in cerebral palsy. Journal of Speech and Hearing Disorders 45: 59–75.

Lybolt J, Netsell R, Farrage F (1982) A Bite-block Prosthesis in the Treatment of Dysarthria. Paper presented at the annual convention of the American-Speech-Language-Hearing Association, Ontario, Canada.

Marsden CD (1982) The mysterious motor function of the basal ganglia. Neurology 32: 515–39.

Mortimer JA, Pirozzolo FJ, Hansch EC, Webster DD (1982) Relationship of motor symptoms to intellectual deficits in Parkinson disease. Neurology 32: 133–7.

Mortimer JA, Webster DD (1978) Relationships between quantitative measures of rigidity and tremor and the electromyographic responses to load perturbation in unselected normal subjects and Parkinson patients. In Desmedt JE (Ed) Cerebral Control in Man: Long Loop Mechanisms, Vol. 4. Basel: Karger.

Netsell RW (1994) Instrumentation and special procedures for individuals with dysarthria. American Journal of Speech-Language Pathology 3(2): 9-11.

Netsell R, Daniel B (1979) Dysarthria in adults: Physiological approach to rehabilitation. Archives of Physical and Medical Rehabilitation 60: 502–8.

Netsell R, Lotz WK, Barlow SM (1989) A speech physiology examination for individuals with dysarthria. In Yorkston KM, Beukelman DR (Eds) Recent Advances in Dysarthria (pp. 3–37) Boston, MA: Little Brown.

Nielson PD, Andrews G, Guitar BE, Quinn PT (1979) Tonic stretch reflexes in lip, tongue and jaw muscles. Brain Research 178: 311–27.

Palmer ED (1974) Dysphagia in Parkinsonism. Journal of American Medical Association 220: 1, 1349.

Phillips CG, Porter R (1977) Corticospinal Neurons. Their Role in Movement. London: Academic Press.

Ramig L, Scherer R, Titze I, Ringel S (1988) Acoustic analysis of voices of patients with neurological disease: a rationale and preliminary data. Annals of Otology, Rhinology and Laryngology 97: 164–172.

Robbins J, Logemann JA, Kirshner HS (1986) Swallowing and speech production in Parkinsons disease. Annals of Neurology 19: 283–7.

Ropper AH (1987) Severe dysarthria with right hemisphere stroke. Neurology 37: 1061–1063.

Rosenbek J, LaPointe LL (1978) The dysarthrias: Description, diagnosis and treatment. In Johns DF (Ed) Clinical Management of Neurogenic Communicative Disorders. Boston: Little, Brown.

Rubow RT (1981) Biofeedback in the Treatment of Speech Disorders. Biofeedback Society of America Task Force Reports.

Rubow RT, Netsell R (1979) EMG biofeedback rehabilitation in facial paralysis: Ten year follow-up of a case study. Proceedings of the Tenth Annual Meeting of the Biofeedback Society of America, San Diego, California.

Sahrman SA, North BJ (1977) The relationship of voluntary movement to spasticity in the upper motor neuron syndrome. Annals of Neurology 2: 460–5.

Schliesser HF (1982) Alternate motion rates of the speech articulators in adults with cerebral palsy. Folia Phoniatrica 34: 258–64.

Shawker TH, Sonies BC (1984) Tongue movement during speech: A real time ultrasound evaluation, Journal of Clinical Ultrasound 12: 125–33.

Shiraki H, Yase Y (1975) Amyotrophic lateral sclerosis in Japan. In Bruyn GW, Vincken PJ, DeJong JM (Eds) Handbook of Clinical Neurology. Vol 2. New York: Elsevier.

Tatton WG, Lee RG (1975) Evidence for abnormal long-loop reflexes in rigid Parkinsonian patients. Brain Research 100: 671–6.

Vincken WG, Gauthier SG, Dollfuss RE, Hanson RE, Darauay CM, Coslo MG (1984) Involvement of upper-airway muscles in extrapyramidal disorders a cause of airflow limitation. New England Journal of Medicine 311: 438–42.

Weitzel H, Schwarting R, Huston JP (1984) Substantia nigra efferents and afferents in the control of the perioral biting reflex. In Bandler R (Ed) Modulation of Sensorimotor Activity During Alterations in Behavioral States. New York: Alan R. Liss.

Wyke B (Ed) (1974) Ventilatory and Phonatory Control Systems. London: Oxford University Press.

Yorkston K, Beukelman D, Bell K (1988) Clinical management of dysarthric speakers. Boston: College-Hill.

Chapter 14
Voice Disorders in Adults

JOSEPH C. STEMPLE

In technical terms, voice is the major element of speech production that provides the speaker with the vibration signal upon which speech is carried. In practical terms, it is much more than this. For voice provides the melody of speech and, beyond the spoken meaning of words, it provides additional expression, intent and mood to our spoken thoughts (Stemple and Holcomb, 1988). We all share an intimate relationship with our voices. The way we feel, both physically and emotionally, will often be reflected in the quality of our voices. In addition, a voice disorder may contribute to significant personal, social and vocational difficulties which may affect the quality of our lives.

The normal voice will fall within a very wide range of acceptability, and thus it is easier to define the abnormal voice. A voice disorder is said to exist when the quality, pitch and loudness differ from those of other persons of similar age, sex, cultural background and geographic location (Stemple, Glaze and Gerdeman, 1994; Aronson, 1980; Boone, 1977; Greene, 1972; Moore, 1971). In other words, if the voice is deviant enough to draw attention to the speaker, a voice disorder is said to be present. The owner of the voice is also very sensitive to vocal changes and may recognize a problem that is not evident to others.

Successful management of the voice disorder will depend upon recognition of the problem by the owner of the voice and acceptance of the need for improvement. The effects of a voice disorder on the lives and livelihoods of individuals will vary considerably. Those with a great need for normal, effective production may be unusually concerned with very minor vocal difficulties. People with low vocal needs may not be greatly concerned with even more severe vocal problems.

Our study will focus on the voice pathologist's role in the evaluation and management of voice disorders commonly seen in the adult population. The role includes identification and modification or elimination of the causes that have led to the development of the voice disorder (if the causes continue as precipitating factors), as well as the evaluation and modification of specific deviant voicing components (i.e. pitch, loudness, breathiness and so on).

Common Causative Factors in Voice Disorders

Discovering the causes of voice disorders is a major first step in the remediation of the disorder. Categories of vocal misuse, medically-related causes, primary disorders and personality-related causes will be discussed here.

Vocal misuse

Vocal misuse refers to functional voicing behaviours that contribute to the development of voice disorders. Indeed, functional misuse of voice is the most common cause for the development of voice disorders. We will divide this category into two major parts, behaviours of vocal abuse and the use of inappropriate voice components.

Vocal abuse

Often, when we think of voice abuse, we focus our attention on children who shout, scream and make unusual vocal noises. Adults also have many opportunities to abuse the voice and demonstrate many vocally abusive behaviours. Vocal abuse occurs whenever the vocal folds are forced to adduct too vigorously causing hyperfunctioning of the laryngeal musculature, which may damage the vocal fold cover. This vocal hyperfunction may take the form of excessive shouting or loud talking such as a mother with her child, cheering at a sporting event, or shouting over noise in a factory. Vocal abuse is also present in screaming, as during an argument, and in excessive harsh crying and laughing.

One of the most prevalent forms of voice abuse in the adults is incessant, habitual, non-productive throat clearing. Throat clearing may be the primary cause of a voice disorder or it may be secondary to the presence of a voice disorder. Coughing is also a vocally abusive behaviour. Because coughing is a symptom of many physical ailments, a persistent cough must always be evaluated medically and is most often treated by a physician.

Inappropriate voice components

The production of voice is dependent upon the balanced relationship of many different components. The major voice components include respiration, phonation, resonation, pitch, and loudness. Any component that is used in a functionally inappropriate manner may be the direct cause of a voice disorder. Let us examine each component.

Respiration

Breathing for speech is dependent upon the appropriate passage of air through the approximated vocal folds. The majority of patients use adequate breathing techniques for the support of speech and voice. Air may be exchanged either through expansion of the thoracic cavity (chest breathing) or through downward diaphragm contraction (diaphragmatic breathing) or a combination of both. Either air exchange method is adequate for providing the necessary respiratory support for voice production. Some patients, however, may use a shallow, thoracic, non-supportive breathing pattern with poor vocal fold adduction. The resultant voice quality will be breathy with a low intensity. Long-term use of poorly supported phonation may lead to laryngeal strain and laryngeal pathology. Another functional breathing pattern which may lead to vocal strain is the habit of speaking on residual air. This occurs when a person continues to speak when the normal tidal expiration has been completed.

Phonation

Inappropriate phonation, as a functional cause of voice disorders, may be present in patients who utilize hard glottal attacks, breathy phonation and glottal fry phonation. A hard glottal attack is accomplished by approximating the vocal folds, building subglottic air pressure, and exploding the folds while phonating initial vowel sounds. When done excessively, this phonatory habit will have a negative impact on the tissue lining of the vocal folds. On the other hand, breathy phonation is accomplished by an incomplete approximation of the vocal folds causing the voice to sound weak and breathy owing to the excessive escape of air. This problem of phonation may also be associated with poor respiratory support.

Glottal fry refers to an aperiodic vibration of the vocal folds in a lower frequency range than the normal pitch of the individual. This sputter-like phonatory pattern causes a grinding of the vocal processes of the arytenoid cartilage and is often produced by persons attempting to demonstrate a deep, authoritative sounding voice and by people experiencing voice fatigue.

Resonation

There is a wide range of acceptable resonation patterns in voice production with acceptability being determined by geographic location. Disturbances of resonation may have a functional or organic basis and be caused by improper coupling of the pharyngeal, oral or nasal cavities or improper positioning of the tongue or larynx.

Hypernasality is present when excessive nasal emission occurs during phonation. This behaviour results when the velopharyngeal port remains open during the production of sounds other than the nasal consonants /m/, /n/, and /ng/. Another form of hypernasality is assimilative nasality. Assimilative nasality occurs when the phonemes adjacent to the three nasal consonants are nasalized along with these sounds. A mild form of hypernasality is called *cul de sac* nasality which occurs with little nasal emission as the voice is resonated in the nasal cavity. Denasality occurs when normal nasal resonance is not present during the production of the nasal phonemes. The acoustic result sounds as if the speaker has a head cold.

A common functional resonation problem is the production of voice with restricted use of the supraglottic vocal tract. This may occur when an individual elevates the larynx and retracts the tongue, thus shortening the vocal tract. The resultant voice quality is pinched and strained. The term back-focus is often used to describe this inappropriate tone focus.

Pitch

Inappropriate use of the voice component of pitch may lead to a voice disorder. Pitch is the perceptual correlate of the fundamental frequency (f_0) of voice, which is the number of times the vocal folds vibrate per second. Misuse refers to pitch levels that are either too high or too low or monotonous during conversational speech. Habitual use of an inappropriate pitch places great strain on the laryngeal musculature.

Habitual pitch is a term that refers to the range that an individual uses the majority of time for conversation. Optimal pitch refers to the most appropriate pitch range for use by an individual. Only when the use of an inappropriate pitch level has been isolated as the primary cause of a voice disorder should therapeutic attempts be made to modify pitch. It is very common for pitch change to be the symptom of a voice disorder and not necessarily the cause. Time spent in direct pitch modification may not be appropriate in this circumstance.

Loudness

Loudness is the perceptual term that relates to vocal intensity which is measured in decibels (dB). The inappropriate use of loudness is demonstrated in voices that are habitually too soft, too loud or monotonous in loudness variability. Vocal intensity is determined by the build-up of air pressure below the approximated vocal folds (subglottic air pressure, p_{sub}) and the amplitude or the lateral excursion of the vibration. Less than adequate air pressure will increase the laryngeal muscle effort to produce voice, leading to a potential voice disturbance. Contrarily, too great a pressure will lead to vocal hyperfunction and a potential voice disorder.

Combination of causative factors

Rarely will a voice pathologist be presented with a voice disorder in which a single voice component is isolated as the primary cause; rather a combination of components will most likely be identified. It must be understood that inappropriate voice components may also be the *result* of laryngeal pathologies that are caused by other aetiological factors. When inappropriate voice components are the result of the pathology, they are recognized as the symptoms of the disorder, such as low pitch, glottal fry phonation, breathiness and so on.

Vocal misuse represents the most common aetiological factor identified in patients with voice disorders. Cooper (1973) found that of 1406 patients, 36.6 per cent had disorders associated with vocal abuse; Brodnitz (1971) reported a figure of 25.8 per cent. Voice therapy is particularly effective in the remediation of voice disorders caused by vocal misuse.

Medically-related causes

Many medical/surgical conditions and situations exist which may lead to the development of a voice disorder. These conditions may be the result of direct or indirect surgeries that affect the larynx such as laryngectomy and thyroid surgery respectively. The causes may also be the result of chronic illness and disorders such as allergies, sinusitis, smoking, alcohol or other substance abuses, and gastro-oesophageal reflux of stomach acids. In addition, a number of other primary medical problems produce vocal difficulties as a secondary symptom along with the major disorder. For example, people who are deaf may not be able to monitor their voices well; people with neurological disorders such as a stroke, Parkinson's disease or Huntington's chorea may have many problems with voice as well as speech.

Personality-related causes

The way we feel, both physically and emotionally, is often directly reflected in the quality of our voices. The tensions and stresses of everyday life may contribute directly to the ineffective functioning of the laryngeal mechanism. One term used to describe the many occurrences in human life that can cause emotional and psychological stresses is environmental stress. Personal, work, school, social or family situations may well create difficulties that increase whole body and laryngeal muscle tension to a level that causes hyperfunction of the voice. This hyperfunction may lead to the development of a voice disorder.

At times, environmental stress may become so severe that avoidance behaviours develop to counteract the stressful situations. These avoidance behaviours, called *psychological conversion reactions*, permit people to draw attention away from the emotional stress and conflict. Conversion behaviours associated with voice disorders include aphonia (whispering), muteness (inability to speak or produce voice), or unusual functional dysphonias.

The final personality-related cause of a voice disorder is that of identity conflict. Persons who experience difficulty in establishing their own identities and personalities may develop specific voice disorders in the presence of normal laryngeal mechanisms. These disorders may include the high pitched voice of the post-adolescent male (functional falsetto) or the weak, thin, juvenile voice of an adult female. The many causes of voice disorders lead to the development of very specific laryngeal pathologies.

Laryngeal Pathologies Common to Adults

We have divided our discussion of laryngeal pathologies into four classifications. These classifications include:

1. congenital laryngeal pathologies;
2. pathologies of the vocal fold cover;
3. neurogenic laryngeal pathologies;
4. pathologies of muscular dysfunction

(Stemple *et al.*, 1994).

Congenital laryngeal pathologies comprise laryngeal abnormalities that are present at birth and therefore will not be discussed in this chapter. Pathologies of the vocal fold cover include those that cause any alteration in the histological structure of the vocal fold mucosal lining. Changes in the mucosal lining will affect the mass, size, stiffness, flexibility, and tension of the vocal folds, as well as the adequate approximation of the folds for phonation. Any one of these vocal fold effects has the potential to change the quality, pitch, and loudness of the voice.

Neurogenic voice pathologies are represented by those voice disturbances that are caused directly by an interruption in the nervous signal supplied to the larynx. In our discussion of primary disorder aetiologies, voice changes associated with other neurological disease processes were described. Under the neurogenic pathology classification, our discussion will focus on the few pathologies that are more or less isolated to vocal function, such as vocal fold paralysis and spasmodic dysphonia.

Pathologies associated with muscular dysfunction include those that occur in the presence of a normal vocal fold cover and without neurologic involvement. These pathologies include the various psychogenic voice disorders as well as those associated with the functional misuse of the laryngeal musculature in the production of voice. Let us examine the various laryngeal pathologies, their causes, and typical treatment modalities.

Pathologies of the vocal fold cover

Acute laryngitis: The term *laryngitis* is used to describe an inflammation of the vocal fold mucosa. Symptoms of acute laryngitis (Figure 14.1) include mild to severe dysphonia, a non-productive cough, and local pain or soreness that is aggravated by phonation. The causes of acute laryngitis may be bacterial infections, inhalation of hot gases or flames, aspiration of caustic solutions, and less commonly, acute vocal abuse. Typical treatments include steam inhalation, anaesthetic lozenges, antibiotic medications and voice rest. Voice therapy is not indicated for acute cases of laryngitis.

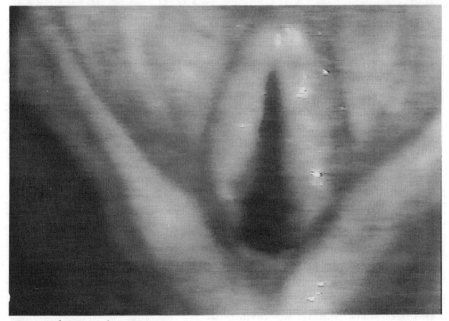

Figure 14.1 Acute laryngitis

Chronic laryngitis: By far the most common form of laryngeal pathology is chronic laryngitis (Figure 14.2). Laryngitis is the laryngeal condition which occurs when the vocal folds are swollen (oedemic) and red (erythema). Chronic laryngitis results from chronic misuse of voice causing fluid to develop in the superficial layer of the vocal folds. Seldom is pain present though the person with the condition will experience hoarseness. People who smoke and drink, shout, talk over noise, and

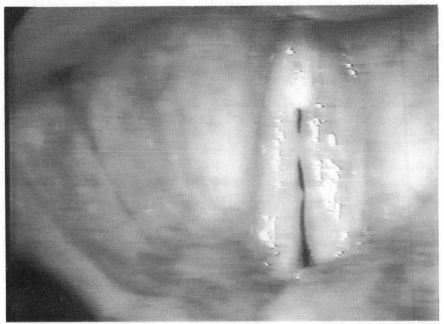

Figure 14.2 Chronic laryngitis

generally misuse their voices, will likely develop this condition. Treatment involves elimination of the misuse of voice.

Vocal nodules: Vocal nodules (Figures 14.3a, b) are a fairly common benign laryngeal growth of the superficial layer of the vocal folds. Sometimes described as vocal fold calluses, singer's nodes or screamer's nodules, these hard fibrous nodules develop as a result of vocal abuse. Vocally abusive behaviours cause friction, which breaks down the normal vocal fold tissue and creates the build-up of layered hard tissue between the anterior one-third and posterior two-thirds of both vocal folds. These hard, fibrous nodules, similar to calluses that might build up on your hands, interfere with the normal vibrations of the vocal folds causing the voice to sound hoarse. Treatment would include elimination or modification of the vocal misuse, training a more appropriate voice production and possible surgical excision of the nodules should therapy not prove successful in their resolution.

Polyps: Another laryngeal pathology, similar in origin to vocal nodules are laryngeal polyps (Figure 14.4). Polyps develop as a result of voice misuse and abuse. They have been described as being similar to blisters in that they are fluid-filled sacs. These sacs may develop as a breakdown of normal vocal fold tissue and occur anywhere along the medial edge of one or both of the vocal folds. Their presence interferes with vibration, causing the voice to be dysphonic. Polyps may resolve with the tissue and fluid being re-absorbed by the normal tissue if the vocal misuse is discontinued. If they do not resolve then they must be surgically excised.

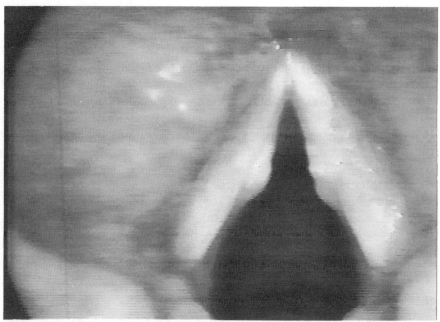

Figure 14.3a Vocal nodules (adducted folds)

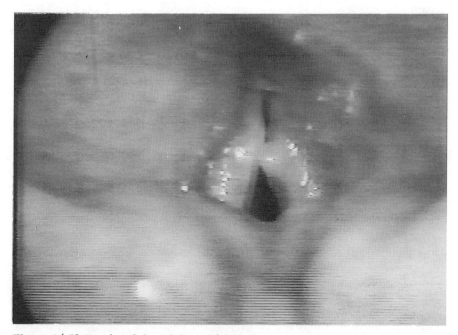

Figure 14.3b Vocal nodules (abducted folds)

Smoking and alcohol abuse, as well as general voice abuse, are implicated in the development of polyps.

Reinke's oedema/polypoid degeneration: This is a diffuse, watery
swelling (Figure 14.5) that may run the entire length of the vocal fold.
Because of voice abuse or other forms of laryngeal irritation, fluid will fill
Reinke's space, giving the fold a floppy, water-balloon appearance. Mild
Reinke's oedema may resolve with the elimination of the causative
behaviours. More severe oedema often requires surgical aspiration of
the affected fold or folds. Diffuse Reinke's oedema seldom occurs in
non-smokers.

Contact ulcers/granulomas: These are illustrated in Figure 14.6 and
are a less common laryngeal pathology than nodules or polyps. Again,
caused by voice misuse, intubation injuries, or reflux of stomach acids,
their development results from a breakdown of the normal mucosal
tissues that course the area around the vocal processes of the arytenoid
cartilages. Voice quality may be hoarse and patients may complain of
pain and a thickness sensation in the throat. A common vocal behaviour
that may lead to the development of contract ulcers is talking while
using a pitch level that is too low. Constant use of a low pitch will cause
the arytenoid cartilages to grind together, thus breaking down the tissue
lining and developing the ulcers. Sometimes the ulcerated tissue will
proliferate, forming granulation tissue. Treatment again will be the identification and modification of voice misuse, medical treatment of acid
reflux, and the possible surgical excision of the ulcerated/granulated
tissue.

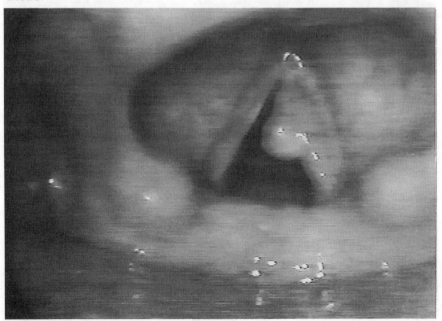

Figure 14.4 Vocal fold polyp

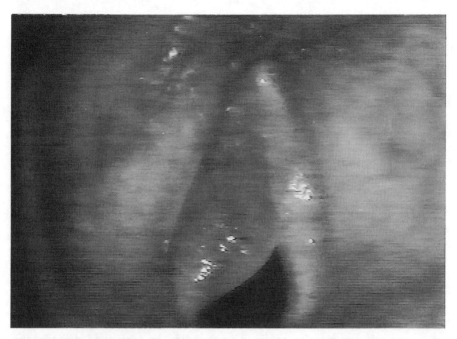

Figure 14.5 Polypoid degeneration

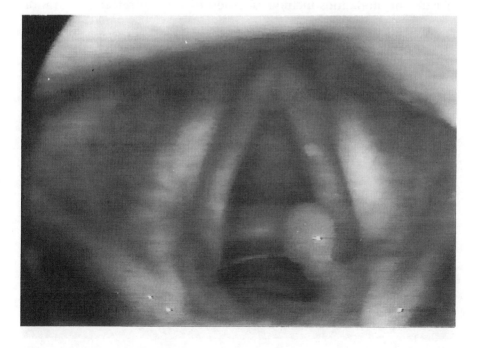

Figure 14.6 Contact granuloma

Leukoplakia and hyperkeratosis: Two pathologies typically classified as premalignant growths are *leukoplakia* (Figure 14.7) and *hyperkeratosis* (Figure 14.8). Causes include the chronic irritations of the chemicals in tobacco smoke, the irritation inherent in alcohol abuse, incessant coughing and throat clearing, and general voice abuse.

Leukoplakia appears as a patchy white membrane and is usually located on the anterior one-third of the true vocal folds. Hyperkeratosis is a layered build-up of keratinized cell tissue. Treatment for both pathologies includes elimination of the irritants and surgical excision of the abnormal tissue. Voice therapy prior to surgery is helpful in reducing behaviours of vocal abuse and for vocal hygiene counselling. Therapy following surgery will aid in re-establishing normal strength, tone, balance and stamina of the laryngeal muscles.

Laryngeal carcinoma: Cancer of the larynx (Figure 14.9) is potentially the most devastating of all laryngeal pathologies because of the life-threatening implications of the disease and the initial devastating effect on communication. The most common symptom of this pathology is persistent hoarseness. There is little if any throat pain or soreness, although either may occur at later stages in the development of the disease and may also be referred to the ears. In advanced disease, the patient may experience both swallowing and respiratory problems.

Laryngeal carcinoma is thought to be caused by chronic irritation to the laryngeal mucosa by such agents as tobacco smoke and alcohol. Treatment modalities include radiation therapy, surgical excision, or

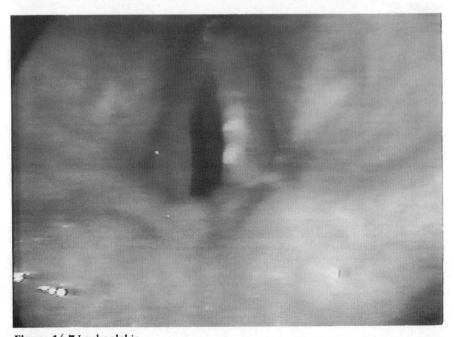

Figure 14.7 Leukoplakia

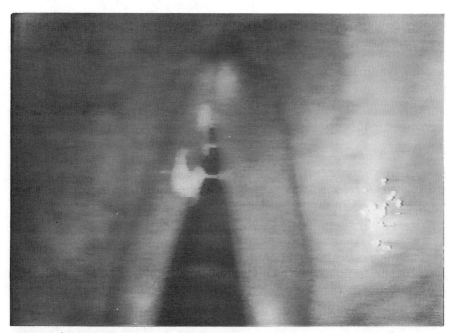

Figure 14.8 Hyperkeratosis

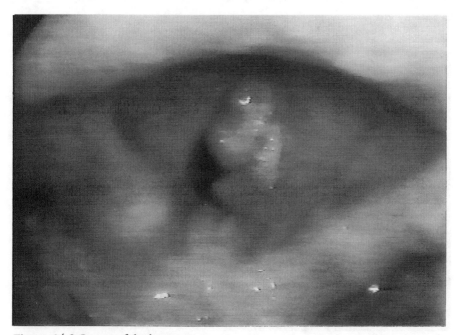

Figure 14.9 Cancer of the larynx

both. Vocal symptoms are characterized by a mild to severe dysphonia depending on the location and the extent of the lesion. The voice pathologist plays an extremely important role in preparing the patient and the family for the consequences of the various forms of surgery and in the subsequent speech rehabilitation.

Neurogenic laryngeal pathologies

Vocal fold paralysis: The symptoms of vocal fold paralysis may vary from no dysphonia (when only one vocal fold is paralysed at the glottal midline) to severe dysphonia (when one or both folds are paralysed in an abducted position). Vocal fold paralysis may be bilateral or unilateral and is typically caused by peripheral involvement of the recurrent laryngeal and, less commonly, the superior laryngeal nerve branches of Vagus.

There are many possible causes of vocal fold paralysis, including indirect surgical trauma, such as thyroidectomy, endarterectomy, and heart, lung, and breast surgeries that may involve the laryngeal nerves. Other causes include cardiovascular disease, neurological diseases, accidental trauma, endotracheal intubation, and bronchoscopy. It is also important to note that the cause of approximately 30 per cent of all vocal fold paralysis is idiopathic. Viral infection is often speculated as the cause of paralysis in these cases, but this cause cannot be proven.

Bilateral abductor paralysis (Figure. 14.10) is the most serious form of vocal fold paralysis in its compromise or respiratory function. With

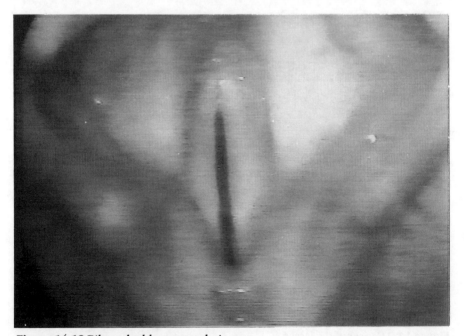

Figure 14.10 Bilateral adductor paralysis

this pathology, both vocal folds are positioned near the midline and are unable to abduct, requiring that an adequate airway be established. This may involve a tracheostomy or a surgical procedure in which one arytenoid cartilage is either removed or tied off laterally in an effort to open the airway. The role of voice therapy, following medical/surgical treatment, is in the establishment of the patient's most efficient voice.

Bilateral adductor paralysis results in both vocal folds resting in a paramedian position, not able to adduct to close the glottis. Individuals with this paralysis will be aphonic or nearly aphonic, but the primary concern is aspiration as the airway protection has been compromised. Within 6 to 9 months the folds may migrate toward the midline position decreasing the severity of the voice and aspiration. However, this migration may create the problems inherent in abductor paralysis. Voice therapy is not effective for bilateral adductor paralysis.

Unilateral adductor paralysis (Figure 14.11) is the most common type of vocal fold paralysis with the paralysed fold resting in the paramedian position while the other fold approximates the midline normally. As might be expected, phonation is characterized by breathiness due to high airflow between the non-approximating folds. The ability to build subglottic air pressure is also impaired, resulting in a decrease of vocal intensity. Patients with this pathology often complain of physical fatigue resulting from the increased effort to approximate the folds for phonation.

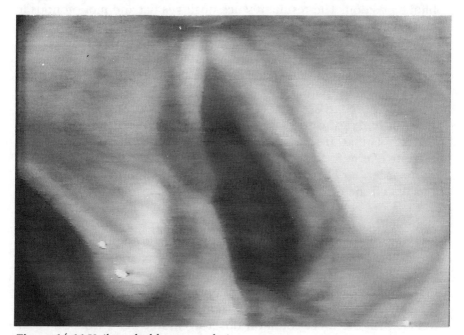

Figure 14.11 Unilateral adductor paralysis

The most common medical treatment for unilateral adductor paralysis involves waiting 9 to 12 months for spontaneous recovery of nerve function. During this time, voice therapy is helpful by providing exercises designed to enhance the efficiency of voice production. When recovery does not occur, the patient may benefit from surgical intervention. Surgery may include Teflon, collagen, or autogenous fat injections into the paralysed fold as a means of bulking that fold and decreasing the glottal gap. More recently, medialization of the paralysed fold has been accomplished through a surgical technique known as thyroplasty. With this technique, a small window is made in the thyroid cartilage on the same plane as the vocal fold. A silastic prosthesis is then inserted into the window and locked in place with the fold medialized in a custom manner. The patient is awake during this procedure permitting the voice to be fine-tuned in surgery.

Bilateral and unilateral superior nerve paralyses occur with involvement of the superior laryngeal nerve, which is much less frequent than paralysis of the recurrent laryngeal nerve due to a much shorter course. Bilateral superior nerve paralysis causes paralysis of the cricothyroid muscles. The voice decreases in pitch and loses the ability to add inflection to the speaking voice or to sing. There is no medical treatment for this pathology. Voice therapy focuses on educating the patient regarding the causes and implications of the pathology.

Unilateral superior nerve paralysis causes an unequal rocking of the cricoid and thyroid cartilage leaving the vocal folds in an overlapped, oblique position. The resultant voice quality is flat and monotonous in pitch, with breathiness and a loss in vocal intensity. Most patients with this pathology complain of vocal fatigue, which results from their efforts to phonate with the obliquely approximated folds. There is no medical treatment. The author has used voice therapy to explain the causes and implications of the pathology and to teach vocal conservation to patients who are required to use their voices daily in their work.

Spasmodic dysphonia: One of the more curious and serious voice disorders is that of spasmodic dysphonia. Spasmodic dysphonia is a descriptive term for a family of strained, strangled voices. The cause of this disorder has been debated for many years. Although early descriptions linked the disorder to a psychoneurosis (Arnold, 1959; Brodnitz, 1976), more recent evidence has demonstrated a neurologic origin (Aminoff et al., 1978; Aronson et al., 1968; Dedo et al., 1978). Blitzer et al. (1988) offered strong evidence that spasmodic dysphonia should be considered a focal dystonia specific to the larynx and similar to other dystonias such as blepharospasm and torticollis.

The incidence of spasmodic dysphonia is unknown, but is thought to be relatively low. The disorder is said to occur equally in men and women with the most common onset in middle age (Aronson et al., 1968; Brodnitz, 1976). We have evaluated patients with onset of the disorder occurring as early as their middle teens. Some patients experience a rapid onset associated with the occurrence of a traumatic event. Others report a more gradual onset following hoarseness associated with an upper respiratory infection. Still others appear to present with an idiopathic spasmodic dysphonia. The severity of the vocal symptoms appears to peak within the first year following the onset of the disorder.

Spasmodic dysphonia is classified in two primary groups: adductor and abductor spasmodic dysphonia. Adductor spasmodic dysphonia is the most common type. The laryngeal behaviour is characterized by an intermittent, tight adduction of the vocal folds creating a strained, forced voicing behaviour. When examined through indirect laryngoscopy, the vocal folds appear normal in structure and function. Intermittent periods of normal phonation may occur during speech production, during both laughter and angry outbursts of speech, and while singing. Some patients are able to reduce the frequency and severity of the spasms when talking at a pitch level that is slightly higher than normal. The majority of patients with adductor spasmodic dysphonia find it difficult to shout.

Many patients with this disorder complain of physical fatigue, tightness of the neck, back and shoulder muscles, and shortness of breath due to their efforts to phonate through the closed glottis. The severity of the symptoms of adductor spasmodic dysphonia vary within and among individuals. Some patients experience only a very mild interruption in normal phonation, while others may be rendered voiceless by the severity of the spasms. In the more severe cases, patients may compensate by whispering or phonating on inspired air. Secondary behaviours similar to those observed in stutterers, such as head jerking, eye blinking, and vocalized starters, may also develop.

Abductor spasmodic dysphonia is a mirror image of the adductor type. Phonation is interrupted by a sudden, involuntary period of aphonia, which is accompanied by a burst of air, as the vocal folds spasm in the abducted position. The vocal fold spasms appear to occur primarily during the production of unvoiced consonants (Aronson, 1980), although Hartman (1980) reported that breathy moments occurred during all positions within words, on whole words, and on several words in succession. Of 13 patients studied by Hartman (1980), eight reported that their voices improved when they were angry, increased their intensity, or altered their pitch. Voice quality worsened when they were anxious or fatigued.

Spasmodic dysphonia is an insidious disorder causing many psychosocial problems for those who display the symptoms of the disorder. We have seen patients who have searched many years, first for a diagnosis of the disorder and then for a treatment to cure or reduce the symptoms. To this end patients have often seen several otolaryngologists, neurologists, psychologists, and speech pathologists. They have gone through voice therapy, psychotherapy, psychological counselling, drug therapies, EMG (electromyographic) and thermal biofeedback, relaxation training, acupuncture, hypnosis, and faith healing. Unfortunately, none of these approaches has proved to be consistently effective in relieving the vocal symptoms. Successful treatment of the symptoms of both forms of spasmodic dysphonia has been found in the injection of botulinum toxin. The toxin causes a temporary paresis or weakness of the vocal folds, thus decreasing the ability of the folds to spasm. Duration of the weakness varies with the average effect of the toxin, lasting three to four months at which time reinjection is necessary to maintain the improved voice production.

Organic (essential) tremor: Essential tremor is a central nervous system disorder that is characterized by rhythmic tremors (4 to 7 cycles/second) of various body parts including the larynx. Tremor may involve the head, arms, neck, tongue, palate, face, and larynx in isolation or in combinations. In some patients, the tremor may only be observed when the affected body part is being used (intentional tremor), whereas other patients will exhibit the tremor behaviour even at rest. The onset of essential tremor is usually gradual, occurring in middle to late middle age. The disorder occurs most frequently in males, is often hereditary, and is often accompanied by other neurological signs (Aronson and Hartman, 1981; Brown and Simonson, 1963; Larsson and Sjogren, 1960).

Laryngeal tremor is most noticeable during prolonged vowels as the rhythm of the tremor is easily discerned. Connected speech may be negatively affected as well. In some cases the tremor is so severe that it causes voice stoppages similar to those of spasmodic dysphonia. Indeed, these two disorders, which may accompany each other, are often mistaken for one another. When in doubt regarding the diagnosis, the clinician is reminded to ask the patient to sustain vowels. Voice therapy is not an effective treatment for organic tremor.

Pathologies of muscular dysfunction

Ventricular phonation: Occasionally a large enough amount of muscle tension is created in the laryngeal area to cause the ventricular folds (false vocal folds) to approximate for phonation (Figure 14.12). Normally the ventricular folds will simply rest quietly while the true vocal folds vibrate. False vocal fold vibration, as a functional behaviour may be caused by physical or emotional tension. This form of voicing has also been used as a compensatory voice when other serious pathologies make it too difficult for the true vocal folds to vibrate. Treatment for functional ventricular phonation involves counselling and vocal re-education through direct voice therapy.

Conversion aphonia and dysphonia: As discussed earlier, some voice disorders may result from environmental stress or out of psychological

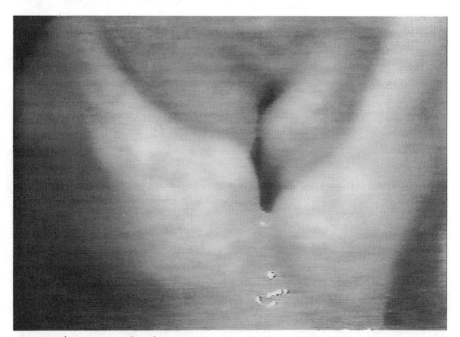

Figure 14.12 Ventricular phonation

needs. The conversion voice problems are evident when a person whispers or produces an inappropriate voice in the presence of normal vocal folds and entirely normal laryngeal mechanism and vocal tract. The conversion voice problems have numerous possible vocal symptoms and the onset is often quite sudden. More women present with conversion problems than men. The conversion pathology is normally the person's unconscious method of avoiding a strong interpersonal conflict that may cause stress, anxiety or depression. Treatment for conversion voice pathologies will involve counselling and direct voice manipulation. It must be noted that people who present with these disorders truly do not believe that they are capable of producing normal voice. They are not joking or malingering and need to be handled delicately.

Functional falsetto/juvenile voice: The laryngeal mechanism goes through a dramatic change in both male and female children during puberty. The male voice lowers about one octave during mutation and the female voice lowers two to three semitones. When this acoustic change does not take place following the normal physical maturation, the male is said to have a functional falsetto and the female a juvenile or child-like voice.

Many causes for functional falsetto have been suggested. They include attempts to resist the natural growth into adulthood; a strong feminine self-identification; the desire to maintain a competent childhood soprano singing voice; and embarrassment when the voice lowers dramatically, perhaps earlier than those of their peers (Aronson, 1980).

We would also suggest that the falsetto voice may also be the result of muscular inco-ordination and dysfunction without other underlying aetiology. The juvenile voice of the post-adolescent female is recognized less commonly than mutational falsetto as the vocal symptoms of this disorder are less dramatic for the female. Women who demonstrate a juvenile voice may have resisted the transition into adulthood or also may have developed a muscular dysfunction. These disorders are well treated through voice therapy.

Assessment Considerations

Prior to being evaluated by the voice pathologist, the patient should have been seen by an otolaryngologist who is an ear, nose and throat specialist. The otolaryngologist will have examined the patient through indirect laryngoscopy, fibre-optic laryngoscopy, a rigid scope, direct microlaryngoscopy or videostroboscopy. This process is necessary to rule out the possibility of life-threatening pathological conditions or conditions which cannot be remedied therapeutically.

The primary objectives of the voice evaluation performed by the voice pathologist are to: (1) identify the causes, (2) describe the present vocal components, and (3) develop an individualized management plan. Secondary objectives include: (1) patient education, (2) patient motivation, and (3) to establish the credibility of the examiner.

The voice evaluation should be viewed not only as a diagnostic tool, but also as a major part of the therapeutic process. It is the first stage of therapy. It helps to establish the rapport and understanding between the therapist and the patient. It serves to develop the patient's awareness and understanding of the disorder and develops the motivation for change.

The typical voice evaluation will be accomplished through a systematic interview including information regarding the history of the development of the problem, associated medical history, information related to personal, work and social lives of the patients, and a formal assessment of the present voice components. When this has been completed, the clinician should have identified all the causes associated with the development of the problem and behaviours which serve to continue to problem. Inappropriate vocal components will be identified and the management plan will be developed. During the interview, your knowledge of anatomy and physiology, causative factors, and pathological conditions becomes extremely important. At the beginning of each evaluation you want to establish that the patient understands the reason for the referral and make sure you know why the patient was referred to you. Therefore, you will develop the patient's knowledge of his or her pathological condition through an explanation of the pathology and common reasons for its development. This will lead the patient to think about his or her own causative factors and help to develop your own credibility.

The history of the disorder as well as the medical and social history of the patient must be systematically evaluated in the interview to learn about the causative and maintaining factors relating to the disorder. Such an interview is followed by the physical oral-peripheral examination and the subjective voice analysis to determine the present state of the various vocal components.

Oral–peripheral examination

The oral–peripheral examination will determine the physical condition of the oral mechanism and the peripheral speech system. At this point the examiner checks for laryngeal area or whole-body tension and difficulties with swallowing. Swallowing difficulties may be present in some patients because of the close relationship between the physical structures associated with voice and swallowing. Laryngeal sensations such as dryness, tickling, aching, burning, soreness or a 'lump in the throat feeling' are also questioned. Some or all of these sensations are often present with laryngeal hyperfunction.

Voice analysis

The subjective voice analysis will then examine each vocal component in detail to determine its appropriateness. At times, a particular voice component, such as pitch, may be used habitually in an inappropriate manner (such as too low) and will be identified as the primary cause of the voice disorder. This cause must then be directly modified. At other times, an inappropriate low pitch may simply be the vocal symptom of the voice disorder and not the actual cause. Often, if the actual cause is eliminated or modified, the voice component will indirectly improve.

To begin the voice analysis, simply jot down the significant voice qualities you heard during the interview. Using a five-point scale, state 'the quality was (1) mild, (2) mild to moderate, (3) moderate, (4) moderate to severe, (5) severe dysphonia characterized by . . .' At this point, list the purely subjective terms that will be meaningful to you at a later time for comparison. These terms may include hoarse, harsh, strident, tinny, breathy, raspy and so on. Then test or comment on the seven major components of respiration, phonation, resonation, pitch, loudness, and rate and rhythm.

Respiration

1. Describe the breathing pattern as abdominal or thoracic and as supportive or non-supportive of voice.
2. Ask the patient to sustain and time the /s/ sound and /z/ sound for as long as possible. The times for both sounds should be fairly equal.

Healthy vocal folds do not require more air to sustain voice on /z/ than to produce the voiceless /s/ (Eckel and Boone, 1981).

3. Ask the patient to sustain and time the /a/ sound for as long as possible. This establishes your respiratory baseline.

Phonation

Report on the presence of (1) hard glottal attacks, (2) breathiness, (3) glottal fry, (4) diplophonia, (5) phonation breaks. If you are not sure from the interview process whether the behaviours are present, simply have the patient recite the alphabet at a moderate loudness level, listen closely and rate the voice production.

Resonation

Report on the presence of (1) hypernasality, (2) hyponasality, (3) assimilative nasality, (4) *cul-de-sac* nasality and (5) back-focused phonation. You may wish to compare contrasting pairs such as: beat/meat, bit/mitt, bait/mate, bet/met, bat/mat.

Pitch

1. Test the present pitch range by asking the patient to sing, in whole notes from the lowest to highest note. Match each note to a pitch pipe or piano and record the note for future reference.
2. Describe adequacy of conversational inflection – monotone, adequate, too great.
3. Subjectively judge where the habitual pitch falls in the present range – bottom, middle, top. We would suggest that an optimum pitch range cannot be identified in the pathological voice.

Loudness

1. Determine whether the voice is too loud, too soft or has appropriate loudness for the speaking situation.
2. Check the patient's ability to shout. This will yield good information regarding the ability of the vocal folds to adequately adduct and build appropriate sub-glottic air pressure to produce voice.

Rhythm and rate

1. Describe whether the rate of speech was too fast, too slow or adequate.
2. Describe any vocal characteristics which may interrupt the normal rhythm of the voice production. These may be frequent voice breaks, hesitations or spasms.

In examining the history of the problem, the medical and social histories, conducting the oral–peripheral examination and subjectively evaluating the vocal components, you have gathered together many pieces of the diagnostic puzzle. Now, examine the pieces and assemble them in the order which identifies the causes of the disorder and describes the present vocal components. Report your results under a section of the evaluation entitled 'Impressions'. Based on these results, under 'Recommendations' develop an individualized management plan that is designed to remedy the problem. In so doing, you will have completed the three major goals of the voice evaluation.

Objective Voice Analysis

The reader should be aware that it is now possible to objectify the voice analysis procedure with special instrumentation. This instrumentation, which depends on computer technology, quickly and objectively analyses both acoustic and aerodynamic parameters of voice. This instrumentation has become more affordable and available. Its use has become a standard component of the voice evaluation. (Details regarding instrumental analysis of voice may be found in Stemple *et al.*, 1994.) Instrumentation, however, will never be able to replace the systematic, detailed patient interview which offers the most important information regarding the psychosocial aspects of the patient's voice disorder.

Theoretical Bases of Intervention

The management of voice disorders by 'speech correctionists' began in the 1930s. Since that early beginning, a rich and interesting history of voice therapy approaches has evolved leading to several philosophical orientations of therapy. These orientations include symptomatic, psychogenic, aetiologic, physiologic, and eclectic voice therapies. The following is a summary of the various orientations as described in Stemple et al. (1994).

Symptomatic voice therapy

The focus of symptomatic voice therapy is on the modification of the deviant vocal symptoms or components that were identified by the voice pathologist during the diagnostic voice evaluation. These symptoms may be breathiness, low pitch, glottal fry phonation, the use of hard glottal attacks, and so on. Boone (1971) was the first voice pathologist to organize previous literature and introduce to the profession the symptomatic therapy orientation. Symptomatic voice therapy is based on the premise that most voice disorders are caused by the functional misuse or abuse of the voice components including pitch, loudness, respiration, and so on. When identified through the diagnostic process, the misuses are eliminated or reduced through various voice therapy *facilitating techniques*. Boone (1971: 11) stated:

In the voice clinician's attempt to aid the patient in finding and using his best voice production, it is necessary to probe continually within the patient's repertoire to find that one voice that sounds 'good' and which he is able to produce with relatively little effort. A **voice therapy facilitating technique** is that technique which, when used by a particular patient, enables him easily to produce a good voice. Once discovered, the facilitating technique and resulting phonation become the symptomatic focus of therapy.... This use of a facilitating technique to produce a good phonation is the core of what we do in symptomatic voice therapy for the reduction of hyperfunctional voice disorders.

Boone's (1971) original facilitating techniques included:

1 altering tongue position
2 change of loudness
3 chewing exercises
4 digital manipulation
5 ear training
6 elimination of abuses
7 elimination of hard glottal attack
8 establish new pitch
9 explanation of the problem
10 feedback
11 hierarchy analysis
12 negative practice
13 open-mouth exercises
14 pitch inflections
15 pushing approach
16 relaxation
17 respiration training
18 target voice models
19 voice rest
20 yawn–sigh approach.

A complete description of each facilitating technique as well as kinds of problems for which the techniques are useful and procedural aspects may be found in Boone and McFarlane (1988). From this list, it may be observed that the main focus of symptomatic voice therapy is direct modification of the vocal symptoms. The voice pathologist constantly probes for the 'best' voice in the presence of the disorder. When the best voice is found, attempts to stabilize that voice with the various facilitating techniques are made. Symptomatic voice therapy assumes voice improvement through direct symptom modification (Stemple, 1993).

Psychogenic voice therapy

Psychogenic voice therapy is based on the assumption of underlying emotional causes for the voice disturbance. The relationship of

emotions to voice production has been well documented in the literature starting as early as the middle 1800's (Goss, 1878; Russell, 1864;
Ward, 1877). West, Kennedy and Carr (1937) and Van Riper (1939)
discussed the need for emotional retraining in voice therapy, while
Murphy (1964) and Brodnitz (1971) presented excellent information
related to the psychodynamics of voice production.

Aronson (1980) first articulated the most complete description of a
psychogenic voice disorder when he stated that:

> A psychogenic voice disorder is broadly synonymous with a functional one
> but has the advantage of stating positively, based on an explanation of its
> causes, that the voice disorder is a manifestation of one or more types of
> psychological disequilibrium – such as anxiety, depression, conversion reac-
> tion, or personality disorder – which interfere with normal volitional control
> over phonation. (p. 131)

Aronson (1990), Case (1984), and Colton and Casper (1990) further
discussed the need for determining the emotional dynamics of the voice
disturbance from the perspectives of emotions as a cause for voice disorders and voice disorders being the cause of emotional disequilibrium.

Psychogenic voice therapy focuses on identification and modification
of the emotional and psychosocial disturbances associated with the
onset and maintenance of the voice problem. When the psychogenic
causes are resolved, so too will there be a resolution of the voice disorder. Voice pathologists must develop and possess superior interview
skills, counselling skills, and the skill to know when the emotional or
psychosocial problem is in need of more intensive evaluation and therapy by other professionals (Stemple, 1993).

Aetiologic voice therapy

Aetiologic voice therapy is based on the reasonable assumption that
there is always a cause for the presence of the voice disorder. If that
cause (or causes) can be identified, then appropriate treatments can be
devised for modifying or eliminating those causes. Once modified, the
voice production has the opportunity to improve or return to normal
(Stemple, 1984). During the diagnostic evaluation, much effort is
focused on identifying the direct and indirect causes of the voice disorder. To be successful, the voice pathologist must understand the many
aetiologic factors that may possibly contribute to the voice disorder.
Once the aetiologic factors are treated, the vocal symptoms often
improve without direct manipulation of the voice components. A
common example may be the reduction of the abusive behaviour of
shouting in children who have vocal nodules. As a result of modifying
the shouting behaviour, the nodules are given the opportunity to resolve
and the voice improves without modification of the voice components

which may have *resulted* from the presence of the nodules (such as lower pitch, breathiness and so on).

Direct symptom modification (i.e. raising the pitch, reducing breathiness, and so on) is reserved for situations where the inappropriate use of a voice component is found to be the primary aetiologic factor. For example, we recently evaluated a patient who attempted to sound more authoritative by using a pitch that was too low with intermittent glottal fry phonation. The use of the inappropriate pitch was found to be the primary cause of the patient's dysphonia and laryngeal fatigue and was therefore modified leading to improved voice production.

Aetiologic voice therapy presumes that every voice disorder has a cause. Once identified, the cause can be modified or eliminated leading to improved voice production. If the primary aetiologic factor is found to be the inappropriate use of a voice component, then direct symptom modification is used to resolve the problem.

Physiologic voice therapy

Physiologic voice therapy is the term used to describe direct voice therapies which have been devised to alter or modify the physiology of the vocal mechanism. Normal voice production is dependent upon a balance among the following: airflow, supplied by the respiratory system; laryngeal muscular strength, balance, co-ordination, and stamina; and co-ordination among these and the supraglottic resonatory structures. In addition, physiologic voice therapy concentrates on developing and maintaining the health of the vocal fold cover. Any disturbance in the physiologic balance of these vocal subsystems may lead to a voice disturbance. As stated by Stemple (1993: 4):

> These disturbances may be in laryngeal muscle strength, tone, mass, stiffness, flexibility, and approximation. Disturbances may also manifest in respiratory volume, power, pressure, and flow. The overall causes may be mechanical, neurologic or psychological. Whatever the cause, the management approach is direct modification of the inappropriate physiologic activity through direct exercise and manipulation.

Physiologic voice therapy strives to balance the physiology of voice production through direct physical exercise and manipulations of the laryngeal, respiratory, and resonatory systems. In addition, special care is taken to account for the health of the vocal fold cover. This care may be related to proper mucosal hydration, attention to voice abuse reduction, or anti-reflux regimens as examples.

Eclectic voice therapy

Eclectic voice therapy is the combination of any and all of the other orientations of voice therapy. Successful voice therapy is dependent upon the voice pathologist using all of the therapy techniques that seem appropriate for individual patients. Many patients may share the same diagnosis, although the aetiologies and personalities, vocal needs and emotional reactions to their voice problems may be very different. Because of these differences, the same pathologies may require very different management approaches. Therefore, the voice pathologist is advised not to adhere to any one philosophical orientation of voice therapy, but rather to learn a broad range of management approaches.

Mainstream Therapy Models

Utilizing a case study presentation, let us now examine how each of these voice therapy orientations would treat the following voice disorder.

Case history

The patient was a 48-year-old woman who was diagnosed by the laryngologist as having moderate bilateral Reinke's oedema with the left fold suggesting a more severe draping, polypoid degeneration. The patient was referred for a voice evaluation and a trial voice therapy programme. Should short-term therapy not prove successful in improving her vocal fold condition and voice quality, then the patient would be scheduled for surgical intervention.

History of the problem

The patient was referred to the otolaryngologist by her internist when, during a regular physical examination, she noticed that the patient's voice quality 'sounded as deep as a man's.' The patient stated that her voice had always been deep and that she really did not think there was much of a problem. However, when the otolaryngologist told her that she had vocal fold polyps, she became concerned enough to throw her cigarettes in the examination room trash can and, by the time of the voice evaluation, had not smoked for two weeks. She reported that her voice quality was essentially the same throughout the day, though it tended to become 'huskier' towards the end of a work day.

Medical history

The patient reported undergoing thyroid surgery 5 years earlier, during which her left thyroid lobe was excised. In addition, she underwent a tonsillectomy and appendectomy as a teenager. In addition to the surgeries, she was hospitalized for chronic depression on two different occasions. The last hospitalization lasted for 3 weeks and occurred 18 months previously. The patient was continuing to be treated for depression with medication and remained in bimonthly counselling.

Chronic medical conditions included asthma and frequent bronchitis, high blood pressure, elevated blood sugar, and rheumatoid arthritis. Daily medications were taken for depression, 'nerves' (a sleep aid), thyroid, high blood pressure, and pain associated with the arthritis. Until 2 weeks prior to the examination, she had smoked 1 1/2 to 2 packets of cigarettes per day for approximately 30 years. Her liquid intake was poor, consisting of approximately three cups of caffeinated coffee and four cans of caffeinated soda per day. Chronic throat clearing was noted throughout the evaluation. The patient indicated that on a day-to-day basis she felt 'fair-to-poor' owing to stress, fatigue, and arthritis pain.

Social history

The patient was married for 29 years, but had presently been separated from her husband for 3 months, causing much stress and tension. She had three grown children. The middle child, a 26-year-old son, had recently divorced and temporarily moved back into the house. Again, the patient pointed to the stress of this situation. The patient was not reticent in talking about her depression and indicated that an unhappy marriage and the feeling of an unfulfilled life were the causes.

The patient had been employed for 6 years by a factory that made latex gloves for medical use. She indicated that her specific job was in the 'powder room' where the gloves were filled with powder and packaged. Apparently the powder dust caused much coughing during the day. In addition, the packaging machines were noisy, requiring the workers to talk loudly to be heard. Most talking on the job was social among the eight people who worked in a large, well-ventilated room.

Non-work activities included walking her two dogs nightly, talking on the telephone with her daughter, and actively shopping with a close friend at yard sales and flea markets. However, all of these activities were curtailed when she did not feel well physically or emotionally.

Oral–peripheral examination

The structure and function of the oral mechanism appeared to be well within normal limits for speech and voice production. The laryngeal sensations of dryness and occasional thickness were reported by the patient. Laryngeal area muscle tension and neck tension were demonstrated by the patient.

Voice evaluation

The patient's voice quality was described as mild-to-moderately dysphonic, characterized by low pitch, inappropriate loudness, and husky hoarseness.

Respiration: s/z = 25 sec/10 sec; Patient demonstrated a thoracic, supportive breathing pattern. She tended to speak on residual air, especially towards the end of phrases.

Phonation: A slight breathiness was noted during conversational voice. Occasional glottal fry was noted toward the end of phrases.

Resonation: Normal

Pitch: Patient demonstrated an unusually low pitch conversationally.

Loudness: Patient spoke unusually loud for the speaking situation.

Rate: Normal.

Acoustic measures and aerodynamic analyses revealed the following:

fundamental frequency	136 Hz
frequency range	106 to 320 Hz
jitter percent: sustained vowels	0.56
shimmer dB: sustained vowels	0.67
intensity (habitual)	76 dB
airflow volume	2300 ml
airflow rate	180 ml/sec, all pitch levels
phonation time	12.7 sec
subglottic air pressure	8.6 cm/H_2O

Laryngeal videostroboscopic observation revealed a moderate bilateral vocal fold oedema, worse left than right. Prominent blood vessels were noted bilaterally. Glottic closure was complete with a mild ventricular fold compression. The amplitude of vibration was moderate-to-severely decreased left and moderately decreased right. The mucosal waves were severely decreased bilaterally. The open phase of the vibratory cycle was slightly dominant, while the symmetry of vibration was irregular by 50 per cent. In short, the patient demonstrated an oedematous, stiff, out-of-phase vocal fold system.

Impressions

The patient presented with a voice disorder secondary to these possible aetiologic factors:

- long-term cigarette smoking
- harsh employment environment in terms of dust and talking over noise;
- poor hydration and large caffeine intake;
- asthma and frequent bronchitis;
- prescription medications causing mucosal drying;
- frequent coughing and throat clearing;

- emotional instability;
- talking too loudly in general conversation;
- using a low pitch;
- laryngeal area muscle tension.

Recommendations

Symptomatic voice therapy. General focus would use facilitating techniques to:

1. raise pitch;
2. reduce loudness;
3. reduce laryngeal area tension and effort.

This direct symptom modification would follow an explanation of the problem and would run concurrently with modification of the vocally abusive behaviours including:

1. smoking;
2. caffeine intake;
3. coughing and throat clearing.

Psychogenic voice therapy. General focus would explore the psychodynamics of the voice disorder. This exploration would include:

1. detailed patient interview to determine the cause and effects of stress, tension, and depression;
2. determination of the exact relationship of emotional problems and voice problem;
3. counselling the patient regarding the effects of emotions on voice problems;
4. reduction of musculoskeletal tension caused by emotional upheaval;
5. support of ongoing psychological counselling.

Secondary focus would deal with modification/elimination of the abusive behaviours including:

1. smoking;
2. caffeine;
3. coughing and throat clearing.

Inappropriate use of pitch and loudness would most likely be viewed as obvious symptoms of the voice problem. As the psychodynamics improve, the voice symptoms would be expected to improve.

Aetiologic voice therapy. General focus would be to identify the primary and secondary causes of the voice disorder and then to modify or eliminate these causes. The primary causes would include:

1. smoking;

2. laryngeal dehydration from poor hydration, caffeine intake, and drugs;
3. voice abuse, such as talking loudly over noise at work, coughing, and throat clearing
4. inhalation of large quantities of powder.

Secondary causes that may be more the result of the problem as opposed to a cause would be:

1. laryngeal area muscle tension due to increased mass and stiffness;
2. low pitch due to increased mass;
3. increased loudness due to effort to force stiff, heavy folds to vibrate.

Therapy would focus on modification or elimination of the primary aetiologic factors. The patient would be supported in her effort to stop smoking, encouraged to begin a hydration programme and to reduce caffeine intake, given vocal hygiene counselling in an effort to reduce the vocally abusive habits, and encouraged to wear a mask to filter her breathing at work. The secondary causes of tension, low pitch and increased loudness, would be expected to spontaneously improve as the primary causes were modified and the vocal fold condition improved.

Physiologic voice therapy. General focus would be to evaluate the present physiologic condition of the patient's voice production and develop direct physical exercises or manipulations to improve that condition. This patient demonstrated increased mass and stiffness of the vocal folds changing the physical dynamics of vocal fold vibration. Indeed, she was required to build greater subglottic air pressure to initiate and maintain vibration, which required a borderline high airflow rate. This increased pressure caused her to speak too loudly in conversation. She also attempted to overcome these problems by making physical adjustments such as increasing supraglottic tension in an effort to maintain her voice. When added to the mucosal and muscular stiffness, vocal hyperfunction was the result. The management programme would therefore include:

1. vocal function exercises designed to restrengthen and balance the laryngeal musculature and to balance airflow to muscular activity and improve supraglottic placement of the tone;
2. hydration programme and decrease in caffeinated products to improve the mucous membrane of the vocal folds;
3. discussion of medications with the patient's physician;
4. elimination of habit coughing and throat clearing ;
5. vocal hygiene counselling for elimination of direct voice abuse.

Eclectic voice therapy. It is obvious in the review of these orientations that each management approach has certain strengths as well as inherent weaknesses. You will be able to best treat your patients with the understanding and use of all of these orientations. Therefore, eclectic voice therapy is obviously the treatment of choice with any voice disordered patient. This patient would best be served when the management plan included:

1. symptom modification;
2. elimination/modification of the causes;
3. attention to the psychodynamics of the problem;
4. direct physiologic exercise and attention to the mucosal covering of the vocal folds.

Effectiveness Measures

In the past, judgement of the effectiveness of the treatment of voice disorders was simply made by the subjective satisfaction of the patient and the clinician. These subjective judgements have now been enhanced by various methods including instrumental assessment of voice, stroboscopic observation of vocal fold vibratory function, and formal outcome surveys completed by the patient at the completion of treatment.

While the best evaluator of voice quality remains the ear of the trained clinician, what our ears hear may now be measured for future reference and comparison by acoustic and aerodynamic instruments. These objective measures, taken prior to the onset of therapy and at the conclusion of treatment, provide the objective data that our ears cannot provide. These measures in no way take the place of the trained ear, but provide an additional assessment tool.

Laryngeal videostroboscopic observation of vocal fold function has provided an extremely valuable tool for the voice pathologist to assess the causes of deviant voice productions and the outcome of treatment. This assessment provides visual data that enhance the data provided by the clinical ear. In addition, videostroboscopy has become a valuable tool for patient education.

Finally, the clinician is only the second best individual to judge the effectiveness of treatment. Indeed, the patient is the best judge of the effectiveness of his or her own voice production. To that end, several outcome tools have been developed which allow the patient to judge the effectiveness of his or her voice therapy programme. These tools help to determine the improvement of voice on both functional and social bases. Indeed, in the USA, the need for patient outcome data has become critical in the present climate of health care reform.

Conclusion

You have now been introduced to the major areas of knowledge necessary for undertaking the treatment of patients with voice disorders. The term 'introduction' is important in this discussion, because your understanding of voice disorders is dependent upon in-depth study of anatomy/physiology, causes of voice disorders, laryngeal pathologies, diagnostic procedures and therapy techniques. Because of space consideration, it is not possible to include more than introductory comments regarding each of these areas of knowledge. Indeed, entire texts are devoted to these topics with many of the texts referenced throughout this chapter. Students are encouraged to read further and to develop the theoretical knowledge necessary for the practical treatment of voice disorders.

Acknowledgements

The author sincerely thanks Singular Publishing Group, Inc., for permission of liberal use of materials from the text *Clinical Voice Pathology: Theory and Management* (2nd ed), 1994, which was referenced within this text.

References

Aminoff M, Dedo H, Izdebski K (1978) Clinical aspects of spasmodic dysphonia. Journal of Neurology, Neurosurgery and Psychiatry 41: 361–5.

Arnold G (1959) Spastic dysphonia I: Changing interpretation of a persistent affliction. Logos 2: 3–14.

Aronson A (1980) Clinical voice disorders: An interdisciplinary approach. New York: Brian C. Decker.

Aronson A (1990) Clinical voice disorders: An interdisciplinary approach (3rd ed.) New York: Brian C. Decker.

Aronson A, Brown J, Litin E, Pearson J (1968) Spastic dysphonia. 1. Voice, neurologic, and psychiatric aspects. Journal of Speech and Hearing Disorders 33: 203–18.

Aronson A, Hartman D (1981) Adductor spastic dysphonia as a sign of essential (voice) tremor. Journal of Speech and Hearing Disorders 33: 52–8.

Blitzer A, Brin M, Fahn S, Lovelace R (1988) Localized injections of botulinum toxin for the treatment of focal laryngeal dystonia (spastic dysphonia) Laryngoscope 98: 193–7.

Boone D (1971) The voice and voice therapy (1st ed) Englewood Cliffs, NJ: Prentice-Hall.

Boone D (1977) The voice and voice therapy (2nd ed) Englewood Cliffs, NJ: Prentice-Hall.

Boone D, McFarlane S (1988) The voice and voice therapy. Englewood Cliffs, NJ: Prentice-Hall.

Brodnitz F (1971) Vocal rehabilitation (4th ed). Rochester, NY: American Academy of Ophthalmology and Otolaryngology.

Brodnitz F (1976) Spastic dysphonia. Annals of Otology, Rhinology, and Laryngology 85: 210–14.

Brown J, Simonson J (1963) Organic voice tremor. Neurology 13: 520–5.

Case J (1984) Clinical management of voice disorders. Rockville, MD: Aspen.

Colton R, Casper L (1990) Understanding voice problems: A physiological perspective for diagnosis and treatment. Baltimore: Williams and Wilkins.

Cooper M (1973) Modern techniques of vocal rehabilitation. Springfield, IL: Charles C. Thomas.

Dedo H, Townsend J, Izdebski K (1978) Current evidence for the organic aetiology of spastic dysphonia. Transactions of Otolaryngology 86: 875–80.

Eckel F, Boone D (1981) The s/z ratio as an indicator of laryngeal pathology. Journal of Speech and Hearing Disorders 46: 147–9.

Goss F (1878) Hysterical aphonia. Boston Medical and Surgical Journal 99: 215–22.

Greene M (1972) The voice and its disorders (3rd ed.) Philadelphia: J.P. Lippincott.

Hartman D (1980) Clinical investigations of abductor spastic dysphonia (intermittent breathy dysphonia). Paper presented at the American Speech-Language-Hearing Association Convention, Detroit.

Larsson T, Sjogren T (1960) Essential tremor: A clinical and genetic population study. Acta Psychiatry and Neurology (Scandinavia) 36 (Suppl. 144): 1–176.

Moore P (1971) Organic Voice Disorders. Englewood Cliffs, NJ:Prentice-Hall.

Murphy A (1964) Functional voice disorders. Englewood Cliffs, NJ: Prentice-Hall.

Russell J (1864) A case of hysterical aphonia. British Medical Journal 8: 619–21.

Stemple J (1993) Voice therapy: Clinical studies. St Louis: Mosby Year Book.

Stemple J (1984) Clinical Voice Pathology: Theory and Management. Columbus, OH: Charles E Merrill.

Stemple J, Glaze L, Gerdeman B (1994) Clinical Voice Pathology: Theory and Management (2nd ed). San Diego: Singular Publishing Group, Inc.

Stemple J, Holcomb B (1988) Effective Voice and Articulation. Columbus: Charles E. Merrill.

Van Riper C (1939) Speech Correction Principles and Methods. Englewood Cliffs, NJ: Prentice-Hall.

Ward W, (1877) Hysterical aphonia. Chicago Medical Journal and Examiner 34: 495–505.

West R, Kennedy L, Carr A (1937) The Rehabilitation of Speech. New York: Harper and Brothers.

Chapter 15
Stuttering in Adults

MARGARET M. LEAHY

Adult stuttering usually has its origins in childhood. When this is so, stuttering is regarded as idiopathic or of unknown causation. There is increasing evidence however that idiopathic stuttering may begin in adulthood, although in some such instances onset may be linked to recent trauma experienced or to psychological states, e.g. depression and anxiety (Stewart and Grantham, 1993; Market et al., 1990). In other instances, acquired stuttering in the adult may have a direct neurogenic origin (Bijleveld, Lebrun and van Dongen, 1994), which is further discussed below.

For adults who have stuttered since childhood, the disruptions that are the central core of the disorder remain, but these may be compounded or truncated with tension and struggle behaviours accompanying the speech effort. In some cases, such features of stuttering may even be hidden by the adult who stutters, but negative feelings and attitudes regarding speech and communication are usual and, indeed, these may be the predominant feature that confronts the therapist.

Definition

The *involuntary* disruption in the flow of speech, experienced as '*loss of control*' is the focal point in several definitions of stuttering (Andrews et al., 1983; Perkins, Kent and Curlee, 1991). Descriptions of stuttering behaviours include the abnormally high frequency of intra-phonemic breaks that disrupt transitions between sounds (Stromsta, 1986); excessive tension and struggle associated with speaking (Van Riper, 1982); and avoidance behaviours (Starkweather, 1987). Cooper (1993: 382) proposes that stuttering be defined as 'a diagnostic label referring to a clinical syndrome characterized most frequently by abnormal and persistent dysfluencies in speech accompanied by characteristic affective, behavioral, and cognitive patterns'.

Dalton and Hardcastle (1989) point out that dysfluency affects not only the segmental aspects of speech but prosodic, syntactic, lexical, and semantic levels of communication. The interaction process may also be disrupted (Krause, 1982) and adults who stutter may experience difficulty with social situations. An important aspect of stuttering is its cyclic or variable nature, i.e. people who stutter will tend to stutter less for long periods or in some situations (Gregory, 1987; Andrews et al., 1983).

Causative Factors

Theories of the origins of stuttering (outlined in Chapter 8) may not bear much relevance to the adult form of stuttering, as the disorder will have grown and changed significantly in its development. It is estimated that as many as 78 per cent of children who have ever stuttered will recover by age 16 (Andrews et al., 1983), but those who persist in stuttering will typically follow patterns of development described by Van Riper (1982) and by Starkweather (1987). These patterns are generally episodic and they provide insight into major influences on stuttering development which are described variously as learning factors (Van Riper, 1982) and as interpreting and responding to construing of events (Hayhow and Levy, 1989).

There is increasing evidence to support theories that consider stuttering to be caused by constitutional differences including, for example, genetic influences (Kidd, 1985) and neurophysiological components (Moore, 1985; Moore and Boberg, 1987). Perhaps the strongest theory of stuttering to emerge to date is that which considers aspects of neuropsycholinguistic dysfunctioning as the basis for stuttering (Perkins et al., 1991). This theory may be considered to extend Sheehan's (1968) theory to an extent (see below) and to provide a basis for understanding 'all forms of disfluent speech flow' (Perkins et al., 1991: 735) by linking together time pressure and speech disruption. There is also evidence that indicates differences in neurophysiological functioning occurring as result of therapy (McFarland and Moore, 1982).

Over the years, elements of learning theories have been applied to the development of the disorder. Among those most often applied are Brutten and Shoemaker's (1967) two-factor learning theory and Sheehan's (1968) approach-avoidance theory. In Brutten and Shoemaker's explanation, the intra-phonemic disruptions of stuttering are influenced and precipitated by classically conditioned negative emotion. In learning to cope with the threat and experience of stuttering, 'helping' or avoiding behaviours which are instrumentally conditioned by reinforcing consequences are used. Thus the secondary behaviours, such as severe blocking and limb movements accompanying stuttering, are learned because they seem to relieve, even temporarily, the core stuttering behaviour. These coping behaviours become part of the stuttering symptomatology.

The approach-avoidance theory centres on the conflict experienced by the speaker when he wants to speak but fears speaking (because of stuttering) and also, he wants to remain silent but fears silence (because of its undesirable consequences, i.e. failure to communicate). The resolving of the conflict lies in one urge becoming stronger than the other and, as the unpleasantness associated with the conflict is reduced, the behaviour ensuing – either stuttering or avoidance – is reinforced. According to Sheehan, the conflict is not only related to speech and speech situations but to the social presentation of the self. So stuttering is more likely when the speaker feels low in self-esteem or when he is in awe of his listener or where he perceives the threat of penalty for stuttering. In this theory, stuttering is self-reinforcing as anxiety levels drop when the stuttering occurs.

Stuttering may also be explained in terms of its own meaning and the functions that it serves. Hayhow and Levy (1989) provide clear demonstrations of the stuttering acquiring a meaning important for the child which is different to the speech disruption itself. In later years, stuttering may take over some social functions, for example, that of identity. It may also serve to rationalize behaviour for adults, e.g. fear of growing up, acting as adult, pursuing particular jobs, etc.

Acquired stuttering in adults

Acquired stuttering, or disfluency reminiscent of stuttering, may follow injury to the central nervous system. It is not considered a unitary disorder, 'anymore than aphasia is a unitary disorder' (Helm-Estabrooks, 1986: 193). Canter (1971) identified three types which he designated as dysarthric, dyspraxic and dysnomic, providing subtypes of dysarthric stuttering. The problem of defining neurogenic stuttering is discussed by Rosenbek (1985), who differentiates it from the disfluencies that occur with any speech-language disorder, stressing the 'involuntary repetition primarily of the correct sounds and syllables any place in a word' (p. 46). Lebrun and his colleagues also describe stuttering as a forerunner of motor-neuron disease (Lebrun, Retif and Kaiser, 1983), following a missile wound (Lebrun, Bijleveld and Rousseau, 1990), and following vascular brain damage without accompanying dysphasic symptoms (Bijleveld et al., 1994). They conclude that for the adult, the symptomologies of acquired and developmental stuttering may closely resemble each other. Despite having different possible aetiologies, approaches to the treatment of acquired and developmental stuttering are strikingly similar (e.g. Market et al., 1990).

Assessment Considerations

Traditionally, speech and language therapists have considered assessment as a dynamic process, often inextricably linked with therapy. Assessment procedures involve the collection of as much relevant information as is necessary to describe and delimit the presenting problem and arrive at a decision regarding therapy. The adult who stutters will be directly involved in the identification and analysis of his stuttering and fluency, although some objective measures of stuttering should also be used (Edwards and Hardcastle, 1987). Ingham and Costello (1984) suggest that there should be at least four once-weekly within- and beyond-clinic assessments of stuttering over the base-rate period, with the rationale of evaluating treatment outcome and terminating therapy. While this may seem time consuming, there is reason to doubt the representativeness of severity ratings estimated from the initial sessions, as clients tend to seek therapy when they are particularly dysfluent (Van Riper, 1982). Whether samples of stuttering are typical may be checked by asking the client directly at intervals during assessment.

Measures of stuttering severity

Minimal requirements for estimating severity of stuttering include sampling speech under different conditions, estimating the frequency of stuttering and rate of speaking, and describing the tension and struggle associated with speaking. Observing extraneous movements during speaking may be included in estimates of struggle. Because of the variability of stuttering, many authors suggest that speech should be sampled in different modes and under different conditions (Ingham and Costello, 1984; Riley, 1982) and if possible using a video recorder. The Stuttering Severity Instrument (Riley, 1982) uses reading and monologue as the base measures, together with a system for estimating tension and degree of struggle and is a most useful assessment instrument.

Exploration as opposed to assessment

Since stuttering is variable in frequency and intensity by nature, usual measurement procedures may not adequately address the implications of the stutter for the client. Exploratory procedures that open up the possibility of discussing the impact of stuttering may for many be more appropriate for some clients. For this reason we use the character sketch (Kelly, 1955; Hayhow and Levy, 1989) and a range of repertory grid techniques (Fransella and Bannister, 1977).

Repertory grids as assessment procedures

The repertory grid was devised as a means of analysing relationships and inter-relationships among constructs and elements in applying Kelly's

(1955) personal construct theory. They have been used successfully in facilitating a delineation of the issues likely to be concentrated on in therapy and as a means of evaluating changes that occur during therapy (Evesham and Fransella, 1985; Leahy and O'Sullivan, 1987), and they are useful for introducing the notion of reconstruction and the possible implications of change for an individual client. Issues highlighted by using grids may be less easily articulated by other means, and points of similarity between members of a group provide an immediate focus for discussion. The role relationship grid and the situations grid (Fransella and Bannister, 1977) allow for development of insight into construing of important roles people play in situations. The use of grids obviates the need to assess attitudes to situations and communication as the construing of events subsumes the notion of attitude and provides immediate data to help in understanding the variation of fluency and stuttering.

Motivation and 'resistance'

Many adults who present for therapy will have attended therapy already and may have experience of failure, as maintaining the gains from therapy may prove too difficult over time. Previously, it was suggested that motivation of both the client and therapist be monitored regularly (Leahy, 1989), but it is questionable whether monitoring motivation *per se* is in effect a prerequisite for successful therapy. Levels of interest and involvement in therapy may fluctuate for both therapist and client, but, if they are continuing to co-operate in the process that is therapy, motivation or desire for *some changes* may be assumed. Both have a vested common interest: both seek to understand better the means of changing the stuttering, and beyond stuttering, changing social presentation and maintaining desired changes for the client. Instead of assuming low motivation or 'secondary gains' from stuttering (considering aspects of stuttering to be rewarding) as the reason for fluctuating levels of co-operation and involvement in therapy, it may be more meaningful to reflect on other factors, e.g. limited understanding of the tasks proposed or the usefulness of such tasks. Changing circumstances either at home or at work may take precedence over assignments undertaken and perhaps over fluency therapy, but the client may be reluctant to opt out of the process entirely. It may be more pertinent to consider threats associated with change and the possible advantages associated with remaining the same (Hayhow and Levy, 1989; Leahy and O'Sullivan, 1987; Leahy and Collins, 1991). Limited involvement in fluency therapy may indicate that stuttering is not the primary problem but perhaps secondary to feelings associated with social situations or relationships. Alternatively, losing an important aspect of self-identity may be too much of a threat to consider and it may emerge that retaining the stutter is preferable to such loss. Such issues are particularly relevant in exploring reasons for relapse after therapy.

Areas directly and indirectly associated with stuttering

Social skills and non-verbal behaviour are integral to successful communication and there has long been an emphasis in the stuttering literature
on specific aspects of these skills, most notably of eye contact and avoidance behaviours. The area of social skills in the broader context of
communication effectiveness has received attention in assessment and
therapy (Levy, 1983). Indications that some people who stutter differ
from non-stuttering counterparts in expression of affect and in the use
of non-verbal behaviours when speaking and when listening (Krause,
1980; 1982) have justified the focus on this area. Rustin and Kuhr (1989)
present useful procedures for addressing such problems.

Avoidance behaviours may be assessed using questionnaires based on
'the Johnson questionnaire' (Johnson, Darley and Spriestersbach, 1963)
and we have also found it useful to assess assertive behaviour with some
clients as it may be directly influenced by avoidance (see schedules
presented by Rathus, 1973, and by Trower, Bryant and Argyle, 1978).

Attitudes

Controversy about focusing on attitudes in stuttering therapy reflects
the unsatisfactory state of attitude assessment (Hayhow, 1983; Ulliana
and Ingham, 1984) as well as the basic controversy about attitude
change and its role in stuttering therapy (Gregory, 1979). The attitude
scale most widely used in stuttering clinics and in research in stuttering
is the S24 (Andrews and Cutler, 1974) or its amended version, the AS24
(Ulliana and Ingham, 1984). In testing the AS24, these authors found
that people who stutter regarded their responses to the scale items as
largely influenced by their judgements about their stuttering and speech
behaviour, and that stuttering frequency was consistently higher in situations associated with item responses implying negative attitudes. Such
findings indicate the need to consider the implications of stuttering
which may be achieved by asking pertinent questions, or with the use of
repertory grids and structured conversations, as described by Hayhow
and Levy (1989).

Theoretical Basis of Intervention

In many therapy approaches, learning and unlearning have played major
roles in therapy for stuttering, regardless of the school of thought
followed about origins of the disorder or the principle approach to therapy. For example, the identification process involves learning, whilst the
use of fluency techniques using slowed speech, DAF procedures or
cancellation, pull-out and preparatory set involve learning, as do the
transfer and generalization phases of therapy. Therapies that derive from

an understanding of stuttering as an operant behaviour provide the theoretical basis for systematic conditioning in stuttering therapy.

Fluency-shaping therapies: underlying principles

The objective of the fluency-shaping therapies is the reduction in frequency, and finally the elimination, of stuttering without direct focus on negative attitudes, feelings or perceptions. Fluency change is brought about mainly by manipulating the consequences of various behaviours in stuttering. Fluency behaviours are reinforced and stuttering behaviours punished and, in some instances, a combination of both reinforcement and punishment has been used (Webster, 1979; Howie, Tanner and Andrews, 1981). Although it is acknowledged that some change in attitude is desirable for change in fluency to be maintained, there is evidence to suggest that attitudes will change as a result of increased fluency (Webster, 1979). The underlying principles of operant conditioning are deftly illustrated by Costello and Ingham (1985: 188), showing possible response contingent arrangements of stimuli that identify operant behaviours and how the frequency of behaviours may be increased or decreased. (More detailed descriptions are provided by Costello, 1982; Shames and Florance, 1986.)

Stuttering modification therapies: underlying principles

The objective of the stuttering modification therapies is change in the form of stuttering with accompanying change in feelings, attitudes and perceptions. This entails direct focus on stuttering with the aim of producing 'fluent stuttering' (Van Riper, 1982) as opposed to fluent speech. But the focus on the person who stutters is no less important than the speech process itself, as adjustment to stuttering, albeit in a more controlled and fluent form, is seen as a major goal in therapy. This adjustment to stuttering has been criticized for producing 'happy stutterers', as some levels of stuttering behaviour are considered acceptable (Stromsta, 1986). However, the stated principle of those who support this approach is that by accepting stuttering, one is in a better position to confront it and to deal constructively with it, as tension and anxiety related to stuttering are reduced.

In other instances however, although learning is considered to be of great importance for changes to be maintained, it is not always the basic premise of therapy.

Mainstream Treatment Practices

Phases in intervention

Typically, intervention procedures for stuttering are described in a series of phases of therapy and this holds true whether the fundamental approach follows fluency shaping, stuttering modification therapies, or perhaps a combination of both. With the possible exception of some programmes based on operant principles, phases are not necessarily rigidly adhered to but they have a function in the organization and orientation of therapy.

Initial contact: interview and information exchange

The initial contact between client and therapist sets the scene for all that follows and is important for instilling in the client a sense of confidence and trust in the therapy process. At the early stages in therapy, it is incumbent on the therapist to be able and willing to provide information to the client as well as collect it. In this way the initial sessions function to exchange information and ideas and this serves to invite the active participation of the client. As well as collecting case history data, including a history of the development of the stuttering and a description of its current status, the therapist can present information regarding experience with stuttering (or lack thereof); various understandings of the problem of stuttering can be discussed and the cyclic nature of the disorder within and without therapy examined. Stromsta (1986) recommends that the complexity of speech and language acquisition be a topic during these early stages. He presents a model of speech production and focuses on the concept of fluent speech as continual movement and co-articulation using examples of sound spectography. Such focus represents for Stromsta the essential aspects of fluency that lead to the development of '... a practical definition of stuttering' (p. 120).

Assessment: identification, analysis and understanding

Assessment and exploratory considerations have already been discussed. It is important to reiterate the client's involvement in identifying and analysing his stuttering, which will be facilitated by knowledge of the speech process and the nature of fluency. Discriminating between core features of stuttering and associated reactive features is necessary, as it leads to a better understanding of the disorder for both parties involved. With the developing understanding, both of the nature of fluency and stuttering and of the nature of therapy, a contract may be drawn up that specifies, among other things, commitment to therapy (including follow-up) and an undertaking to share responsibility in therapy and to dedicate time and attention to change outside the clinic. Fluctuating fluency may also be specified to allow for strategies to be implemented when stuttering increases. Gregory (1987) refers to the initial reluctance of people who stutter to become involved in the analysis of stuttering, but its importance is recognized afterwards as a means of confronting the undesirable nature of stuttering.

Technique selection: trials and practice

Because of the individuality of each person who stutters, as well as the uniqueness of the stuttering presentation, selecting a technique is largely an individual matter. In constructivist terms, technique is considered as part of the experimental process for trying out alternative ways of behaving in order to find one that fits best. Costello and Ingham (1985) recommend the use of probes to help in selecting a technique. Ryan (1986) proposes that a Delayed Auditory Feedback (DAF) programme be used with older clients or those whose stuttering is more severe, and that the Gradual Increase in Length and Complexity of Utterance (GILCU) programme is more suited to younger clients or those whose stuttering is less severe. Composite techniques such as prolonged speech and slowed speech help regulate breathing, pausing, articulatory contact and continuity or co-articulation and allow for the client to develop aspects of the technique that he finds most helpful. Others, such as airflow or easy onset techniques, focus largely on one aspect of behaviour and the development and regulation of that behaviour to reduce dysfluency. The Van Riperian concepts of preparatory set, pullout and cancellation with the emphasis on the stuttering moment and what happens before and after it, can be implemented into a programme of therapy to supplement the primary technique being used. Although the therapist acts as model, teacher, and initially chief monitor of the client's performance, it is the responsibility of the client not only to become proficient in the use of a particular technique but also to learn to evaluate it.

Speech technique (or any different way of speaking, e.g. accent change) carries with it implications for overall presentation of the self that may be threatening for some clients. For example, the person who stutters may feel the imminent loss of an important part of his identity by becoming fluent (or *Kellian guilt*, the 'dislodgement of the self from one's core role structure' Hayhow and Levy, 1989: 45) and for some, that loss may be too much to bear over time. However, by considering alternative, desirable ways of construing the self one can become more comfortable with the process of change. Hayhow and Levy (1989) provide interesting data about conditions that lead to change and some that may obstruct change.

Technique may be considered initially in terms of experimentation, trying out a new way of speaking and checking on the responses received. This may begin within the clinic as the client begins to learn the technique. It is then advanced by changing the composition and size of the audience (speaking with receptionist, within a group, on the telephone) and tried out in some 'safe' situations outside the clinic. Elaborating on the effects of the new way of speaking in terms of expectations and results of trials will help to ease the transition from speaking in the 'old' way (stuttering), to speaking in the more fluent but unfamiliar way (with technique).

Transfer schedules for outside the clinic may be drawn up either from avoidance reports or speaking logs, but in the early stages, situations that are construed as non-threatening, e.g. speaking with selected friends or family, will help the process. As therapy progresses, role play of other more difficult situations outside the clinic can be done in groups and video recorded. Transfer programmes generally exploit behavioural principles to some degree in establishing fluency outside the clinic, but they may also be based on principles of change as specified in constructivist theory. Recognizing the implications of change and dealing with obstacles to successful transfer may need to be a continuing focus of attention. It is often appropriate to consider aspects of relationship and situational concerns that arise for the client through the use of exploratory procedures already discussed. Structured conversations using laddering and pyramiding derived from constructivist ideas, may be useful for looking at the implications of certain constructs (Hayhow and Levy, 1989). Alternative or new ways of behaving can be elaborated and experimented with in role play. The broad spectrum of communication and more effective use of non-verbal skills, including listening skills, are likely to be meaningful as fluency develops and the interaction process no longer centres around the stutter. Self-regulation of fluency with occasional monitoring by the therapist becomes the order of the day during this phase.

Maintenance and preventing relapse

The final phase of therapy is arguably the most important phase as it represents the ultimate goal of fluency therapy: maintenance and development of newly acquired skills and attitudes. Despite this, it is one of the least well researched areas in the literature. Boberg, Howie and Woods (1986: 496) provide a brief overview of four categories of procedures used during this phase. These are:

- regular clinical contact following treatment;
- emphasis on client self-responsibility;
- emphasis on the need for changes in attitudes to speech, self-concept, etc.; and
- intensive 'refresher programmes' or recycling through the initial programme.

Whatever the procedure chosen, a major point of attention is the client's ability to recognize and deal with fluctuations in fluency. Strengthening the fluency and fluency-enhancing behaviours is an important commitment for the client, for as Sheehan (1984: 93) cautions: 'All the stutterer has to do to relapse is to rest on his oars'. Possible reasons for poor practice include the notion of its punishing effect for the client whose fluency has improved dramatically with therapy (Boberg, Howie and Woods, 1979). Spontaneity is lost because of the careful monitoring that is necessary, and feelings of self-acceptance may be reduced. The inherent abnormality of a technique requiring practice may be rejected and the rewards of practice are delayed and not always obvious to the client who is fluent most of the time anyway. Genetic influences may also increase the risk of relapse.

Facing up to failure and admitting defeat is not easy for either client or therapist and relapse may represent failure for both parties. Understanding probable reasons for relapse, however, may be as important as understanding why therapy succeeds and exploration of the implications of change as already described may be of crucial importance.

Kuhr and Rustin (1985) reported an in-patient programme for clients who had failed in 'multiple treatments' and indicated that along with 'booster sessions' with the therapist, help from the social environment of the client, i.e. spouse and friends, was important. The depressing effect of fluency on some participants was also noted as a factor that may influence relapse.

Effectiveness of Therapy

There is no doubt that therapy for stuttering can produce long-term, positive effects with time spent in therapy the single best predictor of outcome (Andrews, Guitar and Howie, 1980; Bloodstein, 1981) but as indicated, neither is there any doubt that degrees of relapse occur for many. In reviewing therapy effects, Andrews et al., (1983) conclude that only the prolonged speech (Perkins 1973, Perkins et al., 1974) and precision fluency shaping (Webster, 1979) strategies have reported sufficient follow-up data on clients to allow claims of success to be made and evaluated. Attitude therapy alone was considered unlikely to be of benefit (Van Riper, 1982; Andrews et al., 1983) and airflow therapy alone, taught over a short term, is also unlikely to have long-term positive effect (Andrews and Tanner, 1982). Nevertheless substantial gains can be made in therapy: the client who receives therapy is more normal speaking than 90 per cent of untreated clients (Andrews et al., 1980). Evaluating effectiveness of therapy was a major theme at the First International Fluency Association Congress in 1994 (proceedings in press) and the specification of factors that affect outcome measures of therapy for stuttering are more clearly defined. Successful outcome of therapy cannot depend on any single phenomenon, but the influence of the therapist will almost always be a major factor.

Although stuttering is probably one of the most researched areas in speech pathology and recent research has greatly improved our understanding of the disorder, there are still unresolved issues and areas of uncertainty which invite and demand further research. It is evident that, although there are divergent opinions about the nature of the disorder and consequently the nature of therapy, every clinician shares the goal of reducing stuttering, increasing fluency and increasing communicative effectiveness.

Working with people who stutter is demanding, inspiring, dynamic, exciting and rewarding; it draws on a wide range of expertise from both therapist and client who work together in a kind of a partnership towards the achievement of an acceptable and controllable level of fluency and communicative effectiveness. The processes of stuttering, and most importantly of working with people who stutter, are better known and understood now than ever before. We have many reasons to be optimistic about future developments in the area of adult stuttering.

References

Andrews G, Craig A, Feyer AM, Hoddinott S, Howie P, Neilson M (1983) Stuttering: a review of research findings and theories c. 1982. Journal of Speech and Hearing Disorders 48: 226–46.

Andrews G, Cutler J (1974) Stuttering therapy: the relation between changes in symptom level and attitudes. Journal of Speech and Hearing Disorders 39: 312–19.

Andrews G, Guitar B, Howie P (1980) Meta-analysis of the effects of stuttering treatment. Journal of Speech and Hearing Disorders 45: 287–307.

Andrews G, Tanner S (1982) Stuttering treatment: replication of the regulated breathing method. Journal of Speech and Hearing Disorders 47: 138–40.

Bijleveld H, Lebrun Y, van Dongen H (1994) A Case of Acquired Stuttering. Folia Phoniatrica et Logopaedica 46.5.94: 250–3.

Bloodstein O (1981) A Handbook of Stuttering (3rd ed). Chicago: National Easter Seal Society.

Boberg E, Howie P, Woods L (1986) Maintenance of fluency: a review. In Shames GH, Rubin H (Eds) Stuttering Then and Now. Columbus, OH: Merrill.

Brutten EJ, Shoemaker DJ (1967) The Modification of Stuttering, Englewood Cliffs, NJ: Prentice Hall.

Canter GJ (1971) Observations on neurogenic stuttering: A contribution to differential diagnosis. British Journal of Disorders of Communication 6: 139–43.

Cooper EB (1993) Red herrings, dead horses, straw men and blind alleys. Journal of Fluency Disorders 18: 275–387.

Costello JM (1982) Techniques of therapy based on operant theory, in Perkins WH (Ed) Current Therapy of Communicative Disorders. New York: Decker.

Costello JM, Ingham RJ (1985) Stuttering as an operant disorder. In Curlee RF, Perkins WH (Eds) Nature and Treatment of Stuttering: New Directions. San Diego, CA: College Hill.

Dalton P, Hardcastle W (1989) Disorders of Fluency and Their Effects on Communication (2nd ed). London: Edward Arnold.

Edwards S, Hardcastle W (1987) Linguistic profiling of stuttering behaviour. In Rustin L, Purser H, Rowley D (Eds) Progress in the Treatment of Fluency Disorders. London: Taylor and Francis.

Evesham M, Fransella F (1985) Stuttering relapse: the effect of a combined speech and psychological reconstruction programme. British Journal of Disorders of Communication 20: 237–48.

Fransella F, Bannister D (1977) A Manual for Repertory Grid Technique. New York: Academic Press.

Gregory H (1979) Controversial issues: Statement and review of the literature in Gregory H (Ed) Controversies about Stuttering Therapy. Baltimore: University Park Press.

Gregory H (1987) Handling relapse. Paper presented at Clinical Management of Chronic Stuttering Conference, Washington DC.

Hayhow R (1983) The assessment of stuttering and the evaluation of treatment. In Dalton P (Ed) Approaches to the Treatment of Stuttering. Beckenham, Kent: Croom Helm.

Hayhow R, Levy, C (1989) Working with Stuttering. Bicester, Oxon: Winslow Press.

Helm-Estabrooks N (1986) Diagnosis management of neurogenic stuttering in adults. In St Louis KO (Ed) The Atypical Stutterer. Orlando, FL: Academic Press.

Howie, P, Tanner S, Andrews G (1981) Short- and long-term outcome in an intensive treatment program for adult stutterers. Journal of Speech and Hearing Disorders 46: 104–9.

Ingham R, Costello J (1984) Stuttering treatment outcome evaluation. In Costello J (Ed) Speech Disorders in Adults. San Diego, CA: College Hill.

Johnson W, Darley F, Spriestersbach DC (1963) Diagnostic Methods in Speech Pathology. New York: Harper Row.

Kelly G (1955) The Psychology of Personal Constructs, Vols. 1 and 2. New York: Norton.

Kidd K (1985) Stuttering as a genetic disorder. In Curlee RF, Perkins WH (Eds) The Nature and Treatment of Stuttering, New Directions. San Diego, CA: College Hill.

Krause R (1980) Stuttering and nonverbal communications: investigations about affect inhibition and stuttering. In Giles H, Robinson WP, Smith PM (Eds) Language: Social Psychological Perspectives. Oxford: Pergamon.

Krause R (1982) A social psychological approach to the study of stuttering. In Fraser C, Sherer KR (Eds) Advances in the Social Psychology of Language. Cambridge: Cambridge University Press.

Kuhr A, Rustin L (1985) The maintenance of fluency after intensive in-patient therapy: long-term follow up. Journal of Fluency Disorders 19: 229–36.

Leahy MM (1989) Adult stuttering. In Leahy MM (Ed) Disorders of Communication: the Science of Intervention (1st ed). London: Whurr.

Leahy MM, Collins G (1991) Therapy for stuttering: experimenting with experimenting. Irish Journal of Psychological Medicine 8:37–9.

Leahy MM, O'Sullivan B (1987) Psychological change and fluency therapy: a pilot project. British Journal of Communication Disorders 22: 245–51.

Lebrun Y, Bijleveld H, Rousseau, J-J (1990) A case of persistent stuttering following a missile wound. Journal of Fluency Disorders 15: 251–8.

Lebrun Y, Retif J, Kaiser G (1983) Acquired stuttering as a forerunner of motor-neuron disease. Journal of Fluency Disorders 8(2): 161–7.

Levy C (1983) Group therapy with adults. In Dalton P (Ed) Approaches to the Treatment of Stuttering. London: Croom Helm.

McFarland DH, Moore WH (1982) Alpha hemispheric asymmetries during an electromyographic biofeedback procedure for stuttering. Paper presented to the annual convention of the ASHA, Toronto.

Market KE, Montague JC, Buffalo MD, Drummond SS (1990) Acquired stuttering: descriptive data and treatment outcome. Journal of Fluency Disorders 15: 21–33.

Moore WH (1985) Central nervous system characteristics of stutterers. In Curlee RF, Perkins WH (Eds) Nature and Treatment of Stuttering: New Directions. San Diego, CA: College Hill.

Moore WH, Boberg E (1987) Hemispheric processing and stuttering. In Rustin L, Purser H, Rowley D (Eds) Progress in the Treatment of Fluency Disorders. London: Taylor and Francis.

Perkins WH (1973) Replacement of stuttering with normal speech: 1 rationale and 2 clinical procedures. Journal of Speech Hearing Disorders 37: 295–303.

Perkins WH, Kent RD, Curlee RF (1991) A theory of neuropsycholinguistic function in stuttering. Journal of Speech Hearing Research 34: 734–52.

Perkins WH, Rudas J, Johnson L, Michael WB, Curlee RF (1974) Replacement of stuttering with normal speech. III. Clinical Effectiveness. Journal of Speech Hearing Disorders 39: 416–29.

Rathus SA, (1973) A 30-item schedule for assessing assertive behaviour. Behaviour Therapy 4: 398–406.

Riley G (1982) The Stuttering Severity Instrument. Tigard, OR: C.C. Publications.

Rosenbek JC (1985) Stuttering secondary to nervous system damage. In Curlee RF, Perkins WH (Eds) Nature Treatment of Stuttering: New Directions. San Diego, CA: College Hill Press.

Rustin L, Kuhr A (1989) Social Skills and the Speech Impaired. London: Taylor and Francis.

Ryan B (1986) Operant therapy for children. In Shames GH, Rubin H, (Eds) Stuttering Then and Now. Columbus, OH: Merrill.

Shames GH, Florance CL (1986) Stutter-free speech: a goal for therapy. In Shames GH, Rubin H (Eds) Stuttering Then and Now. Columbus, OH: Chas C. Merrill.

Sheehan JD (1968) In Gregory H (Ed), Learning Theory and Stuttering. Evanston, IL: Northwestern University Press.

Sheehan JD (1984) Relapse and recovery from stuttering. In Stuttering Therapy: Transfer and Maintenance. Memphis, TN: Speech foundation of America. Publication No . 19.

Starkweather CW (1987) Fluency and Stuttering. Englewood Cliffs, NJ: Prentice Hall.

Stewart T, Grantham C (1993) A case of acquired stammering: the pattern of recovery. European Journal of Communication 28(4): 395–403.

Stromsta C (1986) Elements of Stuttering. Oshtemo, MI: Atsmorts, Publishing.

Trower P, Bryant B, Argyle M (1978) Social Skills and Mental Health. London: Methuen.

Ulliana L, Ingham R (1984) Behavioral and nonbehavioral variables in the measurement of stutterers' communication attitudes. Journal of Speech and Hearing Disorders 49: 83–93.

Van Riper C (1982) The Nature of Stuttering. Englewood Cliffs, NJ: Prentice-Hall.

Van Riper C (1984) The Treatment of Stuttering. Englewood Cliffs, NJ: Prentice-Hall.

Webster RL (1979) Empirical considerations regarding stuttering therapy. In Gregory HH (Ed) Controversies about Stuttering Therapy. Baltimore: University Park Press.

Chapter 16
Surgical Rehabilitation of Adults

JERI A. LOGEMANN

Rehabilitation of the patient with head and neck cancer begins with treatment selection. In laryngeal cancer, radiation therapy or conservation (partial) laryngectomy may cure the cancer while maintaining voice and better function for swallowing than total laryngectomy (DeSanto, 1974; Fletcher and Goepfert, 1981). Patients with smaller lesions of the larynx (that is T1 and T2 lesions) are generally treated with radiotherapy for cure. These patients may exhibit some vocal changes after radiotherapy, but are able to maintain a normal airway and normal swallowing. Voice changes after radiotherapy have been described as mild. Only a few studies, however, have quantified these voice changes (Stoicheff, 1975; Karim et al., 1983; Stoicheff et al., 1983).

Recently, patients with T3 and T4 lesions of the larynx are being treated with organ preservation protocols, i.e. high-dose radiotherapy (6000 to 7000 rads in place of surgery). Cure rates are under study since these treatment protocols have only been used for the last several years. In some facilities patients with the large lesions (T3 + T4) still receive total laryngectomy (Stell and Maran, 1978: Suen and Myers, 1981).

Radio Therapy

Radio therapy to the larynx usually also involves a portion of the pharynx and creates a number of permanent changes, particularly increasing fibrosis involving the pharyngeal constrictors and laryngeal elevators. These tissue changes often create significant swallowing disorders including reduced laryngeal elevation and reduced pharyngeal wall contraction with aspiration after the swallow (Lazarus, 1993). These swallowing problems respond well to swallowing therapy, particularly the super-supraglottic swallow technique, i.e. effortful breath hold (Logemann, 1993). Because the tissue changes after high dose radiation often worsen with time post treatment, these patients may need to use this swallowing therapy technique permanently.

Conservation Laryngectomy – Partial Laryngectomy

In the USA, some patients with T2 and occasionally T3 lesions of the larynx are treated with what is known as a 'conservation' laryngectomy (Goepfert, Lindberg and Jesse, 1981; Ogura and Mallen, 1965; Som, 1951). The term conservation indicates that function is preserved. The conservation laryngectomy procedures are also known as partial laryngectomies and fall into two categories: (1) the vertical or hemilaryngectomy and (2) the horizontal or supraglottic laryngectomy. The surgical procedures in both types of partial laryngectomy vary from patient to patient, depending upon the exact location of the tumour and its size. Thus, the speech and language clinician working with any of these patients on their voice or swallowing must always ask the surgeon to describe exactly what tissues were resected and exactly how the reconstruction was accomplished.

Hemilaryngectomy

Hemilaryngectomy involves removal of one vertical half of the larynx, generally *excluding* the epiglottis, the hyoid bone and the arytenoid cartilages. The hemilaryngectomy resection usually includes one true vocal fold, one ventricle, and one false vocal fold as well as the inner aspect of the thyroid lamina (Som, 1951) . Following this resection, the surgeon generally rotates soft tissue into the surgical defect in order to provide a pad of tissue against which the normal vocal fold may make contact during swallow and voice production. In general, the hemilaryngectomee has few difficulties swallowing, but does have significant changes in voice. Voice after hemilaryngectomy is usually hoarse to some degree, varying from mild to severe. There have been no acoustic studies of voice in hemilaryngectomized patients.

The hemilaryngectomy procedure can also be extended beyond what would be considered a 'narrow-field' hemilaryngectomy. The exact extent of the resection is always dictated by the tumour. Thus, if the tumour is located at the anterior commissure, the resection may be extended around the anterior commissure and well into the opposite vocal fold. Or, if the tumour extends posteriorly to the vocal process of the arytenoid, the resection may include the arytenoid cartilage itself as well as the rest of the vocal fold. In general, the larger the resection, the more severe the hoarseness which results and the longer it takes the patient to relearn to swallow (Ardran and Kemp, 1951, 1967; Aguilar, Olson and Shedd, 1979). The swallowing problems of the hemilaryngectomee involve reduced laryngeal closure. This problem can usually be managed with postural compensations: turning the patient's head to the operated side (which improves airway closure) and by tilting the head forward (which puts the epiglottis in a more overhanging position to protect the airway and narrows the airway entrance (Welch et al., 1993). On average, the hemilaryngectomy patient returns to normal diet in 3 weeks (Rademaker et al., 1993).

Supraglottic Laryngectomy

The supraglottic or horizontal partial laryngectomy involves removal of the epiglottis and aryepiglottic folds, the false vocal folds, and the hyoid bone (Ogura and Mallen, 1965). Removal of the hyoid destroys the foundation of the tongue and the suspension of the larynx. Thus, in the reconstruction procedure, the remainder of the larynx is usually elevated and sutured under the base of the tongue (Calcaterra, 1971). This laryngeal re-elevation is designed to reconstruct the protection for the airway that is provided by the tongue base as it moves posteriorly and the larynx as it elevates under the tongue during the swallow. After a supraglottic laryngectomy, all patients must relearn to swallow by what is known as the 'super supraglottic swallow technique' (Logemann, 1993). In this procedure, patients are taught to hold their breath and bear down at the height of their inhalation, to continue to hold their breath while they swallow, and to follow the swallow with a cough on the exhalation. This technique is designed to close the entrance of the airway, i.e. between the arytenoid cartilage and the base of the tongue, and to expectorate any residue which remains on the vocal folds or around the arytenoids after the swallow. The super supraglottic swallow is an extension of the supraglottic swallow, which closes the airway at the level of the true vocal folds. In a supraglottic laryngectomy, if the airway entrance is not closed, food will enter the airway to the level of the closed vocal folds and be aspirated after the swallow when the patient opens the vocal folds to breathe (Logemann et al., 1995).

Though some patients return to normal eating within several weeks after supraglottic laryngectomy (Logemann, et al., 1995), the average time to return to normal diet for non-extended supraglottics is 4 to 6 weeks.

If the supraglottic laryngectomy resection is extended into the tongue base, or into the arytenoid cartilage, the patient's chances of relearning to swallow are significantly reduced (Rademaker et al., 1993). If a larger amount of tongue base is removed, very often food runs directly off the tongue base and into the airway. If a portion of the arytenoid cartilage is removed, the last sphincter to protect the airway is damaged and the patient must attempt to compensate for this resection by tremendously increased muscle effort. Though the exact extent of resection which results in functional versus non-functional swallowing has not been determined, it is clear that when the arytenoid cartilage and/or tongue base is included in the resection, the chance of the patient relearning to swallow is reduced by at least 50 per cent. Voice quality is also severely impaired.

In theory, the supraglottic laryngectomee should not have a voice problem, since the true vocal folds and arytenoids are left intact. Unfortunately, however, many supraglottic laryngectomees do exhibit some degree of hoarseness, probably related to oedema, to some degree of stiffness in the arytenoid after removal of the surrounding aryepiglottic folds and to possible damage of the superior laryngeal nerve. There are no acoustic studies of voice production after supraglottic laryngectomy.

Clinical Care of the Patient who Receives Radiotherapy or Partial Laryngectomy

Pretreatment counselling regarding effects of radiotherapy or surgery on voice and swallowing should be provided, including the need for speech and swallowing therapy after treatment. After treatment, a radiographic study of the patients' swallowing should be completed, including assessment of the effects of treatment procedures, as needed (Logemann, 1993). Follow up therapy sessions (usually weekly) should be provided until the patient returns to a normal diet.

Total Laryngectomy

Patients with very large laryngeal tumours (T3 or T4), or whose laryngeal cancer recurs after treatment with radiotherapy, generally require total laryngectomy (Harrison, 1972; Stell and Maran, 1978; Suen and Myers, 1981). Total laryngectomy resection includes the hyoid bone, the entire larynx and some portion of the pharynx, and trachea. The exact extent of resection depends on the exact size and location of the tumour. Removal of the hyoid bone eliminates the foundation for the tongue, leaving the patient with slight changes in tongue function. After the entire larynx is removed, the tracheal stump is bent forward to the base of the neck, where a stoma or external hole is created with the tracheal stump sutured to the skin. In reconstruction of the pharyngo-oesophagus in the total laryngectomee, there is generally no attempt made to match fibres of the same muscle in the pharyngo-oesophagus. Once the larynx has been removed with whatever portion of the pharynx is necessary to eradicate the tumour, the remaining pharyngeal and oesophageal tissues are pulled together from each side and sutured. After studying four types of surgical reconstructions of the cricopharyngeal region, Simpson, Smith and Gordon (1972) concluded that re-approximating the cut ends of the pharyngo-oesophageal mucosa was highly correlated with proficiency of oesophageal speech. In many of their patients, the hyoid bone was preserved, unlike most total laryngectomies in the USA, in whom the hyoid bone is taken. It is reasonable to assume that such careful reconstruction might facilitate oesophageal voice learning.

Because the extent of the resection in total laryngectomees varies from patient to patient and there is often no systematic reconstruction of pharyngeal or oesophageal musculature after total laryngectomy, there is wide variability in the location, size and shape of the pseudo-glottis, as demonstrated very clearly by Diedrich and Youngstrom's (1977) work. Their radiographic studies illustrate the variety of heights and configurations of the pseudo-glottis in a large number of total laryngectomies. The exact muscular composition of the pseudo-glottis is not understood. Though the pseudo-glottis is often called the 'pe segment' or 'pharyngo-(o)esophageal segment', there is no clear evidence that the pseudo-glottis is the cricopharyngeus muscle. After total laryngectomy, the pharynx and oesophagus form one continuous soft tissue tube. There is no longer any delineation of the end of the pharynx and the top of the cervical oesophagus. Somewhere along the pharyngo-oesophagus there is usually some flaccid tissue which is adiposed. This tissue comprises the pseudo-glottis, usually capable of vibrating in response to air flowing through it.

Vocal Rehabilitation in Total Laryngectomees

Separation of the airway from the pharyngo-oesophagus leaves no possibility that the patient will aspirate during eating unless a fistula develops in the suture line. Unfortunately, this separation also precludes the patient from driving pulmonary air through the pseudo-glottis in the pharyngo-oesophagus to create a vibrating air stream for speech.

Historically, vocal rehabilitation of the total laryngectomee began soon after the first laryngectomy was completed in 1876. The first attempts to restore voice to the total laryngectomee fell into four categories:

1. artificial larynges;
2. oesophageal voice;
3. surgical restoration methods involving the production of a tunnel or hole connecting the stoma with the oesophagus in order to allow pulmonary air into the pharyngo-oesophagus; and
4. surgical prosthetic methods to bring air from the stoma through a prosthesis and into a fistula in the patient's oesophagus below the pseudo-glottis.

Methods currently in use to rehabilitate laryngectomies still fall into three of these four categories.

Artificial larynges

Artificial larynges provide the patient with an external vibratory (voice) source which is battery driven or pneumatic and is either held to the neck, as in cervical instruments, or introduced into the mouth, as in oral instruments (LeBrun, 1973; Salmon and Goldstein, 1978). Over the years, artificial larynges have improved in design and in vocal quality. Their overall effectiveness, however, is still hampered by their generally mechanical vocal quality, visibility, and the need to use at least one hand to hold the instrument.

Oesophageal voice

Oesophageal voice requires that the patient learn to put air into the pharyngo-oesophagus voluntarily, trap it immediately below the pseudo-glottis and release the air back through the pseudo-glottis to produce voice. Two methods of air intake have been utilized: inhalation and injection (Damste, 1958; Edels, 1983). With the inhalation method of air intake, the patient rapidly expands his thoracic cavity, which drops the intra-thoracic pressure below atmospheric pressure. As the intra-thoracic pressure drops, so does the pressure in the oesophagus. Pressure above the segment (atmospheric pressure) is higher than intra-oesophageal pressure. This causes a suction effect that results in the patient's pulling air into the oesophagus if the pressure in the segment or pseudo-glottis also drops below atmospheric pressure, i.e. if the segment relaxes.

With any of the 'injection' techniques, pre-injection or consonant injection, the patient must increase pressure above the pseudo-glottis sufficiently to overcome the pressure in the pseudo-glottis and, thereby, drive air into the oesophagus. With consonant injection, the patient builds supra-segment pressure during articulation of speech sounds which are characterized by high intra-oral pressures (stops, affricates and fricatives). As the patient articulates these sounds, the intra-oral pressure increases, pushing air into the oesophagus. This air is then released to produce voice. During pre-injection techniques, the patient produces an oral gesture *prior* to speech which compresses air, increases pressure in the oropharynx and pushes air through the pseudo-glottis and into the oesophagus. These pre-speech oral gestures may include compressing the tongue to the palate, closing the lips tightly or pulling the tongue base up and back.

As discussed earlier, there is a large amount of inter-patient variability in the anatomy of the pharynx and the oesophagus after total laryngectomy. Most patients are able to introduce air into the cervical oesophagus through one of these air intake techniques, but not necessarily through all of them. The speech-language pathologist must identify which air intake technique best facilitates a particular patient's introduction of air into the oesophagus for oesophageal voice. As patients become proficient at oesophageal speech, they often use a combination of air intake procedures.

Once air has been put into the oesophagus, the patient must release the air through the pseudo-glottis in the cervical oesophagus to produce voice. This release of oesophageal air is usually, but not always, concurrent with a pulmonary exhalation (Snidecor and Isshiki, 1965; Isshiki and Snidecor, 1965). The pulmonary exhalation exerts pressure on the oesophagus and pushes air upward through the pseudo-glottis, usually creating voice. In general, in the teaching of the act of oesophageal voice, the patient first learns to put air into the cervical oesophagus and then to release that air. With the air release will come sound, if a pseudo-glottis is present. The requirement for a pseudo-glottis is that tissue in the pharyngo-oesophagus must be flaccid enough and adiposed in order to respond to the airflow with vibration, thus creating sound. Occasionally, some laryngectomees, particularly those who have had a large resection, such as cervical oesophagectomy in addition to total laryngectomy, do not have a pseudo-glottis. That is, they do not have sufficient tissue, or tissue which is flaccid enough, to vibrate in response to the air stream. In these cases, digital pressure can be applied to the anterior neck in order to create a temporary pseudo-glottis (Damste, 1958; Duguay, 1979; Shanks, 1983). In some cases, the pseudo-glottis can be created by applying external pressure with a tight collar or elastic band.

Surgical and Surgical Prosthetic Voice Restoration

Because oesophageal voice requires learning and extensive therapy, and does not result in excellent speech in many patients, there have been both surgical and surgical prosthetic attempts to restore voice to the total laryngectomee. Currently, the most successful voice restoration technique, the tracheo-(o)esophageal puncture (TEP), falls into the surgical prosthetic category

Surgical voice restoration

Almost as soon as the total laryngectomy surgery was devised, various surgeons attempted surgical reconstruction for vocal rehabilitation. In all cases, the intent was surgically to create a tunnel or tract to re-introduce pulmonary air into the patient's cervical oesophagus below the level of the pseudo-glottis in order to allow pulmonary airflow to activate the pseudo-glottis and produce voice. To speak, the patient inhaled and covered the stoma with a finger to drive air through the surgically created tract into the oesophagus. The concept, then, was that the patient could drive the pseudo-glottis with pulmonary air and thus produce sustained voicing without having to learn the air intake and release techniques necessary for oesophageal voice. Surgical attempts to create a soft tissue tunnel between the stoma and the oesophagus have been fraught with numerous problems including: stenosis of the tract such that it would no longer conduct airflow; aspiration of liquid and food from the oesophagus to the trachea; surgical complications such as carotid blow-out; and failure to produce consistent voice (Asai, 1965; Conley, DeAmesti and Pierce, 1958; Griffiths and Love, 1978; Guttman, 1935; Komorn et al., 1973).

Other surgical reconstruction procedures have attempted to reconstruct a valve at the top of the tracheal stump. This valve or pseudo-larynx would have to prevent penetration of food into the airway, while shunting air into the pharyngo-oesophagus and serving as the vibratory source (Serafini, 1980; Staffieri, 1980). These surgical reconstructions suffered from the same serious problems as the other surgically created shunts.

Surgical prosthetic voice restoration

The first surgical prosthetic attempts to permit re-entry of air from the stoma into the oesophagus included construction of cutaneous fistulae into the pharynx or cervical oesophagus, which were fitted with prosthetic devices (Edwards, 1980; McConnel, Sisson and Logemann, 1976; Taub and Bugner, 1973). These devices attached from the patient's stoma to the external fistula and served as a conduit for airflow back into the pharyngo-oesophagus.

These surgical prosthetic attempts to construct a cutaneous fistula, to which an external prosthesis would be connected from the stoma, were fraught with problems including: (1) poor prosthetic fit so that the prosthesis dislodged at either the stomal end or the fistula end, (2) leakage of food through the fistula onto the external skin, and (3) aspiration of food through the fistula down the prosthesis and into the stoma. Prosthetic devices tended to have complicated connections and were often awkward in fitting, requiring the patient to change or exchange dressings at least several times per day.

Tracheo-(o)esophageal puncture (TEP) voice restoration

Surgical prosthetic voice restoration attempts culminated in 1980 with the introduction of the tracheo-oesophageal puncture technique (Singer and Blom, 1980), which is the most commonly and successfully used surgical voice restoration technique used today. In this technique, a small fistula tract is created from the posterior wall of the stoma to the oesophagus into which the patient places and wears a soft prosthesis containing a valve at the oesophageal end. This valve allows airflow from the stoma into the oesophagus, but prevents the backflow of food from the oesophagus to the stoma. To speak, the patient merely inhales and occludes the stoma with a finger or valve applied externally to the stoma to direct the exhaled air through the puncture prosthesis and into the oesophagus (Blom, Singer and Hamaker, 1982). Introduced by Mark Singer and Eric Blom (1980), this technique virtually revolutionized the surgical prosthetic voice rehabilitation of total laryngectomees. The puncture can be placed in a short operative procedure after laryngectomy or at the time of the total laryngectomy (i.e. primary puncture). If the patient dislikes the procedure, the puncture site will usually close spontaneously in 8–24 hours, when the prosthesis is removed. To create the puncture or fistula, an endoscope is introduced into the patient's oesophagus to the base of the cervical oesophagus. Another operator applies pressure to the posterior wall of the stoma at 12 o'clock. This pressure is visualized by the operator with the oesophagoscope. When the proper position for the puncture is identified, a hole is created with an No. 18 gauge needle. The tract or fistula is created horizontally or slightly downgoing . A No. 14 French catheter is then placed through the puncture and down into the stomach. This catheter usually remains in place for at least 48 hours, after which the patient can be fitted for the proper length puncture prosthesis.

Since the introduction of the tracheo-oesophageal puncture procedure, the surgical procedure to construct the fistula tract has been modified only slightly by some clinicians (Wolicki, Makielski and Olson, 1985). However, the prosthesis design has changed considerably. Initially, the prosthesis was a cylinder-shaped 'duck bill' prosthesis with a slit at the interior end (Singer and Blom, 1980; Singer, Blom and Hamaker, 1981). In the last few years, the prosthesis has been modified to a flap valve, which reduces the resistance of the prosthesis to the airflow from the stoma into the oesophagus (Weinberg and Moon, 1982; 1984; 1986a, b).

Since the introduction of the Singer–Blom tracheo-oesophageal puncture technique, other head and neck surgeons have designed variations on the procedure (Ossoff, Lazarus and Sisson, 1984; Perry, Cheesman and Eden, 1983; Shapiro and Ramanathan, 1982; Wood et al., 1981). Panje (1981) introduced a similar technique, in which the puncture wound was placed lower in the patient's stoma (just above the lower edge) and the prosthesis was shorter and biflanged to sit in the oesophageal wall. Examination of the resistance characteristics of the Panje prosthesis design indicated that the Panje prosthesis provided much higher resistance to the airflow than that of the Singer-Blom prosthesis and that the Panje prosthesis was highly variable in its quality control (Weinberg, 1982; Weinberg and Moon, 1982, 1984, 1986a; Moon and Weinberg, 1983, 1984; Smith, 1986).

The introduction of the tracheo-oesophageal puncture technique spawned a number of other foci of research. First, a number of investigators began to assess the acoustic and perceptual properties of the voice produced with tracheo-oesophageal puncture speech as compared to oesophageal voice and to normal voice (Baggs and Pine, 1983; Blood, 1984; Monaghan and Murray, 1986; Pauloski, 1987; Robbins, 1982, 1984; Robbins et al., 1984; Trudeau, 1986a, b). Table 16.1 provides a summary of data from this comparative research and earlier work on the acoustic characteristics of oesophageal voice.

These studies indicated that tracheo-oesophageal puncture voice was superior to oesophageal speech in duration and intensity parameters, as well as in intelligibility. These studies have also determined that the range of individual differences in TEP speakers is less than those in oesophageal speakers.

However, candidacy issues are important in all methods of alaryngeal communication. Many patients are unable to learn oesophageal voice because of such learning variables as motivation, ability to follow directions, memory, etc. Some patients are unable to comply with home practice programmes given to them for oesophageal voice, or are simply not compliant in attending therapy sessions. Some of these same patients would also be poor candidates for the puncture procedure. To be a good

Table 16.1 Comparative temporal, acoustic and intensity data on oesophageal and TEP talkers

Measures	Oesophageal Talkers	TEP Talkers
Reading rate	90–124.2 wpm[1]	127.4–144.1 wpm[2]
Fundamental frequency	58.4–87.9 Hz[3]	82.8–109.2 Hz[4]
Per cent periodic	41.6%–59.6%[5]	77.7%[6]
Per cent aperiodic	1.9%–25.0%[5]	11.9%[6]
Per cent silence	29.73%–38.5%[5]	10.5%[6]
Mean phonation time	1.9–4.82 s[8]	10.99–14 s[7]
Mean intensity during sustained vowel	73.8 dB SPL[6]	88.1 dB SPL[6]

[1] Snidecor and Curry (1959, 1960); Curry and Snidecor (1961); Snidecor and Isshiki (1965); Shipp (1967); Hoops and Noll (1969); Robbins et al. (1984).
[2] Robbins et al. (1984); Trudeau (1986a).
[3] Weinberg and Bennett (1972); Smith et al. (1978).
[4] Blood (1984); Robbins et al. (1984); Trudeau (1986).
[5] Curry and Snidecor (1961); Shipp (1967); Weinberg and Bennett (1972); Robbins et al. (1984).
[6] Robbins et al. (1984).
[7] Wetmore, Krueger and Wesson (1981); Baggs and Pine (1983); Robbins et al. (1984).
[8] Berlin (1963); Baggs and Pine (1983); Robbins et al. (1984).

candidate for the TEP procedure, patients need to be able to follow directions, to learn to change the prosthesis and to clean it. They must be motivated to wear a prosthesis and to maintain it, they must have adequate dexterity and vision to take care of the prosthesis and their stoma and they must be compliant to return to the surgeon or speech pathologist should there be any problems.

Reported rates of successful voice acquisition after TEP as a secondary procedure (i.e. as a second surgery following total laryngectomy) range from 37 to 92 per cent (Singer and Blom, 1980; Donegan, Gluckman and Singh, 1981; Johns and Cantrell, 1981; Kerr et al., 1993; Morrison and O'Grady, 1986; Perry et al., 1987)). Success rates after TEP as a primary procedure (i.e. at the time of laryngectomy) are reported between 54 and 77 per cent (Morrison and O'Grady, 1986; Cole and Miller, 1992; Deshmane et al., 1992; Fukutake and Yamashita, 1993). Most patients with successful outcomes can produce voice with little or no therapy, although some investigators have found that intensive speech therapy and patient counselling are necessary for long-term use of tracheo-oesophageal voice (Kerr et al., 1993). In fact, Quer, Burgues-Vila and Garcia-Crespillo (1992) found that 70 per cent of their primary tracheoesophageal puncture patients gave up TEP voice to use oesophageal speech exclusively after receiving oesophageal speech training.

The tracheo-oesophageal puncture procedure has also triggered a group of studies on the anatomy and physiology of the pharyngo-oesophagus and the pseudo-glottis and their relationship to the ability to produce voice. One group of studies has looked at the compliance of the pseudo-glottis in response to airflow (Lewin, Baugh and Baker, 1987; McGarvey and Weinberg, 1984; Schuller et al., 1983). After the puncture had been utilized for several years, it became clear to Blom and Singer, as well as others, that the tracheo-oesophageal puncture did not always result in excellent voice. Some patients exhibited what Singer and Blom (1981) have called 'pharyngo-oesophageal spasm' in the pseudo-glottis. That is, when air was introduced below the pseudo-glottis, the pseudo-glottis went into spasm and failed to vibrate in response to the airflow. Instead of vibrating in response to the airstream, the pseudo-glottis closed tightly and did not allow any air to escape. This 'spasm' was not present during breathing or swallowing. Thus, it was a physiologic response to air, not an anatomic narrowing or stricture. Singer and Blom have called this spasm non-productive to voice restoration and have treated it with one of two procedures, a myotomy or neurectomy (Singer and Blom, 1981; Singer, Blom and Hamaker, 1986). In a myotomy, the pharyngeal constrictors and cricopharyngeal region of the laryngectomee are cut vertically to reduce the tone in this musculature in the pharyngo-oesophagus and prevent the musculature from going into spasm. In neurectomy, the innervation to the pharyngo-oesophagus is cut so that this musculature cannot contract to create the spasm. In both instances, the rationale for the surgical procedure is to produce a pseudo-glottis which is flaccid enough to respond to the airstream and produce voice rather than to contract in spasm and prevent vibration. In a study of normal talkers after introduction of air into the oesophagus, McGarvey and Weinberg (1984) described the spasmodic behaviour of the pe segment as a normal reaction of the oesophagus to the introduction of airflow. These normal data created some controversy regarding the exact nature of the spasmodic activity seen in some laryngectomees in response to air introduced into the oesophagus below the pseudo-glottis. Clearly, however, whether or not this spasm is a normal reaction to the introduction of air or is an abnormal response, in a total laryngectomee spasm prevents the pseudo-glottis from vibrating in response to the airstream and is, therefore, unproductive to the successful acquisition of oesophageal or puncture voice. Thus, it is necessary to manage this spasm in the total laryngectomee in order for the patient to produce voice successfully. At this time myotomy is more broadly used than neurectomy. Both neurectomy and myotomy have been found to relieve spasm and to enable patients to produce continuous voicing without spasmodic interruptions. There has been some indication in the literature that myotomy may in fact be detrimental, secondary to effects on the myoelastic properties of the vibratory segment (Singer and Blom, 1980; Singer et al., 1986; Mahieu et al., 1987). Some investigators have commented on the potential for increased breathiness and reduced intensity of phonation in some myotomized patients (Baugh, Baker and Lewin, 1988; Singer et al., 1986). The resulting voice quality can be relatively easily improved by application of external pressure to a designated portion of the neck. The incidence of this problem is thought to be relatively low (i.e. less than 10 per cent) (Baugh et al., 1988).

Comparison of pilot data from tracheo-oesophageal speakers who received pharyngeal constrictor myotomy for prevention or elimination of pharyngospasms with data from oesophageal speakers from Robbins et al. (1984) indicates that myotomy did not have a detrimental effect on laryngeal voice characteristics (Table 16.2).

Some total laryngectomized patients exhibit a stricture in the pharyngo-oesophagus, in contrast to a spasm. A stricture is an area of narrowing that is anatomically identifiable radiographically and is present at all times, i.e. during respiration, swallowing and phonation. Often, stricture occurs in patients who have had prior radiotherapy or whose surgical resection was large, requiring a tight surgical closure.

The introduction of the tracheo-oesophageal puncture technique has also increased our understanding of oesophageal voice failures, i.e. those patients who attempt to learn oesophageal voice but are unable to do so for previously undetermined reasons (Chodosh, Giancarlo and

Table 16.2 Comparative acoustic and temporal data on oesophageal speakers and myotomized TEP speakers

	Robbins' oesophageal speakers[1]	Finger occlusion TEP plus myotomy[2]	Valve occlusion TEP plus myotomy[2]
f_0 in Hz (vowel)	65(30)	65(27)	66(24)
Maximum phonation time	1.9(0.71)	16.9(4.7)	12.9(4.3)
Percentage periodic phonation (reading)	41.6(11.0)	62.7(18.8)	60.2(24.1)
Percentage aperiodic phonation (reading)	25.0(8.7)	25.2(16.5)	32.6(21.8)
Mean jitter (ms)	4.1(5.2)	1.7(0.91)	1.0(0.72)
Percentage shimmer	2.5(0.70)	2.2(0.87)	1.7(0.91)

[1] Robbins et al. (1984).
[2] Pauloski (1993, private communication). Pilot data

Goldstein, 1984; Gates et al., 1982; Perry, 1983). A number of clinicians have applied the evaluation techniques utilized in assessment of candidates for the TEP to the total laryngectomee who is attempting to learn oesophageal voice. The first of these assessment techniques is what has been called 'the air-blowing' test. First used by Vandenberg and Moolenaar-Bijl (1959) and Sieman (1967) to predict oesophageal voice production from measures of intra-oesophageal pressures, this test was re-introduced by Stanley Taub (1975; 1981), the creator of the Voice-Bak prosthesis, as a way to assess the patient's potential for successful use of his prosthesis. It has been adapted by Singer and Blom (1980) as a test for the successful use of the puncture. In the air-blowing technique, a size 14 red rubber catheter is introduced through the patient's nose and from there down through the oro-pharynx into the thoracic oesophagus. The end of the catheter is positioned below the pseudo-glottis, usually 23–25 cm from the nose. The operator then blows air through the catheter into the patient's oesophagus and subjectively assesses the resulting voice. If the voice is spasmodic rather than sustained, the patient may be unable to produce oesophageal voice because of the abnormality known as 'spasm', discussed earlier. If no voice results, the patient may have a spasm, a stricture or an absent pseudo-glottis. A radiographic study, i.e. videofluoroscopy, is needed to determine which of these problems is present. In 1985, Blom, Singer and Hamaker introduced an improved air-insufflation test in which the patient was able to self-inflate the oesophagus through a special tracheostoma housing fitted to the catheter.

Some investigators have questioned the subjectivity of the air-blowing assessment (Donegan et al., 1981; Panje, 1981; McGarvey and Weinberg, 1984). Variables such as catheter distance into the pharynx and amount and force of airflow needed to initiate and maintain vibration of the pseudo-glottis have created controversy regarding the validity of the test. Lewin et al. (1987) examined intra-oesophageal pressures in 27 laryngectomized patients prior to tracheo-oesophageal puncture in an attempt to predict TEP speech outcome. These investigators objectified the air-blowing test by utilizing compressed air from a Thorpe flow meter at flow rates of 1 and 31 per minute and compared their results with air insufflation by the examiner. The catheter placement was standardized at 23 and 25 cm from the nares. Three groups of speakers were identified during air blowing: fluent speakers, non-fluent speakers, and non-speakers. These groups demonstrated low, intermediate and high intra-oesophageal pressures, respectively. Patients with intermediate and high intra-oesophageal pressures needed myotomy to achieve fluent speech with the TEP. Insufflation by the flow meter and by the examiner were both successful in identifying patients in whom fluent speech would not be achieved without myotomy.

Patients who have undergone extended resection of the larynx, pharynx and cervical oesophagus require the use of tissue from another site to facilitate the reconstruction (Gowgher and Robin, 1954; Ranger, 1964; Bakamjian 1965; Le Quesne and Ranger, 1966; Harrison, 1972; Slaney and Dalton, 1973). If just the cervical oesophagus is resected with the larynx, tissue from the chest wall in the form of a pectoralis or delto-pectoral flap may be introduced to reconstruct the pharynx and cervical oesophagus. Or, tissue from the colon may be introduced to reconstruct the pharyngo-oesophagus. If the entire oesophagus must be resected with the larynx, a stomach pull-up may be utilized to reconstruct the defect. In this procedure, the stomach is freed from its ligaments in the abdomen and stretched vertically until the top of the stomach is at the base of the tongue. The surgeon may attempt to reconstruct an upper gastric valve to prevent reflux of stomach acid or food from the stomach into the mouth. Individuals with a stomach pull-up generally function best when taking four to six small meals a day, rather than three larger meals. They must remain upright after eating to reduce the chance of reflux. Patients who have had these extensive reconstructions are able to learn oesophageal (i.e. gastric or colon) voice or undergo surgical prosthetic voice restoration techniques such as the tracheo-oesophageal puncture. However, their voices are often not as good, perceptually, as patients who have a normal oesophagus. These vocal differences are apparent to the clinician, though they have not been studied objectively. The perceptual differences in voice quality in these patients probably result from the differences in elasticity in the tissues of the colon, the stomach or chest flap as compared to oesophageal mucosa. Those patients with colon reconstruction also exhibit swallowing difficulties because the peristaltic action in the reconstruction is unlike that of the normal pharnyx (McConnel et al., 1986, 1988).

While the tracheo-oesophageal puncture has enabled many total laryngectomees to produce fluent voice and highly intelligible speech, it is clear that some pieces of the puzzle are missing in our understanding of those factors which contribute to the production of excellent vocal quality and fluent speech. Continued research into prosthetic and tissue characteristics, such as flexibility and reaction to airflow within the pharyngo-oesophagus may provide us with additional answers needed to further improve rehabilitation of the total laryngectomee.

Clinical Care of the Total Laryngectomy with Surgical Prosthetic Voice Restoration

Pre-operatively, the patient who is about to undergo a total laryngectomy should receive counselling regarding his/her communication alternatives. In general, these alternatives include oesophageal voice, surgical prosthetic speech rehabilitation and artificial larynges.

At some facilities, patients are offered the option of a primary surgical voice restoration, i.e. the TEP is placed at the time of the total laryngectomy. These patients should meet and talk with another patient who has undergone the procedure.

In primary puncture, the surgeon generally places a catheter (to be used for non-oral feeding) through the puncture site. Thus, the feeding tube is placed through the puncture and down into the oesophagus and stomach, replacing the nasogastric tube. The non-oral feeding is kept in place for approximately two weeks and acts as a stent in the puncture site to keep it open. When the stoma and puncture site have healed adequately and the patient is ready for oral feeding, the catheter is removed and a voice restoration prosthesis is fitted in the same way as is done with secondary puncture procedures. Clinically, a number of speech-language pathologists have noted the psychological difference in patients who receive a primary rather than a secondary puncture. Patients who receive a secondary voice restoration procedure have experienced the frustration of voice loss and the difficulty in learning oesophageal voice and/or using artificial larynges as a communication mode. These patients have become accommodated to the voice quality of oesophageal voice and its limitations in intensity and phrasing. When they receive the surgical prosthetic voice restoration procedure, the improvement in vocal intensity and in phrasing duration is such that they are appreciative of their voice improvement.

Patients who receive the surgical voice restoration procedure as a primary modality with total laryngectomy have never experienced the difficulties of communication with any other alaryngeal modality. They have only their pre-operative voice as a baseline for comparison. Thus, some of these patients do not like the voice quality of the surgical prosthetic voice, perceiving it as abnormally low pitched and rough as compared to their pre-operative voice. Many of them also do not experience the anxiety of voice loss because they know that soon after their surgery they will be able to produce fluent speech. Thus, these patients are often less satisfied with their voice restoration procedure, and some elect to have their puncture closed rather than use that mode of communication. Pre-operative counselling with these patients is extremely important in providing them with examples of surgical prosthetic voice and with the kind of care which the prosthesis requires.

Some patients do not have detailed questions about each of these communication modes pre-operatively, but are content to be aware that a speech-language pathologist will be available post-operatively for assistance in restoring their vocal communication. Generally, pre-operatively, patients are most concerned with their general survival. Immediately following surgery, patients who do not choose or are not offered primary puncture and their families have a number of questions regarding communication alternatives. It is in the first post-operative week that the speech-language pathologist should provide additional counselling, initial training with artificial larynges and discussion of oesophageal voice therapy. In institutions where surgical prosthetic voice restoration is provided as a secondary rehabilitation technique, the patient is usually given 4–8 weeks post-operatively to accommodate to the stoma and its care and to become familiar with the other voice restoration procedures, i.e. oesophageal voice and the artificial larynx. In general, within the first week of hospitalization, the patient should be given a variety of artificial larynges to work with. In that time, with the help of the speech-language pathologist, patients can select the instrument best for them. When the nasogastric tube is removed, the patient can begin oesophageal voice therapy. If no healing problems exist, this therapy usually begins about 10–14 days post-operatively. Thus, by 4 to 8 weeks after surgery, the patient will have had some oesophageal voice therapy, and patient and clinician will be aware of the ease with which the patient is able to put air into the oesophagus, trap the air and release the air with voice.

Radiographic Assessment

Within the first oesophageal therapy session, or perhaps the second, the speech-language clinician should have a good idea of the patient's facility for putting air into the oesophagus and releasing it with voice. If, after trying all of the available techniques, the patient is unable to put air into the oesophagus or to produce sound, it is incumbent upon the clinician to assess the physiology of the total laryngectomy patient's pharyngo-oesophagus. This requires radiographic study of the oral cavity and pharyngo-oesophagus during swallowing and voice attempts. Radiographic assessment should begin with swallows of 1 and 3 cm^3 of liquid barium and paste barium. During the swallows, the clinician should assess the oral and pharyngo-oesophageal transit times of the bolus. Oral transit times should be no more than 1.5 s, while pharyngo-cervical oesophageal transit time should be 3–4 s. There should be no obvious narrowing or obstruction to the flow of food through the oral cavity or pharyngo-oesophagus. If there is an obvious narrowing or stricture, the patient may have difficulty in putting air into the oesophagus. After assessing swallowing physiology, the clinician should examine the patient's pharyngo-oesophagus fluoroscopically while the patient attempts to put air into the oesophagus and release it with voice. On lateral radiographic view, the clinician should be able to see air entering the pharyngo-oesophagus below the adiposed tissue which comprises the patient's vibratory segment. When the patient releases the air with voice, the radiographic image will show the vibratory movement of the pseudo-glottis. If the patient produces oral gestures which are not productive to putting air into the oesophagus, this will be visible radiographically. If the patient puts air into the oesophagus, but the pseudo-glottis goes into spasm and clamps closed tightly in response to the air pressure beneath it, this will also be visible radiographically. If the patient has an anatomic deterrent to the air intake process, such as a structure, this, too, will be visible. Thus, the radiographic assessment of the pharyngo-oesophagus during swallowing and attempts at oesophageal voice production will enable the clinician to assess the patient's physiologic potential for learning oesophageal voice and the patient's potential for surgical prosthetic voice restoration procedures with or without the need for myotomy.

While surgical voice restoration for total laryngectomees has provided improved voice for many patients and has increased our knowledge regarding the physiology of oesophageal voice, it has also opened a number of questions regarding the interaction of airflows, pressures and pharyngo-oesophageal vibration.

References

Aguilar N, Olson M, Shedd D (1979) Rehabilitation of deglutition problems in patients with head and neck cancer. American Journal of Surgery 138: 501–7.

Ardran GM, Kemp F (1951) The mechanism of swallowing. Proceedings of the Royal Society of Medicine 44: 1038–40.

Ardran GM, Kemp FH (1967) The mechanism of the larynx. II. The epiglottis and closure of the larynx. British Journal of Radiology 40: 372–89.

Asai R (1965) Laryngoplasty after total laryngectomy. Archives of Otolaryngology 95: 114–119.

Baggs T, Pine S (1983) Acoustic characteristics: Tracheoesophageal speech. Journal of Communication Disorders 16: 299–307.

Bakamjian V (1965) A two-staged method for pharyngo-esophageal reconstruction with a primary pectoral skin flap. Plastic Reconstructive Surgery 36: 173–84.

Baugh R, Baker S, Lewin J (1988) Surgical treatment of pharyngoesophageal spasm. Laryngoscope 98: 1124–26.

Berlin C (1963) Clinical measurement of esophageal speech: I. Methodology and curves of skill acquisition. Journal of Speech and Hearing Disorders 28: 42–51.

Blom E, Singer M, Hamaker R (1982) Tracheostoma valve for postlaryngectomy voice rehabilitation. Annals of Otology, Rhinology and Laryngology 91: 576–78.

Blom E, Singer M, Hamaker R (1985) An improved esophageal insufflation test. Archives of Otolaryngology 111: 211–2.

Blood G (1984) Fundamental frequency and intensity measurements in laryngeal and alaryngeal speakers. Journal of Communication Disorders 17: 319–24.

Calcaterra T (1971) Laryngeal suspension after supraglottic laryngectomy. Archives of Otolaryngology 94: 306–9.

Chodosh P, Giancarlo H, Goldstein J (1984) Pharyngeal myotomy for vocal rehabilitation post laryngectomy. Laryngoscope 94: 52–7.

Cole I, Miller S (1992) Total laryngectomy with primary voice restoration. Australian and New Zealand Journal of Surgery 62: 279–82.

Conley J, DeAmesti F, Pierce M (1958) A new surgical technique for vocal rehabilitation of the laryngectomized patient. Annals of Otology, Rhinology and Laryngology 67: 655–64.

Curry ET, Snidecor JC (1961) Physical measurement and pitch perception in esophageal speech. Laryngoscope 71: 415–24.

Damste PH (1958) Oesophageal Speech. Groningen: Hoitsema.

DeSanto LW (1974) Selection of treatment for in situ and early invasive carcinoma of the glottis. Canadian Journal of Otolaryngology 3: 552–6.

Deshmane VH, Mehta SA, Chandavarkar RY, Mehta AR (1992) Primary tracheoesophageal puncture – our initial experience. Indian Journal of Cancer 29: 114–6.

Diedrich W, Youngstrom K (1977) Alaryngeal Speech. Springfield, IL: Charles Thomas.

Donegan J, Gluckman J, Singh J (1981) Limitations of the Blom-Singer technique for voice restoration. Annals of Otology, Rhinology and Laryngology 90: 495–7.

Duguay M (1979) Speech problems of the alaryngeal speaker. In Keith RL, Darley FL (Eds) Laryngectomee Rehabilitation. Houston, TX: College Hill.

Edels Y (Ed) (1983) Laryngectomy: Diagnosis to Rehabilitation. London: Croom Helm.

Edwards N (1980) Vocal rehabilitation by external vocal fistula and valved prosthesis: Edwards Method. In Shedd DP, Weinberg B (Eds) Surgical and Prosthetic Approaches to Speech Rehabilitation. Boston: G. K. Hall Medical Publishers. pp 9–16.

Fletcher GH, Goepfert H (1981) Irradiation in the management of squamous cell carcinomas of the larynx. Otolaryngology 5: 1–45.

Fukutake T, Yamashita T (1993) Speech rehabilitation and complications of primary tracheoesophageal puncture. Acta Oto-Laryngologica, Supplement 500: 117–20.

Gates G, Ryan W, Cantu E, Hearne E (1982) Current status of laryngectomy rehabilitation. II. Cause of failure. American Journal of Otolaryngology 3: 8–14.

Goepfert H, Lindberg R, Jesse R (1981) Combined laryngeal conservation surgery and irradiation. Can we expand the indications for conservation therapy? Otolaryngology Head and Neck Surgery 89: 974–8.

Gowgher J, Robin I (1954) Use of left colon for reconstruction of pharynx and oesophagus after pharyngectomy. British Journal of Surgery 42: 283–90.

Griffiths C, Love J (1978) Neoglottis reconstruction after total laryngectomy. Annals of Otology, Rhinology and Laryngology 87: 180–6.

Guttman M (1935) Tracheohypopharyngeal fistulization. Transactions of the American Laryngology, Rhinology and Otology Society 41: 219–26.

Harrison D (1972) Role of surgery in the management of post-cricoid and cervical oesophageal neoplasma. Annals of Otolaryngology, Rhinology and Laryngology 8: 465–8.

Hoops H, Noll J (1969) Relationship of selected acoustic variables to judgments of esophageal speech. Journal of Communication Disorders 2: 1–13.

Isshiki N, Snidecor JC (1965) Air intake and usage in esophageal speech. Acta Otolaryngologica 59: 559–74.

Johns M, Cantrell R (1981) Voice restoration of the total laryngectomy patient: The Singer–Blom technique. Otolaryngology, Head and Neck Surgery 89: 82–6.

Karim A, Snow J, Siek H, Njo K (1983) The quality of voice in patients irradiated for laryngeal carcinoma. Cancer 41: 47–9.

Kerr AI, Demholm S, Sanderson RJ, Anderson SJ (1993) Blom–Singer prostheses – an 11 year experience of primary and secondary procedures. Clinical Otolaryngoly 18: 184–7.

Komorn R, Weyer J, Sessions R, Malone P (1973) Vocal rehabilitation with a tracheo esophageal shunt. Archives of Otolaryngology 97: 103–5.

Lazarus C (1993) Effects of Radiation therapy and voluntary maneuvers on swallow functioning in head and neck cancer patients. Clinics in Communication Disorders 3: 11–20.

LeBrun Y (1973) Neurolinguistics I. The Artificial Larynx. Amsterdam: Swets and Zeitlinger.

Le Quesne LP, Ranger D (1966) Pharyngo-laryngectomy with immediate pharyngo-gastric anastomosis. British Journal of Surgery 53: 105–9.

Lewin J, Baugh R, Baker S (1987) An objective method for prediction of tracheoesophageal speech production. Journal of Speech and Hearing Disorders 52: 212–7.

Logemann JA (1993) A manual for videofluoroscopic evaluation of swallowing (2nd ed) Austin, TX: Pro-Ed.

Logemann JA, Gibbons P, Rademaker AW, Pauloski BR, Kahrilas PJ, Bacon M, Bowman J, McCracken E (1995) Mechanisms of recovery of swallow after supraglottic laryngectomy. Journal of Speech and Hearing Research. In press.

Mahieu HF, Annyas AA, Schutte HK, Van Der Jagt EJ (1987) Pharyngoesophageal myotomy for vocal rehabilitation of laryngectomees. Laryngoscope 97: 451–7.

McConnel FMS, Hester TR, Mendelsohn MS, Logemann JA (1988) Manofluorography of deglutiton after total laryngopharyngectomy. Plastic and Reconstructive Surgery 81(3): 346–51.

McConnel FMS, Mendelsohn MS, Logemann JA (1986) Examination of swallowing after total laryngectomy using manofluorography. Head and Neck Surgery, Sept/Oct: 3–12.

McConnel FMS, Sisson GA, Logemann J (1976) Three years' experience with a hypopharyngeal pseudoglottis for vocal rehabilitation after total laryngectomy. Transactions of the American Academy of Opthamology and Otolaryngology 84: 63–7.

McGarvey SD, Weinberg B (1984) Esophageal insufflation testing in non laryngectomized adults. Journal of Speech and Hearing Disorders 49: 272–7.

Mitchell F, Kirkland R, Morrison W (1981) The Blom-Singer endoscopic technique under local anesthesia for restoration of voice after laryngectomy. Journal of the Tennessee Medical Association 74: 867–9.

Monaghan C, Murray T (1986) Sex identification of laryngeal, esophageal, and tracheoesophageal speakers. Paper presented at ASHA Convention, Detroit, MI.

Moon J, Weinberg B (1983) Evaluations of Blom–Singer tracheoesophageal puncture prostheses performance. Journal of Speech and Hearing Disorders 26: 459–64.

Moon J, Weinberg B (1984) Airway resistance characteristics of Voice Button tracheoesophageal protheses. Journal of Speech and Hearing Disorders 49: 326–8.

Morrison MD, O'Grady (1986) Primary tracheo-esophageal puncture voice restoration with laryngectomy. Journal of Otolaryngoly 15: 69–73.

Ogura J, Mallen R (1965) Partial laryngectomy for supraglottic and pharyngeal carcinoma. Transactions of the American Academy of Opthamology and Otolaryngology 69: 832–45.

Ossoff R, Lazarus C, Sisson G (1984) Tracheoesophageal puncture for voice restoration: Modification of the Blom–Singer technique. Otolaryngology, Head and Neck Surgery 92: 418–23.

Panje W (1981) Prosthetic vocal rehabilitation following laryngectomy: the Voice Button. Annals of Otology, Rhinology, and Laryngology 90: 116–20.

Pauloski BR (1987) A comparative acoustic study of tracheoesophageal speech produced with the Blom–Singer voice prosthesis and the Blom–Singer low pressure voice prosthesis with both digitial occlusion and the Blom–Singer tracheostoma valve. Unpublished doctoral dissertation. Northwestern University, Evanston, IL.

Perry A (1983) Difficulties in the acquisition of alaryngeal speech, in Edels Y (Ed) Laryngectomy: Diagnosis to Rehabilitation. London: Croom Helm. pp 177–91.

Perry A, Cheesman AC, Eden R (1983) A modification of the Blom–Singer valve for restoration of voice after laryngectomy. Journal of Laryngology Otology 96: 1005–11.

Perry A, Cheesman A, McIvor J, Chalton R (1987) A British experience with surgical voice restoration techniques as a secondary procedure following total laryngectomy, Journal of Laryngology Otology 101: 155–63.

Quer M, Burgues-Vila J, Garcia-Crespillo P (1992) Primary tracheoesophageal puncture vs. esophageal speech. Archives of Otolaryngology – Head and Neck Surgery 118: 188–90.

Rademaker AW, Logemann JA, Pauloski BR, Bowman J, Lazarus C, Sisson G, Milianti F, Graner D, Cook B, Collins S, Stein D, Beery Q, Johnson J, Baker T (1993) Recovery of postoperative swallowing in patients undergoing partial laryngectomy. Head and Neck 15: 325–34.

Ranger D (1964) The problems of repair after pharyngolaryngectomy. Proceedings of the Royal Society of Medicine 57: 1099–103.

Robbins J (1982) A comparative acoustic study of laryngeal speech, esopageal, speech, and speech produced after tracheo-esophageal puncture. Unpublished doctoral dissertation, Northwestern University, Evanston, IL.

Robbins J (1984) Acoustic differentation of laryngeal, esophageal, and tracheoesophageal speech. Journal of Speech and Hearing Research 27: 577–85.

Robbins J, Fisher H, Blom E, Singer M (1984) A comparative acoustic study of normal, esophageal, and tracheoesophageal speech production. Journal of Speech and Hearing Disorders 49: 202–10.

Salmon SJ, Goldstein LP (Eds) (1978) Artificial Larynx Handbook. New York: Grune and Stratton.

Schuller DE, Jarrow JE, Kelly DR, Miglets AW (1983) Prognostic factors affecting the success of duck-bill vocal restoration. Otolaryngology – Head and Neck Surgery 91: 396–8.

Serafini I (1980) Reconstructive laryngectomy. In Shedd DP, Wienberg B (Eds) Surgical and Prosthetic Approaches to Speech Rehabilitation. Boston: MA: G.K. Hall Medical Publishers. pp 67–76.

Shanks J (1983) Improving oesophageal communication. In Edels Y (Ed)

Laryngectomy: Diagnosis to Rehabilitation. London: Croom Helm. pp 163–76.

Shapiro M, Ramanathan V (1982) Trachea stoma vent voice prosthesis. Laryngoscope 92: 1126–9.

Shipp T (1967) Frequency, duration, and perceptual measures in relation to judgments of alaryngeal speech acceptability. Journal of Speech and Hearing Research 10: 417–27.

Sieman M (1967) Rehabilitation of laryngectomized subjects. Acta Otolaryngologica 64: 235–41.

Simpson IC, Smith JCS, Gordon MT (1972) Laryngectomy: The influence of muscle reconstruction on the mechanism of oesophageal voice production. Journal of Laryngology and Otology 86: 961–90.

Singer M, Blom E (1980) An endoscopic technique for restoration of voice after total laryngectomy. Annals of Otology, Rhinology and Laryngology 89: 529–33.

Singer M, Blom E (1981) Selective myotomy for voice restoration after total laryngectomy. Archives of Otolaryngology 107: 670–3.

Singer M, Blom E, Hamaker R (1981) Further experience with voice restoration after total laryngectomy. Annals of Otolaryngology, Rhinology and Laryngology 90: 498–502.

Singer M, Blom E, Hamaker R (1986) Pharyngeal plexus neurectomy for alaryngeal speech rehabilitation. Laryngoscope 96: 50–3.

Slaney G, Dalton GA (1973) Problems of viscus replacement following pharyngolaryngectomy. Journal of Laryngology and Otolaryngology 87: 539–46.

Smith B (1986) Aerodynamic characteristics of Blom–Singer low pressure voice prostheses. Archives of Otolaryngology Head and Neck Surgery 112: 50–2.

Smith B, Weinberg B, Feth L, Horii Y (1978) Vocal roughness and jitter characteristics of vowels produced by esophageal speakers. Journal of Speech and Hearing Research 21: 240–9.

Snidecor J, Curry E (1959) Temporal and pitch aspects of superior esophageal speech. Annals of Otology Rhinology and Laryngology 68: 1–4.

Snidecor J, Curry E (1960) How effectively can the laryngectomee expect to speak? Laryngoscope 70: 62–7.

Snidecor J, Isshiki N (1965) Air volume and airflow relationships of six male esophageal speakers. Journal of Speech and Hearing Disorders 30: 205–16.

Som M (1951) Hemilaryngectomy – a modified technique for cordal carcinoma with extension posteriorly. Archives of Otolaryngology 54: 524–33.

Staffieri M (1980) New surgical approaches for speech rehabilitation after total laryngectomy. In Shedd DP, Weinberg B (Eds) Surgical and Prosthetic Approaches to Speech Rehabilitation. Boston, MA: G.K. Hall Medical Publishers. pp 77–118.

Stell PM, Maran AGD (1978) Head and Neck Surgery. London: William Heinemann Medical Books.

Stoicheff M (1975) Voice following radiotherapy. The Laryngoscope 85: 609–18.

Stoicheff M, Campi A, Passi J, Fredrickson J (1983) The irradiated larynx and voice: A perceptual study. Journal of Speech and Hearing Research 26: 482–5.

Suen JY, Myers EN (1981) Cancer of the Head and Neck. Edinburgh: Churchill Livingstone.

Taub S (1975) Air bypass voice prosthesis for vocal rehabilitation of laryngectomees. Annals of Otology, Rhinology and Laryngology 84: 45–8.

Taub S (1981) Air bypass voice prosthesis for vocal rehabilitation of laryngectomees. Ear Nose and Throat Journal 60: 42–54.

Taub S, Bugner LH (1973) Air bypass voice prosthesis for vocal rehabilitation of laryngectomees. American Journal of Surgery 125: 748–56.

Trudeau M (1986a) Characteristics of female tracheoesophageal speech. Paper presented at ASHA Convention, Detroit, MI.

Trudeau M (1986b) Gender identification among female esophageal and tracheoesophageal speakers. Paper presented at ASHA Convention, Detroit, MI

Vandenberg J, Moolenaar-Bijl AJ (1959) Cricopharyngeal sphincter, pitch, intensity, and fluency in oesophageal speech. Practica Oto-rhino-laryngologica 21: 298–315.

Weinberg B (1982) Airway resistance to the Voice Button. Archives of Otolaryngology 108: 498–500.

Weinberg B, Bennett S (1972) Selected acoustic characteristics of esophageal speech produced by female laryngectomees. Journal of Speech and Hearing Research 15: 211–6.

Weinberg B, Moon J (1982) Airway resistance characteristics of Blom–Singer tracheoesophagal puncture prostheses Journal of Speech and Hearing Disorders 47: 441–2.

Weinberg B, Moon J (1984) Aerodynamic properties of four tracheoesophageal puncture protheses. Archives of Otolaryngology 110: 673–5.

Weinberg B, Moon J (1986a) Airway resistance characteristics of Blom–Singer and Panje low pressure tracheoesophageal puncture prostheses. Journal of Speech and Hearing Disorders 51: 169–72.

Weinberg B, Moon J (1986b) Impact of tracheoesophageal puncture prostheses airway resistance on in-vivo phonatory performance. Journal of Speech and Hearing Disorders 51: 88–91.

Welch MW, Logemann JA, Rademaker AW, Kahrilas PJ (1993) Changes in pharyngeal dimensions effected by chin tuck. Archives of Physical Medicine and Rehabilitation 74: 178–81.

Wetmore S, Krueger K, Wesson K (1981) The Singer–Blom speech rehabilitation procedure. Laryngoscope 91: 1109–17.

Wolicki K, Makielski K, Olson N (1985) An improved technique for tracheoesophageal puncture using the urethral filliform and follower, Scientific poster presented at the American Academy of Otolaryngolgy – Head and Neck Surgery Annual Meeting, Atlanta, GA.

Wood B, Tucker H, Rusnov M, Levine H (1981) Tracheoesophageal puncture for alaryngeal voice restoration. Annals of Otolaryngology 90: 492–4.

Index